T0314228

GROUP PSYCHOTHERAPY
in Inpatient, Partial Hospital, and Residential Care Settings

GROUP PSYCHOTHERAPY

in Inpatient, Partial Hospital, and Residential Care Settings

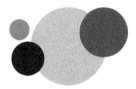

Virginia Brabender AND April Fallon

AMERICAN PSYCHOLOGICAL ASSOCIATION
Washington, DC

Published by
American Psychological Association
750 First Street, NE
Washington, DC 20002
www.apa.org

APA Order Department
P.O. Box 92984
Washington, DC 20090-2984
Phone: (800) 374-2721; Direct: (202) 336-5510
Fax: (202) 336-5502; TDD/TTY: (202) 336-6123
Online: http://www.apa.org/pubs/books
E-mail: order@apa.org

In the U.K., Europe, Africa, and the Middle East, copies may be ordered from
Eurospan Group
c/o Turpin Distribution
Pegasus Drive
Stratton Business Park
Biggleswade, Bedfordshire
SG18 8TQ United Kingdom
Phone: +44 (0) 1767 604972
Fax: +44 (0) 1767 601640
Online: https://www.eurospanbookstore.com/apa
E-mail: eurospan@turpin-distribution.com

Typeset in Goudy by Circle Graphics, Inc., Columbia, MD

Printer: Sheridan Books, Chelsea, MI
Cover Designer: Anne C. Kerns, Anne Likes Red, Inc., Silver Spring, MD

Library of Congress Cataloging-in-Publication Data

Names: Brabender, Virginia, author. | Fallon, April, author.
Title: Group psychotherapy in inpatient, partial hospital, and residential
  care settings / by Virginia Brabender and April Fallon.
Description: First edition. | Washington, DC : American Psychological
  Association, [2019] | Includes bibliographical references and index.
Identifiers: LCCN 2018018028 (print) | LCCN 2018030010 (ebook) | ISBN
  9781433829918 (eBook) | ISBN 1433829916 (eBook) | ISBN 9781433829901
  (hardcover) | ISBN 1433829908 (hardcover)
Subjects: LCSH: Group psychotherapy. | Psychiatric hospital care.
Classification: LCC RC488 (ebook) | LCC RC488 .B7264 2019 (print) | DDC
  616.89/152—dc23
LC record available at https://lccn.loc.gov/2018018028

British Library Cataloguing-in-Publication Data
A CIP record is available from the British Library.

Printed in the United States of America
First Edition

http://dx.doi.org/10.1037/0000113-000

10 9 8 7 6 5 4 3 2 1

CONTENTS

ACKNOWLEDGMENTS

Authors prevail on others' time, resources, and patience. We have piteously prevailed on many and would like to thank these individuals. We acknowledge our debt to other scholars who have contributed richly to the group psychotherapy literature. We would like to recognize in particular the important contributions of our recently departed friend Cecil Rice, whose collection of insightful writings on groups was a boon to our work. Dr. Rice graciously wrote the foreword to our 1993 book, *Models of Inpatient Group Psychotherapy*. We thank our graduate students and psychiatric medical residents who listened to and critiqued our ideas and our 1993 book. Their role in letting us know when we were straying far from clarity was invaluable. Also, our students are placed in such a range of practice situations, including those we feature in this text, that we were able to get a good read on the viability of approaches across contexts. Some graduate students provided extremely capable technical assistance. To three amazingly industrious and competent students, Hailey Bourgeau, Jane Holloway, and Anna Cruz, we offer our sincerest thanks. Widener staff member Patty Nilon also provided very capable and cheerful secretarial support. We also thank the clinician–scholars who read one or more chapters and offered their insights. These individuals include Mary Foley, Elizabeth Foster, Katja Hajek, Michael Long, Frank Masterpasqua, and Mark Richardson. We are grateful to our three anonymous reviewers who provided thoughtful, careful, and detailed feedback, which we applied as the book progressed. We thank Widener University for providing a Provost's Grant that supported this research. We also extend our great gratitude to American Psychological Association (APA) Books. This book is our third with APA Books, and we find the collaboration to be extremely satisfying. A particular note of appreciation goes to acquisitions editor Susan Reynolds, who played a vital role in enabling us to realize the vision of this book. We also thank our development editor, Ida Audeh, for the many helpful ideas she provided that enriched our chapters. Erin O'Brien did a fabulous job as our copyeditor. Our family members (Arthur, Rao, Emile, Gabi, Jacob, Marianna, and Natasha) seem to recognize now that we will always be working on a book and that although the current book might seem to compete with them for our passion, it never really does.

GROUP PSYCHOTHERAPY
in Inpatient, Partial Hospital, and Residential Care Settings

INTRODUCTION

This book describes six group therapy approaches that are appropriate for use in hospitals, partial hospitals, and residential treatment centers. The broad scope reflects changes in group therapy practice in the 25 years since our last book with this general focus was published (Brabender & Fallon, 1993). Since then, the number of models available to the practitioner has increased substantially, and practitioners today may be practicing in settings beyond the inpatient group, namely, partial hospitals, and to a lesser extent, residential treatment settings. The latter sites have emerged more prominently with the decrease in inpatient psychiatric admissions as societies have moved in the direction of health care that is more affordable. By presenting an array of models, we hope readers will see that tremendous variety does exist and will find one that fits their practice settings, the populations served, and their theoretical and technical proclivities. Our aim is to provide

http://dx.doi.org/10.1037/0000113-001
Group Psychotherapy in Inpatient, Partial Hospital, and Residential Care Settings, by V. Brabender and A. Fallon
Copyright © 2019 by the American Psychological Association. All rights reserved.

beginner or midcareer therapists as well as seasoned group psychotherapists with approaches or elements of approaches that will catalyze their group work in a way that makes it more fulfilling and more effective.

IDENTIFYING OUR FEATURED CONTEXTS

The expansion of models is a felicitous development because settings vary widely from one another. We firmly believe that the optimal model a practitioner uses is often not the model encountered during his or her graduate school training or the pet model of a past supervisor. Rather, our view is that the model that will be successful is the one that meshes especially well with the treatment environment. Although this point might appear to be a truism, it is our strong impression, and the research (e.g., Farley, 1998) suggests, that model–context compatibility typically receives little attention in clinical environments and professional training.

The private practitioner who is developing a group has a great deal of control over many variables—where the group will meet, at what time, how many times, and so on. In other words, the private practitioner can select a model and develop a context that will be compatible with it. The group therapist intending to conduct a group that is part of a larger therapeutic program must accept many contextual features as a point of departure. For example, settings often define the time of a group or the duration of the session. The therapist culls group members from a defined population to which the program caters. In other words, the context must precede model selection. Of course, a feature that might be fixed in one setting might be malleable in another. However, overall, groups taking place in a larger treatment environment must be designed with a thorough consideration of context to be both viable and effective. In creating a contrast between groups in a treatment context and stand-alone groups, we recognize that the difference is a matter of degree. Sometimes a group therapist working in an inpatient setting will have a great deal of control over contextual features. It is not unusual for such control to increase along with one's tenure in an institution or organization. It is also true that a private practitioner will be limited by various factors such as the availability of certain types of patients in the community in which he or she practices. Nonetheless, in general, the group psychotherapist operating in a defined context has to give greater deference to context. In doing so, the group psychotherapist can experience the environment supporting his or her work. For example, a model that is comprehensible to other staff is likely to be supported by that staff, as in the case of an aide who notices an opportunity for a member to work on a skill being fostered in the psychotherapy group, on the larger unit, and encourages her to take advantage of it.

The three therapeutic settings that we feature in our text are not the only instances of group psychotherapy in a defined context. Group treatments—for example, in prison settings, schools, and the military—occur in well-defined contexts. Indeed, some of what we talk about in this text applies to these groups, and occasionally we mention these settings. However, our emphasis is on groups located in a broader therapeutic context. The other types of groups have additional challenges and other flexibilities that we do not address.

SELECTING THE MODELS

Probably the biggest decision we had to make beyond the selection of contexts was the identification of particular models we would feature. This decision was challenging because group psychotherapists often combine elements of models and write about them in this fashion. For example, Burlingame, Strauss, and Joyce (2013) wrote about a recent trend in the literature on inpatient, day hospital, and residential groups for individuals with personality disorders, toward the integration of cognitive behavior therapy and psychodynamic theory. This trend is positive in that it represents the therapist's laudable effort to customize a model for his or her setting. Nonetheless, amidst so much variety in combinations and integrations, characterizing models in their pure form was daunting. Still, integrations require a full knowledge of the elements in their essential form; therefore, we felt the effort to undertake this task was worthwhile. Another consideration was our interest in having models with a breadth of application. Today, psychoeducational groups are often used in the settings we feature (see Chapter 2). However, typically, these groups are designed in relation to specific psychological problems and/or characteristics of the patient population. We were interested in models that were sufficiently general as to be applied to a range of human problems, regardless of whether members were formed into symptomatically homogeneous or heterogeneous groupings.

We were also interested for two reasons in featuring models that would have some capability for allowing a focus on process. First, a focus on process (the interactions between and among members and the therapist) is associated with more favorable outcomes. Second, a process focus establishes group psychotherapy as a unique offering in relation to the other formats (including psychoeducational groups) that are popular in treatment programs in the three settings. We believe that the contribution of group psychotherapy should be distinctive rather than duplicative.

Although a focus on group process was important to us, we recognized that some models, such as the interpersonal and psychoanalytic models, are better able than others to accommodate an exploration of process. Whereas interpersonal models focus on dyadic aspects of process, psychoanalytic models lend themselves to looking at process on a subgroup and group-as-a-whole level. We believe that by tapping some of the process elements in the interpersonal and psychoanalytic models, those models that are not naturally oriented toward process can be enriched.

The models we feature were chosen on several grounds:

- The presence of features outlined earlier in this chapter—a model of psychopathology, a statement of goals, and a specification of interventions. This requirement resulted in the exclusion of many contributions that simply proposed techniques or principles.
- The presence of some reasonable level of clinical interest in the model as reflected by the literature on groups over the past 20 years.
- The power of the model to be used in a range of settings and conditions. For example, we excluded from the text some interesting models created for specific diagnostic groups, such as inpatients with chronic combat-related posttraumatic stress disorder (e.g., Southwick, Gilmartin, McDonough, & Morrissey's, 2006, logotherapy model) or eating disorders (Dean, Touyz, Rieger, & Thornton's, 2008, motivational enhancement model). However, those familiar with these models may notice that they have important conceptual links with one or more models presented in the text.
- A breadth and contrast between models. We sought to include models that are highly varied regarding theoretical orientation, goals, techniques, and the demands they place on clinical settings. Once again, our intent here was to increase the likelihood that each reader—given the specificities of his or her setting, population, and person—could find an appropriate model.

We would be remiss if we did not acknowledge that our criteria for inclusion have some arbitrariness. If another team were attempting to organize the theoretical and technical contributions that have been made to group psychotherapy in the three contexts, they would likely have done it in a substantially different but equally descriptive way. This same point applies to our placement of the contributions of various writers in one model category or another. Some writers have ties to a variety of models, and we have endeavored to distill the major emphases of their writings.

SELECTING OUR TARGET AUDIENCE

In presenting the models, we recognized that our target audience is likely to be diverse. According to feedback on the text on which this current book is based (Brabender & Fallon, 1993), we expected that many students would read our book. Students commonly find themselves placed in inpatient hospital programs (IHP), partial hospital programs (PHP), and residential treatment centers (RTC). Often, they are asked to lead groups and are given little direction on how to do so. It is our hope that this book would provide a point of departure for thinking about the group they would like to conduct. To meet students' needs, we provide a fair amount of background on theory and mechanics and do so with the knowledge that many students will enter a placement situation without having had a prior course in group psychotherapy. Of course, if students use our book in this way, we would want them to obtain supervision from a qualified group psychotherapist as they are pursuing their group work. Some students might encounter our book in a graduate course. We have designed the clinical illustrations so that students could act them out in class—an experience our graduate students and psychiatric residents have found to be both edifying and enjoyable.

We also anticipated that our book would be of use to more experienced group psychotherapists who either are finding themselves in one of the three treatment environments for the first time or are interested in learning about new approaches. We recognize that for these group psychotherapists, we probably provide more detail on basic theory and mechanics than is necessary. We invite such readers to adjust how they read the book to their interests and needs.

ROAD MAP OF THE BOOK

Broadly, in the ensuing chapters, we discuss contexts, models, and the interrelationships. In Chapter 1, we argue for the importance of a model framework and delineate the settings that are the scope of this book. In Chapter 2, we characterize the major important contextual dimensions that distinguish one treatment environment from another. All of the dimensions we mention are those that are likely to affect model selection. We then have a set of six chapters that describe the models themselves.

We sequenced the models from the most to the least process-oriented. The first model (Chapter 3) is the popular interpersonal approach, to which most practitioners gain exposure through the writings of Irvin Yalom (Yalom & Leszcz, 2005). Even neophyte practitioners are probably at least somewhat familiar with Yalom's (1983) highly structured versions of an interpersonal approach, which have been applied in many IHP, PHP, and RTC venues. However, in other sites, a more unstructured version can be implemented primarily because of the greater length of group participation. We also cover interpersonal therapy–group (Wilfley, MacKenzie, Welch, Ayres, & Weissman, 2000), which is loosely connected to Yalom's writings but has also been influenced by other theoretical strands. Our chapter aims to capture the richness of all of these contemporary interpersonal applications.

The next chapter addresses the family of psychodynamic models (Chapter 4). Today, an array of psychodynamic models exists that takes into account the realities of contextual group psychotherapy, such as the often-short time frame and the severity of members' pathology. We begin with a consideration of what makes a model psychodynamic and then explore different ways that psychodynamic principles have been used in IHP, PHP, and RTC contexts. We look at a model of group psychotherapy that centers on members' object relations (or internal representations of self and other). The object relations/systems or Kibel (1981, 2003, 2005) model is especially popular in Western Europe. We also describe a newer model that seeks to promote mentalizing in group members (Karterud & Bateman, 2012) to support affect regulation and the development of a cohesive sense of identity.

We then proceed to the cluster of cognitive behavioral approaches (Chapter 5) to contextual group psychotherapy. Increasingly, cognitive behavior therapy (CBT) approaches have drawn on some of the process elements described in the prior two chapters. In the 1980s, the cognitive behavioral approach began as a treatment method for outpatients. Freeman, Schrodt, Gilson, and Ludgate (1993) extended it to the inpatient context, and it continues to garner interest in IHP settings (e.g., Forsey, 2013). More recently, group psychotherapists have developed their applications for PHPs (Neuhaus, Christopher, Jacob, Guillaumot, & Burns, 2007) and RTCs (Armelius & Andreassen, 2007). This chapter also covers schema-focused therapy (McGinn & Young, 1996), which has become an extremely important variation of the cognitive behavioral approaches to group therapy—including IHP, PHP, and RTC—since the publication of our 1993 book. A model that represents a subarea of CBT is dialectical behavioral therapy (DBT; Linehan, 1993). DBT is a highly combinatorial form of treatment, borrowing elements from various schools of thought. Applications of DBT have been developed for IHPs (e.g., McCann, Ball, & Ivanoff, 2000; Swenson, Witterholt, & Bohus, 2007), PHPs (e.g., Simpson et al., 1998; Yen, Johnson, Costello, & Simpson, 2009), and RTCs (e.g., McCann, Ivanoff, Schmidt, & Beach, 2007).

The next two chapters present models that are increasingly established in their own right but have a strong connection to CBT both historically and conceptually. The acceptance and commitment therapy model devised by Hayes (2004) is the focus of Chapter 6. Although this model has many similarities to DBT, it also is distinctive in its greater stress on reducing experiential avoidance and fostering radical acceptance of the full gamut of psychological experiences so that individuals can act in accordance with their goals and values. It shares with CBT and DBT applications the presence of considerable empirical support with the patient populations found in IHP, PHP, and RTC settings.

We then move on to the skill-based interpersonal problem-solving model (Spivack, Platt, & Shure, 1976; Chapter 7) for the treatment of a wide range of psychological and physical problems, which remains the object of considerable empirical inquiry. A strength of this model is its breadth of application with individuals at different levels of ego functioning and its use with children, adolescents, and elderly patients. The last model we present is the social skills training model (Chapter 8), which continues to be used to treat the most severely disturbed patients (e.g., Frey & Weller's [2000] program to treat aggressive behaviors in psychotic and mood-disordered state hospital patients). It is the most concrete of the models presented in this volume and provides the most scripted approach to examining the interactions among members. This model is particularly suited to work with extremely low-functioning group members, although it accommodates a wide variety of presenting problems.

In our final chapter (Chapter 9), we perform a comparative analysis of all six models. We seek to aid the reader in finding a useful model for his or her setting. We reiterate a theme of this book, which is that model selection should be predicated on as much knowledge about the setting, the population, and the therapist as possible. We also underscore the point that we made many times previously that model selection is never a final step because all settings have a uniqueness that must be accommodated for the fit of the model to be optimal. Once this customized model is applied, we stress, it should be continually scrutinized to ensure that it is serving the treatment needs of group members.

In those chapters devoted to the presentation of models, the reader will find that we use a fairly consistent outline. Generally, the topics flow as follows: theoretical suppositions, technical considerations, illustrations, research on the model, contextual requirements (or demands), and a summary. Where we deviate from this order, we do so to accommodate some of the unique features of the model (e.g., we might create a section for a topic covered in the present model but ignored in the others). The illustrations of group sessions are examples of identified therapeutic approaches conducted in specific settings. The patients, their described problems, and their interactions with each other are fictitious composites of the thousands of patients that we and our students have worked with over our decades of clinical work and supervision. They were developed to represent the kinds of populations, problems, and interactions that are likely to occur in each of these settings with the specific model presented. Every setting is unique and every group a different experience. The examples illuminated are successful ones, although we are the first to admit that not all interventions work this well. We, at times, have been humbled by our flops and spurred on by our successes while leading psychotherapy groups. The group therapist may find that his or her context requires a group approach that is in need of considerable fine-tuning and modification to achieve positive results. We encourage the group therapist to recognize that it is a process that is worth the effort.

REFERENCES

Armelius, B. Å., & Andreassen, T. H. (2007). Cognitive behavioral treatment for antisocial behavior in youth in residential care. *Cochrane.* Retrieved from http://www.cochrane.org/CD005650/BEHAV_cognitive-behavioral-treatment-for-antisocial-youth-in-residential-care

Brabender, V., & Fallon, A. (1993). *Models of inpatient group psychotherapy.* Washington, DC: American Psychological Association. http://dx.doi.org/10.1037/10121-000

Burlingame, G. M., Strauss, B., & Joyce, A. (2013). Change mechanisms and effectiveness of small group treatments. In M. J. Lambert (Ed.), *Bergin and Garfield's handbook of psychotherapy and behavior change* (6th ed., pp. 640–689). Hoboken, NJ: Wiley.

Dean, H. Y., Touyz, S. W., Rieger, E., & Thornton, C. E. (2008). Group motivational enhancement therapy as an adjunct to inpatient treatment for eating disorders: A preliminary study. *European Eating Disorders Review, 16,* 256–267. http://dx.doi.org/10.1002/erv.851

Farley, P. N. (1998). *Current practices in general hospital group psychotherapy* (Doctoral dissertation). Retrieved from http://theses.lib.vt.edu/theses/available/etd-3198-142012/unrestricted/dissert.pdf

Forsey, M. (2013). *Brief group therapy for psychosis in acute care* (Unpublished doctoral dissertation). University of Liverpool, Liverpool, England.

Freeman, A., Schrodt, R., Gilson, M., & Ludgate, J. W. (1993). Group cognitive therapy with inpatients. In J. H. Wright, M. E. Thase, A. T. Beck, & J. W. Ludgate (Eds.), *Cognitive therapy with inpatients* (pp. 121–153). New York, NY: Guilford Press.

Frey, R. E., & Weller, J. (2000). Rehab rounds: Behavioral management of aggression through teaching interpersonal skills. *Psychiatric Services, 51,* 607–609. http://dx.doi.org/10.1176/appi.ps.51.5.607

Hayes, S. C. (2004). Acceptance and commitment therapy and the new behavior therapies. In S. C. Hayes, V. M. Follette, & M. M. Linehan (Eds.), *Mindfulness and acceptance: Expanding the cognitive-behavioral tradition* (pp. 1–29). New York, NY: Guilford Press.

Karterud, S., & Bateman, A. W. (2012). Group therapy techniques. In A. W. Bateman & P. Fonagy (Eds.), *Handbook of mentalizing in mental health practice* (pp. 81–105). Washington, DC: American Psychiatric Association.

Kibel, H. D. (1981). A conceptual model for short-term inpatient group psychotherapy. *The American Journal of Psychiatry, 138,* 74–80.

Kibel, H. D. (2003). Interpretive work in milieu groups. *International Journal of Group Psychotherapy, 53,* 303–329. http://dx.doi.org/10.1521/ijgp.53.3.303.42821

Kibel, H. D. (2005). The evolution of group-as-a-whole and object relations theory: From projection to introjection. *Group, 29,* 139–161.

Linehan, M. (1993). *Cognitive behavioral treatment of borderline personality disorder.* New York, NY: Guilford Press.

McCann, R. A., & Ball, E. M. (2000). DBT with an inpatient forensic population: The CMHIP forensic model. *Cognitive and Behavioral Practice, 7,* 447–456.

McCann, R. A., Ivanoff, A., Schmidt, H., & Beach, B. (2007). Implementing dialectical behavior therapy in residential forensic settings with adults and juveniles. In L. A. Dimeff & K. Koerner (Eds.), *Dialectical behavior therapy in clinical practice* (pp. 112–144). New York, NY: Guilford Press.

McGinn, L. K., & Young, J. E. (1996). Schema-focused therapy. In P. M. Salkovskis (Ed.), *Frontiers of cognitive therapy* (pp. 182–207). New York, NY: Guilford Press.

Neuhaus, E. C., Christopher, M., Jacob, K., Guillaumot, J., & Burns, J. P. (2007). Short-term cognitive behavioral partial hospital treatment: A pilot study. *Journal of Psychiatric Practice, 13,* 298–307. http://dx.doi.org/10.1097/01.pra.0000290668.10107.f3

Simpson, E. B., Pistorello, J., Begin, A., Costello, E., Levinson, J., Mulberry, S., . . . Stevens, M. (1998). Focus on women: Use of dialectical behavior therapy in a partial hospital program for women with borderline personality disorder. *Psychiatric Services, 49,* 669–673. http://dx.doi.org/10.1176/ps.49.5.669

Southwick, S. M., Gilmartin, R., McDonough, P., & Morrissey, P. (2006). Logotherapy as an adjunctive treatment for chronic combat-related PTSD: A meaning-based intervention. *American Journal of Psychotherapy, 60,* 161–174.

Spivack, G., Platt, J. J., & Shure, M. B. (1976). *The problem-solving approach to adjustment.* San Francisco, CA: Jossey-Bass.

Swenson, C. R., Witterholt, S., & Bohus, M. (2007). Dialectical behavior therapy on inpatient units. In L. A. Dimeff & K. Koerner (Eds.), *Dialectical behavior therapy in clinical practice* (pp. 69–111). New York, NY: Guilford Press.

Wilfley, D. E., MacKenzie, K. R., Welch, R. R., Ayres, V. E., & Weissman, M. M. (2000). *Interpersonal psychotherapy for group.* New York, NY: Basic Books.

Yalom, I. (1983). *Inpatient group psychotherapy.* New York, NY: Basic Books.

Yalom, I., & Leszcz, M. (2005). *The theory and practice of group psychotherapy* (5th ed.). New York, NY: Basic Books.

Yen, S., Johnson, J., Costello, E., & Simpson, E. B. (2009). A 5-day dialectical behavior therapy partial hospital program for women with borderline personality disorder: Predictors of outcome from a 3-month follow-up study. *Journal of Psychiatric Practice, 15,* 173–182. http://dx.doi.org/10.1097/01.pra.0000351877.45260.70

1

GROUP PSYCHOTHERAPY TODAY

The field of group psychotherapy in its evolutionary process of progressive differentiation has come to recognize the inpatient group as a special arena of treatment. Partial hospitalization and residential treatment groups offer a further differentiation from care developed within the context of a full-time hospital stay. All are forms of *contextual group psychotherapy*—group treatment delivered within a larger treatment environment that simultaneously offers the patient in need of intensive intervention a multiplicity of treatment elements. Group psychotherapy is often one of those elements. In all these situations, the patient is treated not by a single therapist but rather by a multidisciplinary team of individuals who interact with one another. Whereas inpatient groups typically represent brief experiences, in some cases one or two sessions, day (or partial) hospital and residential treatment centers offer groups that range from short term (12 sessions or less) to long term.

In the early days of group psychotherapy, group scholars attempted to distinguish group psychotherapy from individual psychotherapy. Early contributors

http://dx.doi.org/10.1037/0000113-002
Group Psychotherapy in Inpatient, Partial Hospital, and Residential Care Settings, by V. Brabender and A. Fallon

to the inpatient literature, such as Lazell (1921) and Marsh (1935), frequently provided a list of benefits that group participation confers, benefits they saw as absent in individual treatment. Rather than focusing on the unique features of inpatients or other populations, they seemed to be interested primarily in exploring the wonders of this new modality. During the Second World War, Bion (1959), Foulkes (1948), and others invested considerable effort in the identification of those processes that are unique to groups. Although Bion studied both inpatient groups and training groups, he did not critically distinguish between them. The psychoanalytically oriented approaches to group psychotherapy that developed in the 1950s, originally for outpatient groups, were applied to inpatients with little adaptation. As we moved into the 60s, Frank (1963) and others began to underscore that the inpatient and outpatient situations are radically different from one another and require their own goals and methods. This recognition gave rise to the development of principles and techniques specifically designed for the inpatient setting. However, not until the 1980s were these elements organized into more formal approaches that entailed an integration of goals and intervention strategies. Some even referred to their contributions as *models* (e.g., Maxmen, 1984).

We regard a *model* as a guiding conceptual framework. Such a framework includes a set of assumptions about psychopathology, the processes effecting its alteration, a specification of goals for the psychotherapy group, interventions designed to accomplish these goals, and means of measuring the success of the interventions. The model may or may not include a theory of group process.

When we wrote our 1993 book, *Models of Inpatient Group Psychotherapy*, models had just arrived on the inpatient group psychotherapy scene. Since that time, the evidence-based practice movement (Kazdin, 2008) has encouraged the adoption of formal models in conducting treatment in general and inpatient group psychotherapy specifically. Third-party payers, regulatory groups, and clients themselves legitimately question whether the treatment clients are receiving is working—is it producing the positive effects sought by the client in receiving treatment? To demonstrate favorable outcomes, the practitioner has to have a precise way of assessing treatment outcome. A clear delineation of goals helps in the identification of relevant outcome measures. Further, a model specifies the interventions that can link goals with outcomes. In response to this increased accountability, group psychotherapists in all settings have developed models tailored to those settings, and therapists conducting groups on inpatient units, in partial hospital programs, and residential treatment facilities are no exception. Some of these models are highly specific to a particular problem. The ones we have chosen to feature in this text have a reasonable breadth of application. Before introducing these models, we take a closer look at how the use of a model alters in beneficial ways how the group psychotherapist conducts the group.

THE IMPORTANCE OF MODELS

An assumption of this book is that embracing a model facilitates treatment. Although this assertion is far less provocative today than when we wrote our 1993 book—a time when many therapists saw benefit in practicing intuitively and with minimal theoretical constraint—it nonetheless is worth thinking about why having a model is useful. Among the benefits a model provides is its contribution of a system of meaning by which events in a group can be understood. Certainly, any group behavior can be understood from range of perspectives. A member's harsh criticism of another member may be seen as self-defeating social behavior, a projection of the criticizing member's unwanted aspects, an avoidance of intimacy, and so on. The therapist's choice of a system of meaning determines those behaviors and events to which the therapist attends and enables the therapist to intervene systematically rather than haphazardly. That is, the therapist can plan an intervention that is consistent with the chosen system and test the success of the intervention on the basis of what that system would see as the sequelae of a successful intervention. Moreover, the adoption of an interpretive framework facilitates the formulation of timely interventions. The inexperienced therapist, in particular, is handicapped if before devising an intervention, he or she must first settle on an appropriate theoretical framework.

A consistent framework by which events in the group are understood is also helpful because, through it, members can see a thread in all the therapist's interventions. The perception of a clear direction to the therapist's comments enhances members' sense that the group has a purpose. Moreover, a therapist who commits to a particular framework is likely to make interventions with a greater sense of confidence and conviction than the therapist who vacillates among different frames of references. In this vein, Yalom (1983) wrote,

> By developing a cognitive framework that permits an ordering of all the inchoate events of therapy, the therapist experiences a sense of inner order and mastery—a sense that, if deeply felt, is automatically conveyed to patients and generates in them a corresponding sense of mastery and clarity. (p. 122)

The second benefit of a model is that it leads the therapist to limit and make more specific the goals being pursued. This function of models is of special importance for all forms of group therapy but especially in the inpatient setting where the duration of group participation is exceedingly brief in most cases, reflecting the brevity of contemporary hospital stays. One study found, for example, that in Pennsylvania, the average length of stay was 10 days (Lee, Rothbard, & Noll, 2012), and rarely does group occur each day. Although the partial hospital program and residential treatment centers provide more latitude, the inpatient therapist simply does not have the time to pursue an ambitious set of goals. Embracing a model means that some objectives that have importance for patients may go unaddressed. However, the therapist must keep in mind that group psychotherapy is only one of many modalities in which a patient participates. What is important is that the treatment package in the particular setting as a totality addresses all the patients' critical needs; it is not necessary (or possible) for any one modality to do so.

A third benefit of using a model is the provision of a ready set of interventions that are compatible with both the goals of the model and the meaning ascribed to events in the group by the model. Further, the models assist the therapist in anticipating likely events that occur in groups and provide strategies for using these events to members' advantage. For example, many psychodynamic models will use the group's tendency to oppose the leader at some point to help members resolve conflicts toward authority more satisfactorily.

A model also confers benefits beyond the immediate effects of its application during the group sessions. The therapist's use of a model is likely to increase his or her ability to develop a "progroup culture" on the unit (Rice & Rutan, 1987, p. 87; Rice & Rutan, 1981). A *progroup culture* is one wherein the treatment is seen as a valuable component of the patient's treatment package, with all members of the treatment team striving to safeguard its successful operation. The therapist can much more readily engender support for the group when the goals and methods are sufficiently defined to enable other staff to envision where the group fits into the overall therapeutic strategy for a patient. Moreover, when the therapist can identify in highly specific terms what the group can and cannot do, the treatment team is helped in understanding patients' reactions to the group and are less likely to be disappointed by the results of a patient's involvement in the group.

In this age of financial accountability and quality assurance monitoring, practitioners have to specify with a high level of precision what they are endeavoring to achieve with a patient at various points and to what extent they have done so. The concrete and articulated set of goals associated with each model provides the therapist with a framework for defining each member's work and thereby assists the therapist in this task.

Finally, the use of a well-delineated model facilitates research and training activities. With respect to research, the therapist's pursuit of a delimited set of goals and use of a specifiable set of techniques enable the evaluation of the comparative efficacy of that model in relation to other models not only by a primary exponent of the model but also by other practitioner–scientists in other settings who, with a model in hand, are able to replicate (or not) the methodology. Moreover, the concrete description of goals permits the selection of outcome measures that are congruent with the kind of change that the interventions of the model are designed to affect. For example, group psychotherapists can select a model and use measures of the CORE-R battery (Strauss,

Burlingame, & Bormann, 2008) to assess member progress. Vannicelli (2014) noted that new group psychotherapists conducting groups in inpatient settings are greatly in need of supervisory support. We believe these trainees are also aided in facing the challenges of this group work through the use of well-delineated models and close supervision in applying the models. Ideally, they have the opportunity to apprentice with a senior therapist who has achieved expertise with a given model. In the face of the complexity of events of an inpatient group, students are in need of a system of meaning with clear goals, methods of intervening, and means for determining whether their interventions are successful. The intense affect that often characterizes an inpatient group can be confusing and anxiety arousing to students. However, these disturbing feelings are kept in better moderation by students' possession of a cognitive frame to organize their reactions to the affect in the group.

Although many benefits accrue to a therapist's selecting and using a model, models also have disadvantages. These negative consequences of model implementation occur when any given model is applied rigidly. Unless a model has been generated for a very particular context, it is unlikely to mesh perfectly with a practitioner's context. Almost always, some adaptations are warranted. Moreover, many of the models presented in this text have potential to be combined with one another in ways that enable members to pursue a greater range of goals with an expanded set of resources. This benefit is especially likely to be realized when members' tenures in the group last beyond a handful of sessions. As the reader considers each model, he or she might ponder what elements from each might be incorporated into the approach the therapist develops for his or her group. In this framework, no model adoption is so wholesale that it does not allow for the therapist's creative use of it.

THE IMPORTANCE OF CONTEXT

This text shines a light on the contexts in which group therapy is conducted because any given model, to be effective, must be compatible with many aspects of the treatment environment. By *context*, we mean all the features that define a treatment environment. What we have attempted to do is to delineate those contextual features that are likely to have the greatest bearing on any given model's usefulness. We begin at a broad level with a focus on three types of treatment environment: inpatient hospital, day or partial hospitalization, and residential treatment. We have selected these three environments because, in all of them, group psychotherapy takes place alongside a range of other interventions. This fact has a variety of ramifications. We give three examples. First, in selecting a model, the therapist will want to avoid duplicating what is occurring in the rest of the patient's treatment program. At the same time, the therapist must identify an approach that is not at odds with other treatments (e.g., presenting the patient with conflicting views about his or her psychological difficulties). Second, the therapist will necessarily have to cultivate the support of the treatment staff for his or her chosen approach. Third, in evaluating the success of his or her approach, the therapist must recognize that because the group intervention is embedded in a larger treatment program, any changes exhibited might not be due to the group experience exclusively. In this chapter, we provide an overview of these three environments, and in the next chapter, we focus on additional contextual features of these treatment environments that bear upon what types of models are likely to be helpful to the patients being treated in these environments.

. The definitions of inpatient hospitalization, day or partial hospitalization, and residential treatment vary widely, particularly cross-culturally, but even within a given country such as the United States. To the extent that we could capture the consistency in the literature on the use of these terms, we have done so.

Three Types of Context

We offer characterizations of the three contexts that are the focus of this text: inpatient hospital programs (IHPs), partial hospital programs (PHPs), and residential treatment centers (RTCs).

Inpatient Hospital Programs

The inpatient environment offers a full range of medical and psychiatric services on a 24-hour basis. It provides a restrictive environment in which individuals who frequently represent a danger to themselves or others are provided intense treatment that enables their future safe and independent functioning. Inpatients frequently are coping with severe mental disorders potentially alongside comorbid medical conditions. Emphasis is placed on crisis management and stabilizing symptoms. For the safety of inpatients, certain procedures and processes, such as depriving a person of his or her personal belongings, continual monitoring, and restriction of freedom to leave the unit, are put in place and can be stressors in their own right. Inpatient hospitalization can occur within a unit of a general hospital or a freestanding psychiatric hospital. State and county hospitals continue to provide treatment, albeit to a much lesser extent than several decades ago due in large part to the deinstitutionalization movement (Lamb & Bachrach, 2001). They might fill a niche for individuals who have medical problems and chronic difficulties with a behavioral component that cannot be managed in a less-restrictive setting (Fisher, Barreira, Geller, White, Lincoln, & Sudders, 2001).

Inpatient hospitalizations witnessed a sharp decline between 1990 and 2000 with the growth of managed care. However, since that time, an increase has occurred in the rate of hospitalizations for child, adolescent, and nonelderly adult populations (Blader, 2011). Moreover, according to Cook, Arechiga, Dobson, and Boyd (2014), patient admissions in state psychiatric hospitals increased 21% from 2002 to 2005, possibly in part due to the increasing presence of forensic patients, sexually dangerous individuals, and difficult-to-place persons in the state hospital system (Fisher, Geller, & Pandiani, 2009). Notably, 13% of hospitalized individuals will be rehospitalized within a 6-month period of the initial hospitalization (Thompson, Neighbors, Munday, & Trierweiler, 2003), and between 40% to 50% within a year (Bridge & Barbe, 2004).

Psychotherapy groups in other than state and county hospitals are exceedingly brief, with considerable member turnover from day to day. Cook et al. (2014) noted that 3 to 5 days is typical in most inpatient environments. Group members are often highly heterogeneous regarding the level of functioning and symptom presentation. Rarely does the opportunity occur to prepare members for the group experience. The medical emphasis of treatment often leads to interruptions and unexpected absences in the sessions due to the diversion of individual members to other appointments. Cook and Dobson (2018) noted that although these features are common in groups in inpatient environments, considerable variability exists, thereby necessitating the availability of multiple approaches to fit individual settings.

Partial Hospital Programs

A PHP is for individuals who do not require 24-hour medical supervision. Individuals attend the program for periods of time each week but return to their homes. However, not only do the patients leave the treatment setting each day but also, the features of independence and contact with individuals on the outside are frequently incorporated into the design of the program. Relative to the inpatient situation, aside from the features mentioned, *partial hospital* refers to very different treatment entities. Piper, Rosie, Joyce, and Azim (1996) saw the usefulness of distinguishing among three partial hospital formats: day hospital, day treatment, and day care. These forms of partial hospitalization differ, they observed, by the degree of emphasis placed on treatment versus rehabilitation. Whereas *treatment* is designed to effect the fullest restoration of functioning, *rehabilitation* fosters adaptation to the illness—that is, helping the individual to function as well as he or she can, given the illness.

Partial hospitalization is geared to treat acute illness, although some rehabilitative component may be present for patients who have experienced a decline in functioning (Piper et al., 1996). Whereas some of the patients treated in this context would otherwise have been treated in an inpatient setting, others are provided day hospital treatment as a transition from the inpatient to the outpatient environment. Still others are treated in this setting when intensification of outpatient treatment is sought while avoiding the life-disrupting aspects of inpatient hospitalization (Kennair, Mellor, & Brann, 2016). Sometimes these programs are offered in the evening so that participants can continue to work. With day treatment, the more chronic population receives fairly comparable proportions of treatment and rehabilitation. Typically, these programs are designed to treat specific diagnostic groups, such as individuals with borderline personality disorder (Bateman & Fonagy, 2005), within a limited time frame. Day care programs are centered on a more chronic population still, one that benefits more fully than the others from a strong rehabilitation emphasis.

Access to both the program and their everyday environment is typically built into the design of many programs for PHP participants. Participants frequently identify this feature as a major aspect of how such programs can be helpful. Mörtl and Von Wietersheim (2008) asked clients in a partial hospital facility in Ulm, Germany, to describe the experiences that had been helpful during their program participation. Patients, all women, were interviewed three times: during Week 4 of treatment, the second to the last week of therapy, and 3 months after therapy. The interview focused on identifying factors that were helpful to patients, somewhat along the lines of Yalom's therapeutic factors (Yalom & Leszcz, 2005). Among the sets that emerged prominently in the interview were *transfer factors*, which captured the synergy between participation in each of the environments, home and program. Participants indicated program experiences transferred in favorable ways to their home settings. For example, some clients said that they helpfully transferred structural elements of the program to their home environments. Some participants such as Christine tried out learning from the program in their home environments,

> But it actually was important to me that I could implement the stuff at home that I had learned here. And when problems occurred, in the evenings or on weekends, that I could come here again and talk about the problems immediately. (Mörtl & Von Wietersheim, 2008, p. 289)

Her comment also suggests that home experiences provided "grist for the mill" within the day hospital program, enabling the refinement of skills or their enhanced coordination.

Residential Treatment Centers

RTCs are like inpatient environments in that the individual is supervised on a 24-hour basis. For the residents, activity is more restricted relative to partial hospitalization but less restricted than inpatient hospitalization. In residential treatment facilities, a full medical staff is typically not available on a 24-hour basis, and so the individual must have achieved greater psychiatric stability than the inpatient. What establishes the need for residential treatment is the inability of the person to function in the community regardless of whether the inability is acute or chronic. Although RTCs traditionally involved treatment that was long term (i.e., a year or beyond) because of managed care's influence, the time frame of treatment in RTCs currently varies greatly from several weeks to multiple years, both for adolescent and adult populations (Brodsky, 2012; Burns, Hoagwood, & Mrazek, 1999). The ambience of an RTC is more homelike than medical. As in the case of day hospitals, individuals may enter RTCs as a step down from hospitalization. Some patients enter an RTC when intensive outpatient treatment has proven insufficient to enable the individual to function adequately. In some cases, whether an individual goes to a PHP or RTC depends on where an opening exists. Fortunately, though, research is accruing to assist practitioners in ascertaining which format may be optimal according to the individual's needs (e.g., see Chiesa, Fonagy, Holmes, & Drahorad, 2004).

RTCs are a common treatment venue for children and adolescents who have a complex set of psychological problems. According to a survey of such centers in the United States (Mauch, Krumholz, & Robinson, 2008), youth admitted to RTCs exhibit *barrier behaviors* (e.g., disruption in the community, difficulties such as extreme aggression and self-injury) that prevent the child from remaining in the community. Of these programs, 90% involve some form of group psychotherapy. A hallmark of RTCs for children and youth is that residents and their family members are actively engaged in their own treatment planning.

Contrasts With Outpatient Groups

In this text, we draw attention to the differences between groups being conducted in the three featured settings (inpatient, partial, and residential) regarding their implications for model use. However, it must be recognized that a variety of common features that do not occur in a broader therapeutic context distinguishes these groups from outpatient groups. An exemplar of the latter is the private practice outpatient group. In such a group, the therapist typically has a high degree of control over contextual factors such as composition, duration of group participation, location, and so on. With this greater degree of control, the therapist can adjust the external environment to accommodate the requirements of a chosen model, a luxury rarely experienced by therapists in inpatient, partial, and residential treatment settings.

Another feature differentiating the private practice group from the other three concerns the boundary between the group and the group's immediate environment. The notion of a *boundary* is derived from general systems theory (von Bertalanffy, 1950). A boundary demarcates a subsystem from the system in which it is embedded. A boundary can have different levels of porousness with its immediate, external environment. With highly porous boundaries, the various elements present in the external environment easily enter the group and shape its character. This circumstance exists for our target trio of settings. With highly impermeable boundaries, information exchange is minimal, a situation more characteristic of a private practice group. Therefore, the therapist in one of the three settings will have to be thoughtful about how the group will manage information entering the group. For example, if members enter the group affected by an event that occurred on the unit or in the program, the therapist will unlikely be able to ignore the emotional load group members are carrying. For the private practice therapist, external events that might influence important aspects of the group's functioning are less immediate and pressing. Occasionally, exceptions exist and the external environment might insinuate itself into the outpatient group's process and content. For example, after the 9/11 terror attacks, Americans ubiquitously experienced stress reactions (Schuster et al., 2001), and these reactions tended to enter all group settings, including psychotherapy groups. For the most part, however, the private practice group has insularity, with external influences operating on individuals rather than the group as a whole.

Whereas individuals in a private outpatient group might be working with other practitioners, patients in the three settings are always doing so and typically on a daily basis. Therapists in the three settings must concern themselves both with the compatibility of the group model with these other interventions and with the attitude of the staff toward the members' work in the group. This point is developed further in Chapter 2. Because for the outpatient private patient therapist other therapeutic experiences often do not occur in close spatial and temporal proximity, the demands to attend to these alternate experiences are less intense and ongoing.

One factor that all three types of settings have in common is that they are expensive relative to outpatient treatment. Consequently, they are regularly under scrutiny to determine whether the investment yields adequate returns (Bettmann & Jasperson, 2009), both on a holistic and component level. That is, third-party payers and regulatory groups, as well as the patients themselves, expect treatment to be evidence based, including each element of the treatment package. Hence, group psychotherapists practicing in these settings have an obligation to show how the model is underpinned by evidence and has demonstrated effectiveness within the therapist's setting given all its particulars. However, because of the concurrence of the group experience with other interventions, often, it is difficult for the group psychotherapist to parcel out the effects of this single intervention. For private practice settings, favorable changes that are observed across members can more easily be attributed to the psychotherapy group, particularly when other types of concurrent therapy experiences vary from member to member.

Table 1.1 summarizes some of the major differences between private practice outpatient groups and inpatient, partial, and residential groups using the contextual dimensions that are introduced in Chapter 2.

TABLE 1.1
Differences Between Types of Groups: Private Practice/Community Versus Inpatient Hospital Program, Partial Hospital Program, and Residential Treatment Center Contexts

Dimension	Contexts	
	Private practice/community	IHP, PHP, RTC contexts
Philosophical context	The individual practitioner's philosophy and values are primary drivers of model selection, but therapist must harmonize his or her chosen approach with the ethos of the communities from which clients are drawn.	Group therapists must achieve congruence between the values and treatment philosophy of the setting and those of the selected model.
Relationship to other program components	The group psychotherapist must coordinate with individual therapists and other treatment providers. The effects of other modalities on group psychotherapy are highly variable.	Coordination is extensive given the multiplicity of other interventions. A high likelihood exists that given their proximity in time and space, developments in other modalities infuse the content and affective tenor of the psychotherapy group.
Temporal variables	Sessions tend to be weekly or semi-weekly and last between 60 and 120 minutes.	Sessions tend to last between 30 and 90 minutes and occur daily.
Size	Generally, 6 to 12 members.	Six to 10 members for higher functioning groups; 4 to 7 for lower functioning groups.
Member composition	Members are more likely to be self-referred and self-motivated and, although covering a broad range of functioning, are higher functioning and capable of more independent functioning.	Members are skewed toward mid and lower range of functioning. The development of their motivation to participate in the group might require considerable therapist attention.
Therapist variables	Requires the ability to coordinate care, often in the absence of natural contact opportunities, and a capacity to work without immediate team support. Other demands are created by the specific population the therapist serves and the model used.	Requires the ability to function as a team member, serve as advocate for group in the broader system, cope emotionally with rapid patient turnover, form caring relationships quickly, and maintain active posture throughout sessions.

Note. IHP = inpatient hospital program; PHP = partial hospital program; RTC = residential treatment center.

The common challenges faced by inpatient, partial, and residential groups are the basis for examining them together in this text. Although we often focus on the differences among them, in fact, the similarities are great.

DOES GROUP PSYCHOTHERAPY IN INPATIENT, PARTIAL, AND RESIDENTIAL CONTEXTS WORK?

In our 1993 book, we reported on individual studies that had been conducted to examine the effectiveness of inpatient group psychotherapy, particularly regarding a particular model. Some models, such as cognitive behavioral and problem solving, had a considerable corpus of empirical support, whereas others, such as the object relations/system model, had little. Since the publication of *Models of Inpatient Group Psychotherapy* (Brabender & Fallon, 1993), two developments have occurred. First, with the widespread recognition of the importance that treatment must be evidence based, additional studies have accrued, particularly for some of the newer models used in inpatient, partial hospital, and residential settings. A severe limit to the usefulness of data rendered from these studies is that many involve a pre–post design in the absence of a comparison group, and investigators frequently fail to report the pre–post correlation between scores that would enable the calculation of trustworthy effect sizes (Kösters, Burlingame, Nachtigall, & Strauss, 2006). In addition, the treatment involved a greater number of sessions than is possible in current inpatient environments, and the patients were less ethnically diverse than the population at large. Still, extant studies can teach us something about contextual group effectiveness, particularly when effect sizes are corrected through statistical means. Second, researchers have increasingly used meta-analyses to summarize effectiveness across a range of studies. Before reporting these findings, we must state one significant caveat. All the groups we study exist within a treatment context with other components. What all these outcome studies show is the effectiveness of group psychotherapy when it is part of a larger treatment package (Dinger & Schauenburg, 2010). This factor distinguishes it from studies of outpatient groups; the outpatient group might be the only intervention the client is receiving.

Inpatient Hospital Settings

To date, researchers have conducted several meta-analyses either using setting as a variable with "inpatient" as a level of the variable or restricting the meta-analysis to studies on inpatient groups. Burlingame, Fuhriman, and Mosier (2003) provided an example of the former. An analysis of six inpatient studies found that outpatient groups produced greater positive change

studies (e.g., Bateman & Fonagy, 1999; Chiesa et al., 2004; Greenfield et al., 2004; Karterud et al., 1992) being conducted in these settings have focused on the overall effectiveness of the program rather than different treatment components. The findings of these studies have relevance to group psychotherapy because, in most PHPs, group psychotherapy is a major part of the treatment package. Because the findings of those studies that do explicitly concern group psychotherapy have not been integrated via meta-analyses, we describe them as they are relevant to the models we describe in subsequent chapters.

SUMMARY

In this chapter, we characterized and contrasted three intensive treatment contexts in which psychotherapy groups are commonly conducted: inpatient, partial hospital, and residential treatment center settings. Psychotherapy groups in these settings have distinctive features in relation to private practice and community groups, particularly in the areas of the duration of group participation and therapist control over composition. Although the research evidence for the effectiveness of psychotherapy groups in the three settings is still nascent, what exists is promising, especially research on inpatient groups.

REFERENCES

Bateman, A., & Fonagy, P. (1999). Effectiveness of partial hospitalization in the treatment of borderline personality disorder: A randomized controlled trial. *American Journal of Psychiatry, 156*, 1563–1569. http://dx.doi.org/10.1176/ajp.156.10.1563

Bateman, A., & Fonagy, P. (2005). *Psychotherapy for borderline personality disorder: Mentalization-based treatment.* Oxford, England: Oxford University Press.

Bettmann, J. E., & Jasperson, R. A. (2009). Adolescents in residential and inpatient treatment: A review of the outcome literature. *Child & Youth Care Forum, 38*, 161–183. http://dx.doi.org/10.1007/s10566-009-9073-y

Bion, W. R. (1959). *Experiences in groups.* London, England: Tavistock.

Blader, J. C. (2011). Acute inpatient care for psychiatric disorders in the United States, 1996 through 2007. *Archives of General Psychiatry, 68*, 1276–1283. http://dx.doi.org/10.1001/archgenpsychiatry.2011.84

Brabender, V., & Fallon, A. (1993). *Models of inpatient group psychotherapy.* Washington, DC: American Psychological Association.

Bridge, J. A., & Barbe, R. P. (2004). Reducing hospital readmission in depression and schizophrenia: Current evidence. *Current Opinion in Psychiatry, 17*, 505–511. http://dx.doi.org/10.1097/00001504-200411000-00015

Brodsky, M. (2012). Residential treatment—When to consider it, what to look for. *Social Work Today, 12*(2), 8. Retrieved from http://www.socialworktoday.com/archive/031912p8.shtml

Burlingame, G. M., Fuhriman, A. J., & Mosier, J. (2003). The differential effectiveness of group psychotherapy: A meta-analytic perspective. *Group Dynamics: Theory, Research, and Practice, 7*, 3–12. http://dx.doi.org/10.1037/1089-2699.7.1.3

Burlingame, G. M., MacKenzie, K. R., & Strauss, B. (2004). Small group treatment: Evidence for effectiveness and mechanisms of change. In M. J. Lambert (Ed.), *Bergin and Garfield's handbook of psychotherapy and behavior change* (5th ed., pp. 647–696). New York, NY: Wiley.

Burns, B. J., Hoagwood, K., & Mrazek, P. J. (1999). Effective treatment for mental disorders in children and adolescents. *Clinical Child and Family Psychology Review, 2*, 199–254. http://dx.doi.org/10.1023/A:1021826216025

Chiesa, M., Fonagy, P., Holmes, J., & Drahorad, C. (2004). Residential versus community treatment of personality disorders: A comparative study of three treatment programs. *The American Journal of Psychiatry, 161*, 1463–1470. http://dx.doi.org/10.1176/appi.ajp.161.8.1463

Cook, W. G., Arechiga, A., Dobson, L. A. V., & Boyd, K. (2014). Brief heterogeneous inpatient psychotherapy groups: A process-oriented psychoeducational (POP) model. *International Journal of Group Psychotherapy, 64*, 180–206. http://dx.doi.org/10.1521/ijgp.2014.64.2.180

Cook, W. G., & Dobson, L. A. V. (2018). "Revolving doors and brief encounters: Dare we do inpatient groups?" Reflections on being an AGPA conference panelist. *International Journal of Group Psychotherapy, 68*, 261–264. http://dx.doi.org/10.1080/00207284.2017.1412263

Dinger, U., & Schauenburg, H. (2010). Effects of individual cohesion and patient interpersonal style on outcome in psychodynamically oriented inpatient group psychotherapy. *Psychotherapy Research, 20*, 22–29. http://dx.doi.org/10.1080/10503300902855514

Fisher, W. H., Barreira, P. J., Geller, J. L., White, A. W., Lincoln, A. K., & Sudders, M. (2001). Long-stay patients in state psychiatric hospitals at the end of the 20th century. *Psychiatric Services, 52*, 1051–1056. http://dx.doi.org/10.1176/appi.ps.52.8.1051

Fisher, W. H., Geller, J. L., & Pandiani, J. A. (2009). The changing role of the state hospital. *Health Affairs: At the Intersection of Health. Healthcare Policy, 28*, 676–684.

Foulkes, S. H. (1948). *Introduction to group-analytic psychotherapy*. London, England: Heinemann.

Frank, J. D. (1963). Group therapy in the mental hospital. In M. Rosenbaum & M. Berger (Eds.), *Group psychotherapy and group function* (pp. 453–468). New York, NY: Basic Books.

Greenfield, L., Burgdorf, K., Chen, X., Porowski, A., Roberts, T., & Herrell, J. (2004). Effectiveness of long-term residential substance abuse treatment for women:

Findings from three national studies. *The American Journal of Drug and Alcohol Abuse, 30,* 537–550. http://dx.doi.org/10.1081/ADA-200032290

Karterud, S., Vaglum, S., Friis, S., Irion, T., Johns, S., & Vaglum, P. (1992). Day hospital therapeutic community treatment for patients with personality disorders: An empirical evaluation of the containment function. *Journal of nervous and mental disorders, 180,* 238–243. http://dx.doi.org/10.1097/00005053-199204000-00005

Kazdin, A. E. (2008). Evidence-based treatment and practice: New opportunities to bridge clinical research and practice, enhance the knowledge base, and improve patient care. *American Psychologist, 63,* 146–159. http://dx.doi.org/10.1037/0003-066X.63.3.146

Kennair, N., Mellor, D., & Brann, P. (2016). Curative factors in adolescent day programs: Participant, therapist, and parent perspectives. *International Journal of Group Psychotherapy, 66,* 382–400. http://dx.doi.org/10.1080/00207284.2016.1149412

Kösters, M., Burlingame, G. M., Nachtigall, C., & Strauss, B. (2006). A meta-analytic review of the effectiveness of inpatient group psychotherapy. *Group Dynamics: Theory, Research, and Practice, 10,* 146–163. http://dx.doi.org/10.1037/1089-2699.10.2.146

Lamb, H. R., & Bachrach, L. L. (2001). Some perspectives on deinstitutionalization. *Psychiatric Services, 52,* 1039–1045. http://dx.doi.org/10.1176/appi.ps.52.8.1039

Lazell, E. W. (1921). The group treatment of dementia praecox. *Psychoanalytic Review, 8,* 168–179.

Lee, S., Rothbard, A. B., & Noll, E. L. (2012). Length of inpatient stay of persons with serious mental illness: Effects of hospital and regional characteristics. *Psychiatric Services, 63,* 889–895. http://dx.doi.org/10.1176/appi.ps.201100412

Leichsenring, F., & Leibing, E. (2003). The effectiveness of psychodynamic therapy and cognitive behavior therapy in the treatment of personality disorders: A meta-analysis. *The American Journal of Psychiatry, 160,* 1223–1232. http://dx.doi.org/10.1176/appi.ajp.160.7.1223

Marsh, L. C. (1935). Group therapy in the psychiatric clinic. *Journal of Nervous and Mental Disease, 82,* 381–393. http://dx.doi.org/10.1097/00005053-193510000-00002

Mauch, D., Krumholz, A., & Robinson, G. (2008). *Characteristics of residential treatment for children and youth with serious emotional disturbances.* Cambridge, MA: Abt.

Maxmen, J. S. (1984). Helping patients survive theories: The practice of an educative model. *International Journal of Group Psychotherapy, 34,* 355–368. http://dx.doi.org/10.1080/00207284.1984.11491390

Mörtl, K., & Von Wietersheim, J. (2008). Client experiences of helpful factors in a day treatment program: A qualitative approach. *Psychotherapy Research, 18,* 281–293. http://dx.doi.org/10.1080/10503300701797016

Piper, W. E., Rosie, J. S., Joyce, A. S., & Azim, H. F. A. (1996). *Time-limited day treatment for personality disorders: Integration of research and practice in a group program.* Washington, DC: American Psychological Association. http://dx.doi.org/10.1037/10208-000

Rice, C. A., & Rutan, J. S. (1981). Boundary maintenance in inpatient therapy groups. *International Journal of Group Psychotherapy, 31,* 297–309. http://dx.doi.org/10.1080/00207284.1981.11491709

Rice, C. A., & Rutan, J. S. (1987). *Inpatient group psychotherapy: A psychodynamic perspective.* New York, NY: Macmillan.

Schuster, M. A., Stein, B. D., Jaycox, L., Collins, R. L., Marshall, G. N., Elliott, M. N., . . . Berry, S. H. (2001, November 15). A national survey of stress reactions after the September 11, 2001, terrorist attacks. *The New England Journal of Medicine, 345,* 1507–1512. http://dx.doi.org/10.1056/NEJM200111153452024

Strauss, B., Burlingame, G. M., & Bormann, B. (2008). Using the CORE-R battery in group psychotherapy. *Journal of Clinical Psychology, 64,* 1225–1237. http://dx.doi.org/10.1002/jclp.20535

Thompson, E. E., Neighbors, H. W., Munday, C., & Trierweiler, S. (2003). Length of stay, referral to aftercare, and rehospitalization among psychiatric inpatients. *Psychiatric Services, 54,* 1271–1276. http://dx.doi.org/10.1176/appi.ps.54.9.1271

Vannicelli, M. (2014). Supervising the beginning group leader in inpatient and partial hospital settings. *International Journal of Group Psychotherapy, 64,* 144–163. http://dx.doi.org/10.1521/ijgp.2014.64.2.144

von Bertalanffy, L. (1950, January 13). The theory of open systems in physics and biology. *Science, 111,* 23–29.

Yalom, I. (1983). *Inpatient group psychotherapy.* New York, NY: Basic Books.

Yalom, I., & Leszcz, M. (2005). *The theory and practice of group psychotherapy.* New York, NY: Basic Books.

2

CONTEXTUAL DIMENSIONS

Group psychotherapy is conducted, always, within a context. For an outpatient group, whether that group takes place in an outpatient clinic versus a private practice setting will bear on the group's functioning in myriad ways. For example, in an outpatient clinic, it may be necessary to place new members in a group quickly—without the opportunity to prepare existing members. The private practice group typically would not have this limitation—that is, the group psychotherapist would have greater control over the session in which a member is introduced to the group. In this book, we focus on groups that are thoroughly embedded in the broader treatment context and derive their character from this context. For this reason, we use the term *contextual group psychotherapy* to underscore this point. In contextual group psychotherapy, the group member has the benefit of a treatment team and a host of other therapeutic elements. He or she is likely to have myriad relationships with other group members and the therapists, including relationships that take place outside the group. All of these factors can help or hinder

http://dx.doi.org/10.1037/0000113-003
Group Psychotherapy in Inpatient, Partial Hospital, and Residential Care Settings, by V. Brabender and A. Fallon

what occurs within the group. The broad context can either abet or hinder the application of particular models of treatment.

In the prior chapter, we characterized the three contexts that are the focus of this text: inpatient units in general medical hospitals or psychiatric hospitals, partial hospitals, and residential treatment settings. In this chapter, we expand on the notion of context by identifying other contextual dimensions that frequently must be considered in deciding on a treatment approach that is likely to be effective in that setting. These include the clinical mission of the care setting, system perception of the group, temporality (e.g., session length), size, group composition, and developmental status. We end our coverage of variables with a consideration of the person of the therapist and how the therapist's cognitive and emotional proclivities can make a difference in what model is likely to be effective.

In thinking about these dimensions (or clusters of variables), the group therapist who is designing a group for a particular setting should ascertain the degree to which any given variable can be altered. Some variables within a setting are unchangeable. Frequently, they are definitional features of the organization or institution in which the psychotherapy group takes place. For example, a residential treatment center might have a particular patient population that it seeks to serve. The group psychotherapist has to fashion the group around this fixed element. Other features of the setting are moderately alterable—that is, capable of modification if the therapist can identify effective strategies and allocate sufficient time to this effort. Many of these features represent administrative conveniences to other staff. For instance, the psychotherapy group may meet only twice a week so that other activities can be scheduled. To achieve a change in the direction of greater frequency, at a minimum, the therapist has to work with staff to educate them on its benefits. Still other features are more or less accidental and are readily subject to modification. In a partial hospital setting, for instance, group psychotherapy may be scheduled at the end of the treatment day. The therapist might recognize that an alternate temporal placement of the group may be more auspicious. Once again, carrying this proposal requires that the therapist develop an argument that is compelling to other staff.

Whether a feature is fixed, moderately modifiable, or highly plastic is relevant to determining whether that feature controls the selection of a model. Unmodifiable features have the most limiting effects on whether a particular group model can be effective in a setting. The features that are alterable are important because their consideration enables the therapist to use a model under the most optimal conditions possible in that setting. For example, a number of models demand that the group take place in a setting that is strongly supportive of its goals and methods. With some effort, the therapist can effect a significant shift in staff members' attitudes toward the therapist's approach to the group. However, failure of the therapist to attend to the staff members' view of the group could lead to unsupportive staff behaviors that would render the group less effective than it might be.

CLINICAL MISSION OF THE CARE SETTING

Philosophy and Theoretical Orientation

Whereas values, goals, and philosophy are interwoven, theoretical orientation can stand apart from these guiding notions. In some settings, however, all four systems are related.

Philosophy and Related Values and Goals

In this context, we see *values* as broad aspiration principles that the setting establishes and *goals* as targets of change consistent with a set of values. For example, in an institution that embraces the value of training, the goal of locating funds for staff training is likely to be pursued. If group psychotherapy is perceived to be an important training area, those staff members who conduct groups will be offered resources (e.g., money for continuing education events) to improve their group work. In such a setting, staff members are better equipped to use those models that place greater demands on their training. Another example is a hospital that places minimal emphasis on coordinating treatment among professionals who use different modalities because the administration regards time spent in such activities as cost-ineffective. A number of models in this book, such as dialectical behavior therapy and the object relations/systems approach, demand a high level of coordination between the group psychotherapist and other members of the treatment team. The use of these models would be, at best, hampered and, at worst, precluded in such a setting.

Large systems are rarely simple from a values perspective. A large day treatment program, say, may have subsystems that have competing values and priorities. One faction may support the institution's development of its reputation as a training facility. Another faction may privilege maintenance of solvency. These subsystems may reflect a conflict within the organization-at-large about what values should be preeminent. Organizations resolve conflicts in various ways. One way may be to allow one powerful subsystem with a particular set of values to dictate policy. A group psychotherapist embedded in such an organization must be concerned not only with a model's compatibility with the values of the organization but also with its compatibility with those of the powerful subsystem. This point was potently made in a recent study (Lean et al., 2015) in which staff members on a British National Health

Service rehabilitation unit were given in-service training to improve patient engagement in the services on the unit. At the end of training, staff gave evidence of having acquired the skills that were the target of the training, skills that appeared to be accepted by the staff as valuable. However, as soon as the trainers left, staff reverted to earlier modes of interacting with patients. The authors drew the useful conclusion that they had insufficiently attended to the values and priorities of senior staff in introducing the training.

Settings differ, too, in their expectations of what kinds of change should occur in the patient as a function of treatment. Some institutions see themselves as treating patients in a holistic fashion. Although the patient presents with specific psychological complaints, the hospital views its mission as assisting the individual with any interpersonal, financial, or physical problem that emerges during the course of his or her involvement with the institution. In contrast, some settings define their tasks in narrower terms, focusing on only the target complaints themselves. Of course, the extent to which an institution has a global versus a narrow focus ranges in degrees. The more holistic a setting, the greater is the range of models that can be successfully applied.

Theoretical Orientation

Institutions vary regarding the theoretical orientation that predominates within the setting. For example, some hospitals in the United States have outstanding reputations for being bastions of psychoanalytic thought. The group therapist who attempts to use behavioral techniques in such places invites the risk of having his or her group work seen as trivial. Although many other factors within a system might compel the therapist to use a behavioral approach, the institutional image of what constitutes therapy cannot be safely ignored.

In one institution, a group psychotherapist wished to use a gestalt model in a primarily psychodynamic-oriented institution. She provided regular in-services to unit staff in which she translated gestalt concepts in psychoanalytic terms. Although her approach required more effort than using an approach that was familiar to the staff, she was successful in creating a progroup climate (Rice & Rutan, 1981), as defined in Chapter 1. Hence, the therapist who is willing to go against the theoretical grain of an institution must be committed to investing energy in creating a friendly home for the group within the institution or organization.

Discerning Values, Philosophies, and Theoretical Orientations

The process of determining a model's fit with an institution's values, mission, and so on, is not as simple as reading that institution's official statement of purpose that perhaps appears on its home webpage. Institutions and organizations frequently have unarticulated agendas and goals. Consider the following example:

> A psychiatric hospital known for serving affluent patients was under pressure by the surrounding community to increase the number of admitted public assistance patients. Eventually, in the interest of preserving its reputation, the institution not only agreed to expand the number of beds for persons on Medicaid but also, with great fanfare, announced the creation of special programs that would be tailored to the needs of this population—needs that hospital administrators saw as different from those of its more long-standing population. Many specialists were hired, one of whom was a group psychotherapist who had worked in institutions that had served primarily economically disadvantaged individuals. The therapist designed a group with an interpersonal focus; it was not that different from groups run elsewhere in the hospital. The therapist believed the similarity was auspicious: it would lead others to understand and support the group. However, the therapist was surprised to encounter various types of staff resistance. Patients were often unable to attend group because of conflicting appointments with medical specialists. Frequently, an insufficient number appeared to make the group session viable. When the session did occur, staff would intervene in various ways to make difficult his establishment of an interpersonal focus. For example, staff would urge patients to bring somatic problems to group and to discuss there the unpleasant side effects of medication.

What the puzzled and dismayed group therapist failed to discern was that the institution's stated mission was not at one with its real mission. The institution regarded the community's demand as a threat to its integrity as an organization. The effort of the organization was to place the threat within the organization where it could be managed (and subdued) more easily (see Hirschhorn, 1988). By identifying this new population as having radically different needs and resources than their more affluent patients, and by seeing the new population as being treatable by biological interventions only, the institution cordoned off that population. Through this maneuver, the institution continued to keep individuals drawn from the warded-off population on the periphery of the organization in a way that would be less apparent to the community. The group therapist's approach to conducting the group was at odds with the institution's effort to maintain the status quo. Although the therapist's theoretical orientation was similar to that of staff working with the more long-standing, more valued patient population, the similarity was detrimental. It implied some commonality between the old and new populations, a position at odds with the classist perspective of those holding power within the institution. Had the group therapist been cognizant of the institutional dynamics, he might have decided to either adopt an alternative model, use an interpersonal approach in a way that would take into account the staff's resistance to it, or not accept the position altogether.

In the example just discussed, the psychotherapy group was affected by the institution's effort to contain an external pressure. In some instances, external pressures lead institutions to operate in ways that may be at odds with their long-held values. For example, Gabbard (1992) commented on how the demands on hospitals to satisfy regulatory groups have diminished the opportunities of treatment team members to have meaningful discussions with one another. He wrote,

> The required documentation of treatment plans and justification for treatment being delivered has shifted the focus of staff meetings from the processing of transference–countertransference developments to the tedious writing of accounts that will satisfy surveyors and lead to accreditation. (p. 16)

Here, too, the psychotherapy group will be affected. Even if staff members philosophically recognize the value of communication and treatment coordination, their efforts to satisfy external bodies will hinder the application of those models that are especially dependent on such interaction. The task of the group therapist is to determine how the tensions between both an institution's actual and stated goals and the institutional and sociocultural systems in which it is embedded are likely to affect the viability of different models in that setting (Karterud & Urnes, 2004).

THE GROUP IN RELATION TO THE BROADER THERAPEUTIC PROGRAM

Unlike the circumstance of the therapist running a stand-alone group, the therapist who is designing a group that is part of a larger therapeutic program must consider the other elements in that program. Currently, a primary offering in many therapeutic programs is the *psychoeducational group* (PEG). As the name implies, these groups emphasize the acquisition of knowledge and skills (Cowls & Hale, 2005); they are designed to increase functionality by imparting specific information to a particular audience. For example, there are PEGs for depression (Aagaard, Foldager, Makki, Hansen, & Müller-Nielsen, 2017), first episode psychosis (Petrakis & Laxton, 2017), schizophrenia (Matsuda & Kohno, 2016), alcoholism (Yeh, Tung, Horng, & Sung, 2017), and bipolar disorder (R. Chen et al., 2018; Scott et al., 2009). PEGs have also been designed for relatives of patients with depression (Frank et al., 2015) and schizophrenia (Bäuml, Froböse, Kraemer, Rentrop, & Pitschel-Walz, 2006; Mino, Shimodera, Inoue, Fujita, & Fukuzawa, 2007). Topics are typically selected to improve functionality in such areas as parenting (Sullivan, Deutsch, & Ward, 2016), identifying warning signs of relapse (Duman, Yildirim, Ucok, Er, & Kanik, 2010), or compliance with medication (Matsuda & Kohno, 2016). The skills often fostered in PEGs might be traditional mental health topics, such as raising self-esteem, but they might also involve the cultivation of leisure-time pursuits such as cooking and exercise. These groups are highly structured and have specified content for a particular audience (Cowls & Hale, 2005). In PEGs, it is typically the leaders who impart information, but the term also can refer to groups in which information is imparted primarily through video or film (von Maffei, Görges, Kissling, Schreiber, & Rummel-Kluge, 2015). Although there are models in which process is explored (e.g., Cook, Arechiga, Dobson, & Boyd, 2014), the overwhelming majority of them are structured, and process receives minimal attention. Although some leaders solicit input from the group, often, the interaction of the leader with his or her audience is limited to questions at the end. In that way, the sessions can appear similar to a lecture. Leaders can range from mental health professionals to individuals outside the profession who have particular expertise in a content area. In some cases, former patients might participate in the leadership of these groups (Rummel-Kluge & Kissling, 2008).

Cowls and Hale's (2005) study of participants in PEGs in an inpatient setting found that what participants value in such groups is the activity itself rather than the verbal processing of group experiences. Consistent with this finding, Yalom (1983) has repeatedly made the point that groups conducted in a more inclusive treatment program should not duplicate other activities. From Yalom's perspective, then, the psychotherapy group tends to make its greatest contribution when it is not duplicating the activity focus of a PEG. The value of these models is that they can be tailored to a specific group of patients to convey specific information. Professional time can be minimized and both small and large audiences can be accommodated without varying the format. Because these groups are so specific to the problem at hand and, at the same time, so varied regarding structure, they are not easily captured in a set of principles. Thus, we chose to encourage group leaders interested in this form of treatment to pursue the specific literature on these groups.

Although, in general, one would not want the therapy group duplicating the contribution of a PEG or any other type of intervention, in some cases, different types of groups or other program components work strategically toward the same ends. An example is a circumstance in which a community meeting is run according to the same principles as the psychotherapy group to make these principles salient to patients. In such a case, one modality can potentially increase the potency of another. Another good example of the collaboration of PEGs with the more traditional group therapy is the use of the PEG to explain the value and use of a thought record, which would then be used in a cognitive behavioral group in which patients learn the relationship between precipitating events, automatic thoughts, and resulting depressed or anxious feelings. What is particularly undesirable is when components of a program work at cross-purposes, such as when staff on the unit deliver a message that patients should attempt to move away from negative feelings, and other components of the program, such as the psychotherapy group, take the stance that members should accept such feelings and know that they are part of the palette of human experiences. At times, contradictions between the aims of modalities might be more apparent than real, but in these cases, patients have to be helped to make the appropriate differentiations ("In here, we are working on having you reckon with your feelings, but when you leave here, you have an opportunity to focus on other parts of yourself").

TEMPORAL VARIABLES

The family of temporal variables includes how long a member participates in a group, whether the group is closed-ended or open-ended, and the number of sessions per week.

Length of Group Participation

In inpatient hospital programs (IHPs), partial hospital programs (PHPs), and residential treatment centers (RTCs), one of the most important factors in model selection is the length of time a member is likely to be in a group. The variable of length of time of group participation is important in at least two respects, one of which pertains to the individual and the other to the group as a whole. As the length of time in the group increases, the array of goals an individual could potentially achieve expands. The achievement of particular goals requires the member's mastery of successive mini-steps en route to the goal. For example, in the social skills training model, the achievement of a skill such as greeting another person involves a series of accomplishments, each of which is fostered in the group. This process requires a considerable amount of time. However, other goals require the deployment of processes that are only available once members have had an opportunity to get to know one another and work through a series of issues. For example, the rich self-disclosures that are necessary for members to rid themselves of feelings of shame often occur only once members have achieved trust in one another and a sense of the group as a place where they can be helped and where taking risks does not bring on great peril. That is, self-disclosures at a deep level require a group that has had an opportunity to develop, and group development takes time (Brabender & Fallon, 2009; Wheelan, 1997). Likewise, early in the life of a group, members are far less likely to see each other in highly differentiated terms relative to members who have had the time to move beyond superficial relating. This greater refinement in perceptions of one another makes possible the exchange of high-quality feedback that is crucial to many models of group psychotherapy. However, if members do not have the luxury of time, they can use their stint in group to learn about the feedback process and have some fledgling experience with it. This experience can support later, more sustained therapeutic involvements with more significant, life-altering outcomes.

Enhancing one's appreciation of time in group psychotherapy is knowledge of group development, which is a core concept of group psychotherapy. Those developmental stages outlined in the American Group Psychotherapy Association's guidelines for the practice of group psychotherapy (Bernard et al., 2008) are similar to our model of group development (Brabender & Fallon, 2009). Both consist of five stages. The first stage involves members' establishment of trust in one another and the group's accomplishment of a sense of cohesion. In the second stage, members address their feelings toward, and dependency on, authority, as well as the differences between and among one another. In the third stage, members approach feelings of intimacy toward one another. Stage 4 provides the opportunity for members to do interpersonal work as they tackle the problem of how to stay connected to others while retaining their individualities. The final stage concerns dealing with loss, a challenge stimulated by the loss of the group and of one another. As Spivack (2008) noted, in short-term settings such as the IHP unit, the group is likely to spend much of its time in Stages 1 and 2.

Different models place different demands on a group's development. Some models, to be implemented, fully require that members move beyond the earliest two stages of development. Other models make no such presumption and can accommodate a group's unvarying residency in the earliest stage of development. The models presented in this group represent a range of demands on this score. Although model designers are not explicit about developmental demands, we attempt to construe and share what each model tends to be expecting regarding group development.

Closed-Ended Versus Open-Ended Groups

Most groups in IHPs, PHPs, and RTCs are open-ended. That is, members enter and leave the group on an ongoing basis. An alternative format is one in which once the group begins, no new members are added, and all members end the group at the same time. Relative to their open-ended counterparts, closed-ended groups, not having to withstand the disruptive effects of membership turnover, are likely to achieve a higher level of cohesiveness and trust (Henderson & Gladding, 2004), both of which promote the group's development beyond the earliest stages. Closed-ended groups also provide members with a well-defined time limit. In these groups, members' work is galvanized by the knowledge of a precise ending date, which highlights the disparity between what they have and have not accomplished (Spitz, 1996). Although many therapeutic advantages accrue to closed-ended groups, often they are not feasible in many settings because they demand the presence of cohorts who are beginning and ending treatment at the same time. None of the models we present in this text require a closed-ended structure. When sources of stability are built in, open-ended structures can achieve some of the strengths of closed-ended groups. For example, in some settings, new members join on a particular day of the week. When members are slated to leave the group, some advance notice is given to the group. These efforts to enhance the predictability of comings and goings strengthen the membership boundary, which in turn fosters group cohesion.

Number of Sessions per Week

Frequency of sessions supports the movement toward the group goals. When groups meet infrequently (e.g., twice a week), the therapist is handicapped in using any model that demands a high level of group cohesion or a capacity to connect present with past group events. Frequency is a feature over which the therapist might have little control. The structure of some settings may preclude frequent sessions. For example, PHPs meet at different times, including evenings and weekends. Fortunately, some models require only that degree of cohesiveness that can be reached in a single session. Such models do not entail the group's consideration of its history across sessions. However, other models require that fairly complex learning be carried from one session to the next, a process aided when sessions are in close temporal order.

Staff continuity and session frequency often work at odds with one another. That is, to have sessions that are highly frequent, it is often necessary to have multiple, changing staff lead the group. This instability can also detract from group cohesion. In the absence of any solid research on the effects of this trade-off, it falls on the local clinicians to make this assessment for their groups. In any case, the introduction of a changing therapy team requires a high level of communication among the therapists conducting the groups, perhaps with the exception of the problem-solving model.

Also, although some groups may meet frequently, even daily, if the group member's stay in the treatment setting is extremely brief, that group member may fail to benefit from the sense of continuity that frequently meeting groups can provide.

SIZE OF THE GROUP

The size of the group is an important consideration for several reasons. First, size affects the extent to which each member can actively participate in the sessions. All else being equal, the larger the group, the less time each member has to respond and to obtain a response. Some models emphasize the importance of individually centered interventions as when, for example, a model requires that the session begins with a go-around in which each member reviews his or her homework from the past session. In a group of 12 members meeting for 60 minutes, it would be nearly impossible for the group to complete the specified steps for a session in which each member formulated an individual agenda. The second reason is that as the group size increases, members frequently have a diminished sense of responsibility for the group's work. *Social loafing*—individuals in a group are less productive than working solo—is a well-established social psychological phenomenon (Kassin, Fein, & Marcus, 2014). Social loafing increases as group size increases (Liden, Wayne, Jaworski, & Bennett, 2004). Third, when groups become extremely small, the needed diversity among members in personality and interpersonal style may be insufficient to use the therapeutic processes on which a particular model depends. For example, interpersonal models tend to require some diversity in interpersonal style, and an extremely small group might not provide it. Fourth, when groups are extremely large—a phenomenon not unusual in PHP and RTC groups—members may experience a lack of safety that could discourage their involvement. *Milieu therapy*—which can broadly be construed as a type of group psychotherapy—is different in that, typically, not only are all the patients of a unit present but also all the staff.

GROUP COMPOSITION

Of all of the variables that define a group, compositional variables have received the most attention in the research literature regarding the extent to which they interact with different models' effectiveness. The cardinal compositional variables are explored in this section.

Level of Ego Functioning

The continuum of ego functioning can roughly be divided into four levels: psychotic, borderline, neurotic, and normal (Kernberg, 1967; Lingiardi & McWilliams, 2017). Individuals whose *ego functions*—mechanisms that foster adaptation to one's internal and external environment—are severely compromised populate the lowest level of ego functioning. Examples of such ego functions are reality testing, coherent thinking, capacity to regulate feelings, and capability to persist in the course of purposive behavior. These individuals are generally diagnosed as psychotic. Individuals in the next level are ones who have moderate to severe deficits areas of ego functioning. These individuals are commonly deemed as having severe personality disorders. This segment also includes some persons with persistent depressive disorder and bipolar disorder. Moving up the continuum still is a level in which fall individuals whose ego functioning disturbances are in the mild to moderate range. Some areas of ego functioning are likely to be intact. The more theoretical level of normal individuals are those persons with only mild and temporary lapses in ego functioning, individuals who are comfortable with themselves and adapting well to their environments.

Leopold (1976) was an early writer on inpatient group psychotherapy who held that the group format and leadership style should be predicated on the level of the member's ego functioning. For the highly regressed, psychotic patient, Leopold recommended approaches that emphasize a high level of support, warmth, and individual attention from the therapist. He saw it as important to provide the patient with a highly positive emotional experience to help the patient be less anxious and more trusting of others. For less regressed group members, he advocated those approaches that require the members' tolerance of some anxiety in the sessions as they learn about their dysfunctional interpersonal behaviors. Such an approach, he suggested, might include exploratory elements to assist the member in discovering some of the internal feelings, thoughts, and impulses underlying relational problems.

Although many subsequent writers since Leopold have concurred with his observations, few studies have directly compared individuals at different levels of functioning across different formats. Those studies that have been done are fairly old. For example, Coché and Polikoff (1979) observed that a high level of self-disclosure was associated with good outcomes in high-functioning inpatients and poor outcomes in their lower functioning counterparts. Leszcz, Yalom, and Norden (1985) found that lower functioning inpatients were more likely than highly functioning inpatients to see as helpful those therapeutic processes that are supportive rather than exploratory. In particular, lower functioning group members saw instillation of hope and the reception of advice as key to their progress in the group. The research also suggested that the lower group members' ego functioning, the more they are helped by a high level of structure. Greene and Cole (1991) found that psychotic patients had better outcomes in a highly structured task group, whereas borderline patients had better outcomes in a less-structured interactional group. Recently, a set of approaches, such as dialectical behavioral therapy (Linehan, 2014; Linehan & Wilks, 2015), schema-focused therapy (Martin & Young, 2010), and mentalization-based treatment of borderline personality disorder (Bateman & Fonagy, 2004, 2005), has been developed for individuals with severe personality pathology. These approaches have been applied in IHPs, PHPs, and RTCs. Although they contain elements of exploration, they vary regarding depth and the extent to which more structured elements are introduced. These approaches have shown positive outcomes but not necessarily on the same set of outcome variables. That is, the outcome measures selected are typically predicated on the goals of the model.

Although the research has not, for the most part, provided direct comparisons of individuals at different levels of ego functioning within our three settings of interest—or any settings for that matter—the limited comparative research that does exist, as well as the research conducted on different populations separately, does seem to justify some conclusions. Group members at the lowest rung of ego functioning are likely to benefit from models that (a) are highly supportive, (b) encourage a low or moderate but never high level of self-disclosure or exploration of private experience, (c) do not require the tolerance of more than minimal anxiety in the session, and (d) provide a structured session enabling members to anticipate the flow of events. As the reader will see, a number of existing models have these characteristics. Members in the second tier of ego functioning that we described can tolerate a greater level of anxiety during the sessions than their psychotic counterparts. For example, some models require members' tolerance of the anxiety associated with hearing negative observations about themselves. Other models entail that members accept the verbal expression of anger in the sessions. However, all proponents of these and other models for members occupying this second tier of ego functioning emphasize the necessity of both titrating the amount of anxiety to which group members are subject and providing a good measure of emotional support.

The preceding discussion of levels of ego functioning assumes that the setting allows for patient groups that are relatively homogeneous in this area. In some settings, particularly those in which only a single group might be available, the inclusion of members at different levels of ego functioning in the same group is necessary. This situation frequently occurs in small psychiatric units of general hospitals. In such instances, the therapist must appraise the flexibility of any given model. Models that work particularly well are those developed for members at the lowest level of ego functioning with the potential for some adaptation for higher functioning members. At times, with an appropriate model, the inclusion of higher functioning members can serve to catalyze the level of lower functioning individuals (Kealy, Ogrodniczuk, Piper, & Sierra-Hernandez, 2016).

Diagnostic Status

Diagnosis relates to the specific combinations of symptoms presented by the patient. In inpatient, partial, and residential settings, psychotherapy groups differ from one another by whether a group is homogeneous or heterogeneous in terms of diagnosis and the particular diagnoses of individuals who compose the group. Pertinent to the first source of variability are the practical factors that often necessitate that diagnostically heterogeneous individuals be placed in the same group. Unless the broader setting itself is devoted to the treatment of a particular type of symptom—for instance, an eating disorders unit—often, the critical mass needed for a group is not reliably present. Even if a sufficiency of candidates with a particular diagnosis were available, a homogeneous group might deprive other patients in the setting of a group experience. Consequently, in many settings, the group therapist will find individuals present together who are depressed, anxious, afflicted with eating or substance abuse disorder or compulsions, and so on. Fortunately, in terms of model selection, heterogeneity of diagnoses is not a highly limiting factor. Most models presented in this text are *transdiagnostic*—that is, constructed with a symptomatically heterogeneous group in mind. However, with minimal or no adaptation, many of them can accommodate symptomatically homogeneous groupings of members. Alternatively, the reader can turn to the broader literature to find a model developed for a specific symptom pattern. Examples are group treatment for individuals with trauma associated with traumatic brain injury (Delmonico, Hanley-Peterson, & Englander, 1998), chemical dependence (Santa Ana, Wulfert, & Nietert, 2007), posttraumatic stress due to child sexual abuse (Palmer, Stalker, Gadbois, & Harper, 2004), eating disorders (Tasca, Flynn, & Bissada, 2002; Tchanturia, 2015), agoraphobia (Hoffart, Øktedalen, Svanøe, Hedley, & Sexton, 2015), and schizophrenia (Kanas, 1996). Burlingame, Fuhriman, and Mosier (2003) conducted a meta-analysis of 111 studies and found that homogeneous groups are associated with more favorable outcomes relative to heterogeneous groups.

When the group psychotherapist has the option of whether to establish a heterogeneous or homogeneous member group, several factors should be considered:

- For groups that are extremely short term, homogeneous symptom groupings can enable the establishment of quick cohesion. Members can discern immediately that others understand their afflictions in a way that family and friends might not. Burlingame, McClendon, and Alonso (2011) conducted a meta-analytic review of 40 studies based on the outcome patterns of 3,323 patients. They found that as cohesion increased, symptoms decreased. These investigators also found that, with time, cohesion builds but often requires 12 sessions to achieve an optimal level. Their meta-analysis revealed that cohesion is particularly important for outcomes in adolescent groups. In 2010, Dinger and Schauenburg demonstrated the relationship between cohesion and outcome with groups of 327 inpatients. Typically, the inpatient group psychotherapist does not have the benefit of time and, consequently, other means of achieving cohesion become important.

- In interpersonally oriented groups, the therapist relies on some diversity in members' interpersonal styles for the group to perform its work. For example, members who share the features of passivity and reticence may not even recognize them sufficiently to label them when they are manifest in the group. The therapist in such groups should seek to use whatever selection tools are available to ensure this type of diversity is present. The therapist should be mindful of the fact that particular personality features may accompany symptom patterns (e.g., individuals with eating disorders often exhibit perfectionistic tendencies). The therapist must consider how these features may play out in the group if a significant subgroup of the members is in possession of them.

- An advantage of homogeneity of symptoms is that the therapist can identify specific and sensitive outcome measures to test the effectiveness of a given model with that population. Because these measures are highly focused, they tend to be fairly brief. Therapists should take advantage of this potential to ensure that a model that makes good theoretical sense also makes practical sense given the specificities of the setting.

Identity Variables

Group members' experiences are shaped by all that defines them as individuals and how they are the same or different from one another on important identity variables. Gender, gender identity, sexual orientation, generation, religion and spirituality, and socioeconomic and immigration status, among others, constitute the individual member's cultural self. All will figure into that member's capacity to work in the group. Hence, the therapist must be attuned to these identity elements and the lens they offer a given member. Two considerations in relation to group members' identities are pertinent to model selection.

First, in some treatment settings, members are likely to be relatively homogeneous regarding a given identity variable. For example, both of us have had the experience of working in inpatient settings that were predominantly female. It was not unusual for a group of eight to include only a single male member. Such extreme lopsidedness is likely to be lost on neither the members of the majority or the minority. Members of both subgroups are likely to wonder, often privately, whether the dominant topics will have relevance to minority members. Often, these private questions turn public as members of both the majority and minority groups question whether this group is the most appropriate placement for the latter. To avoid precipitous departures from the group, the therapist must have means of addressing this issue with the members. Some models are more conducive to addressing such issues than others. For example, the therapist using an interpersonal model could point out how members make assumptions about one another's thoughts and feelings based on such factors as gender, sexual orientation, and so on, but group provides an opportunity to ascertain whether other members' experiences match these assumptions.

Second, some identity statuses are associated with stigma. As Herek (2009) noted, stigma takes various forms, all of which are applicable to the workings of a psychotherapy group. Key forms are structural stigma, enacted stigma, felt stigma, and internalized stigma.

Structural Stigma

Structural stigma is society's valuation of particular features of a person (e.g., particular body types) and groups (e.g., particular ethnicities or religions). Structural stigmas are likely to inform stigmatization patterns in institutions such as hospitals, the units that compose those institutions, and the subunits, such as psychotherapy groups. Knowledge of structural stigma can provide hypotheses to the group psychotherapist about the stigmatizing activity he or she is likely to see in the psychotherapy group.

Enacted Stigma and Microaggressions

Enacted stigma is the local translation of structural stigma. It occurs when a person or group exhibits discrimination, bullying, or some other adverse action against a person or group based on that person's category of membership. In a psychotherapy group, an example of enacted stigma is a member being discouraged from speaking based on his or her minority group status. Enacted stigmas are also termed *microaggressions* (Sue, 2010) and frequently occur on an unconscious basis; that is, the aggressor is unaware of his or her aggressive impulses toward the targeted member. This unconscious aspect makes the microaggression elusive. However, it is far more modifiable in a therapeutic context in which a focus is placed on identifying unconscious motivators of behavior than in everyday social interactions. However, the models featured in this text vary greatly in the extent to which they focus on the identification of unconscious processes and, hence, some would be more suited to recognizing microaggressions than others.

Felt Stigma

Felt stigma is the awareness of the likelihood of enacted stigma by stigmatized and nonstigmatized individuals alike, as well as the particular contextual factors that control stigmatizing behavior. In a psychotherapy group, felt stigma would occur were a member to hide his or her minority status to avoid some adverse treatment, a phenomenon known as *passing*. All the models in this text seek to create a sense of safety wherein members are increasingly able to share parts of themselves, including parts rejected by others in past social environments. Groups that last beyond a few sessions are better equipped to provide experiences enabling members to challenge their fears about social interactions that lead them to hide from others.

Internalized Stigma

Internalized stigma occurs when the individual makes part of the self a negative view of his or her membership in a given category. For example, were a group member to experience shame in the group on the basis of his or her sexual orientation, gender identity, race, ethnicity, and so on, that member would be in the thrall of internalized stigma. Internalized stigma can also be developed in relation to the presence of psychological problems. Society regards individuals with psychological diagnoses with great suspicion, and those with such diagnoses can readily internalize this negative view. According to Lysaker, Roe, and Yanos (2007), approximately one third of individuals with severe psychological difficulties show evidence of internalized stigma and, consequently, it must be a focus of the group psychotherapist working with this population. Lysaker et al. saw the source of the stigma as the patient's severe mental illness. However, if the individual is also a member of a sexual or racial minority, the individual bears a double stigma, with a corresponding increase in stress. Sibitz, Provaznikova, Lipp, Lakeman, and Amering (2013) demonstrated in a PHP that participation in a range of groups ameliorated internalized stigma in a group of schizophrenic patients. However, whether particular therapeutic components played a more critical role in producing this effect could not be determined from these data. Increasing attention to the use of group psychotherapy to address internalized stigma is seen in the development of specific protocols for this purpose. For example, Yanos, Roe, West, Smith, and Lysaker (2012) developed a protocol for the treatment of internalized stigma among persons with severe mental illness, and Heilman (2018) created a format for the treatment of internalized homophobia in gay men.

Table 2.1 provides examples of how these kinds of stigma might manifest in IHP, PHP, and RTC groups.

Implications for Conducting Groups

It is essential that the therapist be poised to address stigma within the group because many of the patients in IHP, PHP, and RTC settings have experienced trauma in their lives. Without the therapist's ready response to emerging victimization, members are at increased risk of adverse outcomes. These include, but are not limited to, leaving the group prematurely, seeing therapy as something threatening, becoming more symptomatic, or at worst, being retraumatized within the group. At the level of the group-as-a-whole, Agazarian (1997) argued that when members are locked into a process of seeing one another stereotypically, they are severely impeded from doing significant psychological work in the group. Of course, in any group, issues related to stigma can arise, and these issues may be far ranging and to some extent unpredictable. However, the therapist also does well to anticipate what types of stigma might be most common in the population from which he or she draws, how pernicious the effects of the stigma are likely to be, and finally, how the therapist might address them within the confines of any selected model.

For example, on a psychiatric unit of an urban hospital, it may be the case that whereas the majority of patients are both heterosexual and conservative in their views, the group regularly includes a gay man or lesbian who may be at various degrees of being out. The leader might sense that this variation is a source of tension. Perhaps the members who are in the sexual majority exhibit veiled or overt negative attitudes toward the gay or lesbian member in the form of microaggressions, or the sexual minority member does not feel comfortable in discussing concerns that may be related to his or her status on this dimension. Some models easily lend themselves to addressing such issues. Bateman and Fonagy's (2004) mentalization model can facilitate members in understanding the psychological experiences of other members, including those who are different themselves. In this approach, members who stigmatize other members can achieve a sense of the feelings that are generated by their treatment of that member. Reciprocally, the stigmatized member can learn something about the fears of the other members that are rooted in felt stigma (i.e., "If I relate positively to this member, I will be stigmatized in a similar manner"). Other models, such as the social skills training model, may require greater creativity on the part of the therapist in providing the means for performing this crucial diversity work. Acceptance

TABLE 2.1
Manifestations of Types of Stigma in Inpatient Hospital Program,
Partial Hospital Program, and Residential Treatment Center
Groups and Potentially Constructive Therapist Responses

Type of stigma	Example of manifestation	Potentially[a] constructive response
Structural	The group psychotherapist, members, or both base their perception of a group member on how society generally regards the group to which that member belongs.	Therapist's awareness of societal perceptions of particular groups to know when these perceptions are manifested in the session. Identifying linkages between member biases and broader societal pressures.
Enacted	A therapist or member expresses hostility or some other negative state to a group member based on the group member's identity.	• Rapid protection of stigmatized member (e.g., deflecting the aggression from the member to the therapist). • Consideration and possibly exploration of the function of the enacted stigma within the group in the present moment. • Consideration of the extent to which group dynamics might be a reflection of stigmatizing dynamics within the unit or program. Address with treatment staff unhelpful program-level dynamics. • Help members to bond on the basis of shared issues rather than demographic categories.
Felt	A member assumes that he or she has been or will be subjected to negative treatment by virtue of that member's identity or membership in a cultural group.	Assist the member in testing the perception while acknowledging any component that is rooted in other members' behavior toward that member. If felt stigma is at odds with behavioral data, help member recognize roots in structural stigma.
Internalized	Members by virtue of their identity feel unacceptable to themselves, a reaction that represents an internalization of societal values.	• Aid members in recognizing that the self-condemnation involves an act of internalization. • Help member to reality test the self-perception. Group feedback might be valuable in this regard. • Integrate protocols that have been developed to address internalized stigma in the psychotherapy group setting (e.g., Heilman, 2018).

Note. [a]Whether a given strategy is helpful depends on a variety of factors. For example, if the group is reflecting program dynamics, the openness of staff on the unit affects whether the therapist can pursue the modification of the dynamics in the broader system.

and commitment therapy (S. C. Hayes, 2004) works to lessen experiential avoidance. One means of experiential avoidance is to project self-disliked qualities onto others, a common underpinning of stereotyping. The problem-solving model reduces the tendency to see the other as the problem. The model fosters the concrete description of the problem and the search for solutions.

Although many of the models in this text have some capabilities for addressing diversity, for the most part, the literature specifically covering models' technical considerations have not made them explicit. For example, none of the model developers have addressed sexuality diversity in the group or even sexuality, for that matter, a problem in the group psychotherapy literature at large (Nitsun, 2012). Therefore, it will require active exploration on the part of the therapist using the model to discover means by which members can work constructively with all of the diversities that present in IHP, PHP, and RTC groups.

If a chosen model does not easily provide the means to dismantle stereotyping, therapists might use pretraining for this purpose. That is, the therapist can cultivate members' openness to interacting with those who may be different from themselves. Helpful in this process is the therapist's knowledge of the identity characteristics of his or her group members, knowledge that is easier to achieve in PHPs and RTCs versus IHPs, given the rapid turnover in the latter. It is also important, regardless of the model selected, that the therapist, in an ongoing way, collects feedback on group members' perceptions of the group (e.g., through use of the measures of the CORE-R battery, developed by the American Group Psychotherapy Association, 2007). The therapist through this means can capture member reactions that are not clearly displayed.

Fortunately, the burgeoning awareness of the importance of identity statuses to individuals' behaviors in, and capacity to derive benefit from, group psychotherapy is giving rise to research on linkages between members' perceptions of one another's identities and group behavior. For example, Garcia (2017) found that when members see one another as sharing an identity status, they are poised to recognize similarities between them. Conversely, when they believe they are in a different racial or gender identity category, they are primed to see differences between them. Garcia pointed out that therapists leading groups of members who have salient identity differences might have to work more actively to assist them in seeing commonalities. This notion is especially relevant to a time-limited group (e.g., a typical inpatient group) in which members do not have the luxury to discover shared experiences slowly. Garcia suggested that, in some cases, it might be useful for members to interact initially with one other group member to catalyze their discernment of commonalities.

When most group members identify as members of a minority or a group that is structurally stigmatized, it is recommended that therapists learn all they can about the experience of that group in their community. When the therapist shares the minority identity, group members often express an increased sense of safety in the group and may be able to articulate their struggles related to experienced victimization (Ibrahim, Kamsani, & Champe, 2015; Stacciarini, O'Keeffe, & Mathews, 2007).

THERAPIST VARIABLES

The research of the past 25 years supports the value of a positive therapeutic relationship (i.e., a strong therapeutic alliance) as a factor associated with the effectiveness of treatment (Norcross & Lambert, 2010). Meta-analytic studies have shown that empathy (Elliott, Bohart, Watson, & Greenberg, 2011), genuineness (Kolden, Klein, Wang, & Austin, 2011), capacity to repair ruptures (Safran, Muran, & Eubanks-Carter, 2011), and the ability to manage one's reactions as therapist (J. A. Hayes, Gelso, & Hummel, 2011) contribute to favorable outcomes. All these findings tell us that the individual who delivers the treatment or implements the model is a critical factor in the patient's capacity to benefit from treatment. This is no less so for group psychotherapy. Yet, as Greene (2017) pointed out, "We have just scratched the surface in identifying personal qualities and capabilities of therapists that make a difference across groups and within specific group treatments" (p. 12). This point is no less true with respect to group approaches designed for IHPs, PHPs, and RTCs. Research on therapist variables in group psychotherapy is particularly important to advance treatment in the three settings of IHP, PHP, and RTCs This section addresses three considerations in which different models of group psychotherapy in their application in our three featured contexts might place demands on the therapist. These include leader role, training in group psychotherapy, and the structure of the group leadership (cotherapy or solo leadership).

Leader Role

Therapists come to the group with a defined set of personality characteristics and preferences for different types of activity. To the extent that a match occurs between the therapist's natural proclivities and what the model asks of the therapist, the delivery of a model is likely to be successful. The models featured in this book place very different demands on the activity of the therapist. Whereas some models (e.g., the problem-solving and the social skills training models) entail the therapist's continual structuring of the session, other models, such as the object relations approach, require that the therapist avoid structuring the session but nonetheless respond with alacrity and sensitivity to emerging material. As Edwards and Bess (1998) pointed out, the self-knowledge of the therapist is key to the therapist's recognition of how he or she can work most effectively and use the self most actively.

Training

As Vannicelli (2014) stated, therapists, including those in training, must have skills and knowledge that pertain to any model. Examples are the capacity to set consistent boundaries, the ability to establish a clear purpose for the group, the capacity to develop a map for each session, and the ability to work within a multicultural system. However, each model places different levels of demand on the training of the therapist. Some models require the therapist's mastery of a particular, perhaps complicated, theoretical approach to human psychology, psychopathology, and group process, as well as a set of interventions congruent with this approach. Other models make limited demands on the therapist's grasp of theory. This factor is important in circumstances in which a wide variety of professionals at different levels of training participate in delivering group psychotherapy or in which the same model is adopted for the unit and the group.

For example, the social skills training model is one that could be implemented easily with staff at different levels of training. Thompson, Gallagher, Nies, and Epstein (1983) demonstrated that professional, paraprofessional, and nonprofessional people were able to master the basics of this model after a 12-hour course. Of course, the more extensive one's background is in the principles and techniques of group psychotherapy, the more effectively any of these models are likely to be applied. No model precludes the emergence of group dynamics or group-level resistances, and knowledge of how to address them is at many junctures indispensable.

Therapists also require training in model selection. Farley's (1998) research on group psychotherapy practiced on psychiatric units of general medical facilities indicated that therapists working in such venues do not proceed through any systematic process of selecting models but do so by happenstance—that is, applying what models they know or feel competent to deliver. In part, this text is designed to provide the therapist with essential information to select the model with the most optimal fit. However, even with this information on different models, the therapist has to proceed through a process of systematically exploring the characteristics of the site as they align with the characteristics of the available model. Sites would be well served by providing new group psychotherapists the time, space, and mentorship to engage in this all-important process.

Clinical Load

All approaches described in this text make some demands on the therapist's time, energy, and attention. However, some models require more investment on the therapist's part than others. Taylor, Coombes, and Bartlett (2002) described a study in which researchers tracked the various indicators of the success of inpatient group psychotherapy in four acute wards in various locations in southeast England. The group psychotherapists used a model that is described in the text, Yalom's (1983) interactional agenda model. They found that over time, the quality of the groups deteriorated apparently not because of the value of the model itself but because the staff was so overburdened that their ability to deliver the model eroded. It is possible that in those venues no model would have been successfully used. What their study showcases, though, is the importance of the group psychotherapist in designing a group to consider his or her activities in his or her group role against the backdrop of all other professional responsibilities.

Leadership Structure: Solo Versus Cotherapy

Models of group psychotherapy, including those featured in this text, vary regarding the type of demands they place on the leadership structure. In general, whereas a solo therapist might be feasible with some of the models we describe, cotherapy is the optimal arrangement for many of them. The four classes of leadership function, identified by Lieberman, Yalom, and Miles (1973) and broadly discussed by others (Bernard et al., 2008; Brabender, Fallon, & Smolar, 2004), facilitate characterization of IHP, PHP, and RTC leadership of psychotherapy groups.

The *executive function* involves the therapist's engagement in those administrative tasks that provide safety (e.g., the setting of boundaries) and establish a purpose for the group (communicating the goals to members). In IHP, PHP, and RTC groups, this function is crucial because many members cannot perform particular executive activities on their own. For example, members may confuse feelings with action ("If I feel anger, it means I must be hurting someone"). *Emotional stimulation* involves members' attention to the thoughts, feelings, and impulses stimulated by the here and now. In some groups in these settings, the emotional intensity can be at a level that is unmanageable for group members, and for other groups, the use of defenses such as primitive denial reduces emotionality to level that leads members to feel disengaged from the group. The group therapist in these settings carries the responsibility of modulating the level of intensity so that it is in the zone optimal for work. *Caring* is the demonstration of positive feeling on the part of the therapist toward the members. Frequently, members come into the group with a perception, real or imagined, of the absence of caring figures in their lives. Although, ultimately, members require a sense of being cared about by their peers, it is the therapist whose warmth is critical to members' willingness to invest in the group experience. Finally, *meaning attribution,* members' ability to understand their internal and external lives, is a vital therapist function. For individuals in IHP, PHP, and RTC settings, experiences are typically incoherent, fragmented, and chaotic. The therapist's capacity to assist members in sorting reactions out and understanding the connection between their reactions and events in their life (particularly, interpersonal events) aids members in achieving the sense of control that brings confidence in tackling life tasks.

The high level of vigor at which all four core functions of the therapist in IHP, PHP, and RTC settings must be performed often necessitates the presence of two professionals who can share in the responsibilities and possibly have different emphases. For example, while one therapist is checking to see where Mr. Jones went when he ran out of the session (executive function), the other therapist can assist the group in processing (meaning attribution) Mr. Jones's departure. However, often, the therapy pair need not be two professionals who function at an expert level. The three settings are fertile and commonly used training grounds for students of group psychotherapy. These trainees benefit greatly from being in a support role vis-à-vis the senior therapist, an arrangement that Roller and Nelson (1991) termed a *nequipos.* Cotherapy provides another benefit beyond the ability to manage a range of leadership responsibilities and training of students. Cotherapy can be an antidote to the high level of stress that accompanies leading psychotherapy groups with individuals with considerable difficulties. Therapists usually value the opportunity to clarify their perceptions about the group and obtain support for the difficult events and personalities they encounter in sessions.

Identity Status of the Therapist

Therapists are informed by the cultures in which they grew up and their current cultures. Cultural elements of the therapist's identity can and will figure in important ways in how the therapist reacts and behaves in the sessions. Consider in this regard the following example:

> Nora was a new staff member of a hospital that drew heavily from the surrounding community. This community was composed of many individuals who were first-generation Russian immigrants. Nora, herself, was a second-generation Russian American. One component of Nora's responsibilities was leading a psychotherapy group. In the sessions, she found herself feeling irritated when the group members talked about their distress and sense of betrayal when their children left home at an

early age. Nora's parents had not responded negatively to her decision to live independently on the completion of her graduate education. For this reason, she was puzzled that she would be annoyed by what she saw as members "whining." Fortunately, she had a supervisor who helped her recognize that she had internalized a cultural prescription that she was violating by her self-sufficient, independent behavior. Some of the group members were articulating the prescription and thereby elicited her guilt for having separated from her parents at what would be seen as an early point in her life.

In this case, it was not the respect in which her culture was different from that of the group members but, rather, the cultural elements she shared with them that was at issue. Like all group psychotherapists, therapists in inpatient, partial hospital, and residential settings must be reflective about the facets of their identity and how differences and similarities give rise to at least some of the reactions therapists have in sessions. In looking at identity status, group therapists should be as comprehensive as possible. Ethnicity, sexuality orientation, gender identity, religion, military status, generation, socioeconomic and immigration status are just a subset of the identity variables that can shape the therapist's group experiences.

CONTEXT COMPATIBILITY ANALYSIS

We recommend that, in deciding on a particular model, the therapist perform a context compatibility analysis in which all relevant features of the setting are considered in relation to the demands of the model. This process entails consideration of where the flexibilities exist regarding both the model and the setting. The group psychotherapist might also outline for him- or herself what action steps will be needed to take advantage of a particular type of flexibility. For example, the therapist might ascertain that a model's application would flourish with a relatively small group size. The therapist might have to approach the treatment team to determine whether a relatively small group would be feasible given the needs of the unit. To facilitate the accomplishment of this task, we offer a Context Compatibility Checklist (CCC), which appears in Figure 2.1.

To illustrate the application of this model, we might take the case of a new inpatient therapist whose primary responsibility in the setting is conducting psychotherapy groups on a locked unit consisting primarily of psychotic patients. Use of the CCC will enable the therapist to consider whether a particular model is likely to be successfully used in that setting. Suppose that the director of the unit expressed interest in the therapist's running an acceptance and commitment therapy (ACT) group (see S. C. Hayes, Strosahl, &

Model _____

Setting variables	Model demands	Setting demands	Possible resolution	Action steps
Philosophy and values				
Theoretical orientation of setting				
Other components of therapeutic program				
Temporal factors 1. Average number of sessions 2. Length of session 3. Frequency				
Size of group				
Member characteristics 1. Ego functioning 2. Diagnosis 3. Identity				
Therapist characteristics				
Other				

Figure 2.1. Context compatibility checklist.

Wilson, 2011). The therapist herself had a strong interest in ACT applications and, therefore, found the suggestion enticing. In our experience, many therapists would run straightaway into the formation of one or more ACT groups. The CCC requires that the therapist linger longer in the model consideration stage.

In surveying the list, the therapist might alight on the institution's treatment philosophy, although the therapist could begin with a different contextual dimension. From interviewing staff, the therapist might learn that the institution has a strong belief that the most efficacious interventions are biological. Nonetheless, the therapist senses that some openness exists to other mediums, as signified (among other manifestations) by the site's investment in a range of PEGs and the director's seeking out an ACT therapist for this therapeutic component. She realizes, though, that were she to move forward with an ACT approach, a significant commitment would have to be made to communicating with the staff, including upper administration, about the approach and considering how this intervention might work together with others. Her presentation might benefit from research showing that ACT provides value added in relation to the typical medication regime. She might discuss with staff that when patients are driven to focus wholly on symptoms, it can have a paradoxical effect of intensifying them (Pankey, 2003). This presentation, and other educational efforts with the staff about the ACT model, would constitute the Action Steps in the CCC.

Early on in the analysis, the therapist should visit the temporal dimension, which, as noted previously, consists of a group of variables. For many models, a key temporal variable is number of sessions. The therapist learned that most patients would be available for five to eight sessions. The lower limit would not preclude the use of an ACT group, although five sessions would be less than ideal. Also, the expectation was that, in every session, new members would be added to the group. She considered designing the group in such as a way that each session would to a large extent stand alone. She also thought that the large number of members who would visit the unit in the context of repeated hospitalizations would derive benefit from multiple group experiences with the ACT model. The typical session length for various activities on this unit was 45 minutes, a reasonable length of time for an ACT session.

With respect to the size of the group, the therapist learned that typically on this unit, the upper limit for members was eight, but the therapist had the leeway to set the group at six members. She thought this latter number might be suitable, particularly given the level of functioning of the members.

The characteristics of the potential group members was a somewhat set feature because the group was to draw from a unit composed primarily of psychotic individuals. The therapist was aware that ACT had been used with this patient population, and specific protocols were available to aid her in designing session formats. From an identity perspective, the therapist knew from consultation with the staff that a subset of the population had experienced homelessness due to the conjunction of poverty and psychotic symptoms. These individuals sometimes experienced discrimination on the unit when facets of their history were known.

The therapist carefully considered whether ACT could accommodate cultural differences in the form of class dynamics within the group. She thought that an important design feature of the group would be to say at the beginning of each session that each member comes to the group with different reactions based in part on their cultural backgrounds. This suggestion is consonant with the counsel of many writers in the area of multiculturalism (e.g., E. C. Chen, Kakkad, & Balzano, 2008) that when members are prepared for diversity in the group, they tend to respond less defensively to emerging differences. Had she had time to screen members individually, she would have been able to provide more substantial preparation for experiences in diversity. For example, she could have followed the suggestion of Haley-Banez and Walden (1999) that the entering member be given a chance to anticipate how he or she might respond to certain types of differences. The therapist also recognized that she must pay careful attention to manifestations of these tensions in the sessions. She reminded herself that projecting onto others self-rejected qualities is a form of experiential avoidance, which the model can address directly. The therapist also was assured that if she needed a cotherapist, she could draw from various other staff that had a background in group psychotherapy but not necessarily ACT. She reasoned that she could fairly easily train another group-savvy staff member to support her in applying the ACT model. She also determined that the clinical load for staff on the unit was not so great as to compromise the delivery of an ACT group approach.

These are the major variables the therapist should consider in performing a context compatibility analysis for a model under consideration. This therapist's analysis led to the conclusion that the ACT model could be feasibly implemented. Still, one or more other models might be equally or more compatible with the setting than ACT. For this reason, it is often useful for the therapist not to engage in the common practice described by Farley (1998) of homing in on one model to the exclusion of all others in designing a new group. Also, broadening the set of models considered might lead to a consideration of ways in which desirable features of one model might be integrated into the model that is ultimately selected.

SUMMARY AND COMMENT

Clinical environments distinguish themselves from one another on a variety of dimensions, and a particular environment's status on all key dimensions should be considered in the selection of a model. In this chapter, we highlighted the following dimensions: values, goals, and philosophy; theoretical orientation; other program components; temporal variables; size of group; group composition; and therapist variables. These dimensions are ones we deem to be important across settings, but for any one setting, other factors may be important. Furthermore, as we learn more about the features of the setting, including the features of the patient population, we will be better able to consider what variables should figure into model selection. For example, research is accruing on the interaction between members' personality characteristics and group features as they determine the outcome. Dinger and Schauenburg (2010) found, for instance, that highly dismissive patients benefit from higher cohesion and highly affiliative patients from lower cohesion. As the research base on personality expands, this set of variables may be important to consider with different types of groups being developed for group therapy candidates with particular personality styles.

In the chapters that follow, for each model we present, we describe the demands it places on the treatment context. No setting is likely to satisfy the demands of any given model perfectly. Rather than making an easy and obvious match between a model and a setting, the practitioner most typically faces the challenge of ascertaining which model is more congruent with the setting than others. Usually, the selection process entails a determination of which incongruities between the setting and a model can be minimized through either a change in the model or a change in the setting.

Ultimately, the group psychotherapist must reckon with the reality that his or her clinical context is unique. Any one of the models presented in this book may be an excellent point of departure for a suitable model for a setting. It is important for the clinician to keep in mind that all these models were developed for some setting other than that in which the clinician is practicing. The most effective model will invariably be one that is tailored to all the features of a setting.

REFERENCES

Aagaard, J., Foldager, L., Makki, A., Hansen, V., & Müller-Nielsen, K. (2017). The efficacy of psychoeducation on recurrent depression: A randomized trial with a 2-year follow-up. *Nordic Journal of Psychiatry, 71*, 223–229. http://dx.doi.org/10.1080/08039488.2016.1266385

Agazarian, Y. M. (1997). *Systems-centered therapy for groups.* New York, NY: Guilford Press.

American Group Psychotherapy Association. (2007). *Practice guidelines for group psychotherapy.* Retrieved from http://www.agpa.org/home/practice-resources/practice-guidelines-for-group-psychotherapy

Bateman, A., & Fonagy, P. (2005). *Psychotherapy for borderline personality disorder: Mentalization-based treatment.* Oxford, England: Oxford University Press.

Bateman, A. W., & Fonagy, P. (2004). Mentalization-based treatment of BPD. *Journal of Personality Disorders, 18*, 36–51. http://dx.doi.org/10.1521/pedi.18.1.36.32772

Bäuml, J., Fröböse, T., Kraemer, S., Rentrop, M., & Pitschel-Walz, G. (2006). Psycho-education: A basic psychotherapeutic intervention for patients with schizophrenia and their families. *Schizophrenia Bulletin, 32*, S1–S9. http://dx.doi.org/10.1093/schbul/sbl017

Bernard, H., Burlingame, G., Flores, P., Greene, L., Joyce, A., Kobos, J. C., . . . Feirman, D. (2008). Clinical practice guidelines for group psychotherapy. *International Journal of Group Psychotherapy, 58*, 455–542. http://dx.doi.org/10.1521/ijgp.2008.58.4.455

Brabender, V., & Fallon, A. (2009). *Group development in practice: Guidance for clinicians and researchers on stages and dynamics of change.* Washington, DC: American Psychological Association. http://dx.doi.org/10.1037/11858-000

Brabender, V., Fallon, A., & Smolar, A. (2004). *Essentials of group therapy*. New York, NY: Wiley.

Burlingame, G. M., Fuhriman, A., & Mosier, J. (2003). The differential effectiveness of group psychotherapy: A meta-analytic perspective. *Group Dynamics: Theory, Research, and Practice, 7*, 3–12. http://dx.doi.org/10.1037/1089-2699.7.1.3

Burlingame, G. M., McClendon, D. T., & Alonso, J. (2011). Cohesion in group therapy. *Psychotherapy, 48*, 34–42. http://dx.doi.org/10.1037/a0022063

Chen, E. C., Kakkad, D., & Balzano, J. (2008). Multicultural competence and evidence-based practice in group therapy. *Journal of Clinical Psychology, 64*, 1261–1278. http://dx.doi.org/10.1002/jclp.20533

Chen, R., Xi, Y., Wang, X., Li, Y., He, Y., & Luo, J. (2018). Perception of inpatients following remission of a manic episode in bipolar I disorder on a group-based psychoeducation program: A qualitative study. *BMC Psychiatry, 18*, 26. http://dx.doi.org/10.1186/s12888-018-1614-1

Coché, E., & Polikoff, B. (1979). Self-disclosure and outcome in short-term group psychotherapy. *Group, 3*, 35–47. http://dx.doi.org/10.1007/BF01547028

Cook, W. G., Arechiga, A., Dobson, L. A. V., & Boyd, K. (2014). Brief heterogeneous inpatient psychotherapy groups: A process-oriented psychoeducational (POP) model. *International Journal of Group Psychotherapy, 64*, 180–206. http://dx.doi.org/10.1521/ijgp.2014.64.2.180

Cowls, J., & Hale, S. (2005). It's the activity that counts: What clients value in psychoeducational groups. *Canadian Journal of Occupational Therapy/Revue Canadienne D'Ergothérapie, 72*, 176–182. http://dx.doi.org/10.1177/000841740507200305

Delmonico, R. L., Hanley-Peterson, P., & Englander, J. (1998). Group psychotherapy for persons with traumatic brain injury: Management of frustration and substance abuse. *The Journal of Head Trauma Rehabilitation, 13*(6), 10–22. http://dx.doi.org/10.1097/00001199-199812000-00004

Dinger, U., & Schauenburg, H. (2010). Effects of individual cohesion and patient interpersonal style on outcome in psychodynamically oriented inpatient group psychotherapy. *Psychotherapy Research, 20*, 22–29. http://dx.doi.org/10.1080/10503300902855514

Duman, Z. C., Yildirim, N. K., Ucok, A., Er, F., & Kanik, T. (2010). The effectiveness of a psychoeducational group program with inpatients being treated for chronic mental illness. *Social Behavior and Personality, 38*, 657–666. http://dx.doi.org/10.2224/sbp.2010.38.5.657

Edwards, J. K., & Bess, J. M. (1998). Developing effectiveness in the therapeutic use of self. *Clinical Social Work Journal, 26*, 89–105. http://dx.doi.org/10.1023/A:1022801713242

Elliott, R., Bohart, A. C., Watson, J. C., & Greenberg, L. S. (2011). Empathy. In J. C. Norcross (Ed.), *Psychotherapy relationships that work* (2nd ed., pp. 132–152). New York, NY: Oxford University Press. http://dx.doi.org/10.1093/acprof:oso/9780199737208.003.0006

Farley, P. N. (1998). *Current practices in general hospital group psychotherapy* (Doctoral dissertation). Retrieved from http://theses.lib.vt.edu/theses/available/etd-3198-142012/unrestricted/dissert.pdf

Frank, F., Wilk, J., Kriston, L., Meister, R., Shimodera, S., Hesse, K., . . . Hölzel, L. P. (2015). Effectiveness of a brief psychoeducational group intervention for relatives on the course of disease in patients after inpatient depression treatment compared with treatment as usual—Study protocol of a multisite randomised controlled trial. *BMC Psychiatry, 15*, 259. http://dx.doi.org/10.1186/s12888-015-0633-4

Gabbard, G. O. (1992). The therapeutic relationship in psychiatric hospital treatment. *Bulletin of the Menninger Clinic, 56*, 4–19.

Garcia, R. L. (2017). Perceived self-to-other similarity as a mediatory of the effects of gender and racial composition on identification in small groups. *Group Dynamics: Theory, Research, and Practice, 21*, 220–233. http://dx.doi.org/10.1037/gdn0000075

Greene, L. R. (2017). Group psychotherapy research studies that therapists might actually read: My top 10 list. *International Journal of Group Psychotherapy, 67*, 1–26. http://dx.doi.org/10.1080/00207284.2016.1202678

Greene, L. R., & Cole, M. B. (1991). Level and form of psychopathology and the structure of group therapy. *International Journal of Group Psychotherapy, 41*, 499–521. http://dx.doi.org/10.1080/00207284.1991.11490677

Haley-Banez, L., & Walden, S. L. (1999). Diversity in group work: Using optimal theory to understand group process and dynamics. *Journal for Specialists in Group Work, 24*, 405–422. http://dx.doi.org/10.1080/01933929908411446

Hayes, J. A., Gelso, C. J., & Hummel, A. M. (2011). Managing countertransference. *Psychotherapy, 48*, 88–97. http://dx.doi.org/10.1037/a0022182

Hayes, S. C. (2004). Acceptance and commitment therapy, relational frame theory, and the third wave of behavioral and cognitive therapies. *Behavior Therapy, 35*, 639–665. http://dx.doi.org/10.1016/S0005-7894(04)80013-3

Hayes, S. C., Strosahl, K. D., & Wilson, K. G. (2011). *Acceptance and commitment therapy: The process and practice of mindful change.* New York, NY: Guilford Press.

Heilman, D. (2018). The potential role for group psychotherapy in the treatment of internalized homophobia in gay men. *International Journal of Group Psychotherapy, 68*, 56–68. http://dx.doi.org/10.1080/00207284.2017.1315585

Henderson, D. A., & Gladding, S. T. (2004). Group counseling with older adults. In J. L. De Lucia-Waack, D. A. Gerrity, C. A. Kalodner, & M. T. Riva (Eds.), *Handbook of group counseling and psychotherapy* (pp. 469–478). Thousand Oaks, CA: Sage. http://dx.doi.org/10.4135/9781452229683.n34

Herek, G. M. (2009). Hate crimes and stigma-related experiences among sexual minority adults in the United States: Prevalence estimates from a national probability sample. *Journal of Interpersonal Violence, 24*, 54–74. http://dx.doi.org/10.1177/0886260508316477

Hirschhorn, L. (1988). *The workplace within: The psychodynamics of organizational life.* Cambridge, MA: MIT Press.

Hoffart, A., Øktedalen, T., Svanøe, K., Hedley, L. M., & Sexton, H. (2015). Predictors of short- and long-term avoidance in completers of inpatient group interventions for agoraphobia. *Journal of Affective Disorders, 181,* 33–40. http://dx.doi.org/10.1016/j.jad.2015.04.015

Ibrahim, N., Kamsani, S. R., & Champe, J. (2015). Understanding the Islamic concept of usrah and its application to group work. *Journal for Specialists in Group Work, 40,* 163–186. http://dx.doi.org/10.1080/01933922.2015.1017067

Kanas, N. (1996). *Group therapy for schizophrenic patients.* Washington, DC: American Psychiatric Association.

Karterud, S., & Urnes, Ø. (2004). Short-term day treatment programmes for patients with personality disorders. What is the optimal composition? *Nordic Journal of Psychiatry, 58,* 243–249. http://dx.doi.org/10.1080/08039480410006304

Kassin, S., Fein, S., & Marcus, H. R. (2014). *Social psychology* (9th ed.). Belmont, CA: Wadsworth.

Kealy, D., Ogrodniczuk, J. S., Piper, W. E., & Sierra-Hernandez, C. A. (2016). When it is not a good fit: Clinical errors in patient selection and group composition in group psychotherapy. *Psychotherapy, 53,* 308–313. http://dx.doi.org/10.1037/pst0000069

Kernberg, O. (1967). Borderline personality organization. *Journal of the American Psychoanalytic Association, 15,* 641–685. http://dx.doi.org/10.1177/000306516701500309

Kolden, G. G., Klein, M. H., Wang, C. C., & Austin, S. B. (2011). Congruence/genuineness. *Psychotherapy, 48,* 65–71. http://dx.doi.org/10.1037/a0022064

Lean, M., Leavey, G., Killaspy, H., Green, N., Harrison, I., Cook, S., . . . King, M. (2015). Barriers to the sustainability of an intervention designed to improve patient engagement within NHS mental health rehabilitation units: A qualitative study nested within a randomised controlled trial. *BMC Psychiatry, 15,* 209. http://dx.doi.org/10.1186/s12888-015-0592-9

Leopold, H. S. (1976). Selective group approaches with psychotic patients in hospital settings. *American Journal of Psychotherapy, 30,* 95–102.

Leszcz, M., Yalom, I. D., & Norden, M. (1985). The value of inpatient group psychotherapy: Patients' perceptions. *International Journal of Group Psychotherapy, 35,* 411–433. http://dx.doi.org/10.1080/00207284.1985.11491425

Liden, R. C., Wayne, S. J., Jaworski, R. A., & Bennett, N. (2004). Social loafing: A field investigation. *Journal of Management, 30,* 285–304. http://dx.doi.org/10.1016/j.jm.2003.02.002

Lieberman, M. A., Yalom, I. D., & Miles, M. B. (1973). *Encounter groups: First facts.* New York, NY: Basic Books.

Linehan, M. M. (2014). *DBT skills training manual* (2nd ed.). New York, NY: Guilford Press.

Linehan, M. M., & Wilks, C. R. (2015). The course and evolution of dialectical behavior therapy. *American Journal of Psychotherapy, 69,* 97–110.

Lingiardi, V., & McWilliams, N. (Eds.). (2017). *Psychodynamic diagnostic manual* (2nd ed.). New York, NY: Guilford Press.

Lysaker, P. H., Roe, D., & Yanos, P. T. (2007). Toward understanding the insight paradox: Internalized stigma moderates the association between insight and social functioning, hope, and self-esteem among people with schizophrenia spectrum disorders. *Schizophrenia Bulletin, 33,* 192–199. http://dx.doi.org/10.1093/schbul/sbl016

Martin, R., & Young, J. (2010). Schema therapy. In K. S. Dobson (Ed.), *Handbook of cognitive-behavioral therapies* (3rd ed., pp. 317–346). New York, NY: Guilford Press.

Matsuda, M., & Kohno, A. (2016). Effects of the nursing psychoeducation program on the acceptance of medication and condition-specific knowledge of patients with schizophrenia. *Archives of Psychiatric Nursing, 30,* 581–586. http://dx.doi.org/10.1016/j.apnu.2016.03.008

Mino, Y., Shimodera, S., Inoue, S., Fujita, H., & Fukuzawa, K. (2007). Medical cost analysis of family psychoeducation for schizophrenia. *Psychiatry and Clinical Neurosciences, 61,* 20–24. http://dx.doi.org/10.1111/j.1440-1819.2007.01605.x

Nitsun, M. (2012). Sexual diversity in group psychotherapy. In J. L. Kleinberg (Ed.), *The Wiley-Blackwell handbook of group psychotherapy* (pp. 397–408). West Sussex, England: Wiley.

Norcross, J. C., & Lambert, M. J. (2010). Evidence-based therapy relationships. In J. C. Norcross (Ed.), *Evidence-based therapy relationships* (pp. 1–4). Oxford, England: Oxford Scholarship Online. Retrieved from https://nrepp.samhsa.gov/Legacy/pdfs/Norcross_evidence-based_therapy_relationships.pdf

Palmer, S., Stalker, C., Gadbois, S., & Harper, K. (2004). What works for survivors of childhood abuse: Learning from participants in an inpatient treatment program. *American Journal of Orthopsychiatry, 74,* 112–121. http://dx.doi.org/10.1037/0002-9432.74.2.112

Pankey, J. (2003). Acceptance and commitment therapy for psychosis. *International Journal of Psychology & Psychological Therapy, 3,* 311–328.

Petrakis, M., & Laxton, S. (2017). Intervening early with family members during first-episode psychosis: An evaluation of mental health nursing psychoeducation within an inpatient unit. *Archives of Psychiatric Nursing, 31,* 48–54. http://dx.doi.org/10.1016/j.apnu.2016.07.015

Rice, C. A., & Rutan, J. S. (1981). Boundary maintenance in inpatient therapy groups. *International Journal of Group Psychotherapy, 31,* 297–309. http://dx.doi.org/10.1080/00207284.1981.11491709

Roller, B., & Nelson, V. (1991). *The art of co-therapy.* New York, NY: Guilford Press.

Rummel-Kluge, C., & Kissling, W. (2008). Psychoeducation in schizophrenia: New developments and approaches in the field. *Current Opinion in Psychiatry, 21,* 168–172. http://dx.doi.org/10.1097/YCO.0b013e3282f4e574

Safran, J. D., Muran, J. C., & Eubanks-Carter, C. (2011). Repairing alliance ruptures. *Psychotherapy, 48,* 80–87. http://dx.doi.org/10.1037/a0022140

Santa Ana, E. J., Wulfert, E., & Nietert, P. J. (2007). Efficacy of group motivational interviewing (GMI) for psychiatric inpatients with chemical dependence. *Journal of Consulting and Clinical Psychology, 75,* 816–822. http://dx.doi.org/10.1037/0022-006X.75.5.816

Scott, J., Colom, F., Popova, E., Benabarre, A., Cruz, N., Valenti, M., . . . Vieta, E. (2009). Long-term mental health resource utilization and cost of care following group psychoeducation or unstructured group support for bipolar disorders: A cost–benefit analysis. *The Journal of Clinical Psychiatry, 70,* 378–386. http://dx.doi.org/10.4088/JCP.08m04333

Sibitz, I., Provaznikova, K., Lipp, M., Lakeman, R., & Amering, M. (2013). The impact of recovery-oriented day clinic treatment on internalized stigma: Preliminary report. *Psychiatry Research, 209,* 326–332. http://dx.doi.org/10.1016/j.psychres.2013.02.001

Spitz, H. I. (1996). *Group psychotherapy and managed mental health care: A clinical guide for providers.* New York, NY: Brunner/Mazel.

Spivack, N. (2008). Subgrouping with psychiatric inpatients in group psychotherapy: Linking dependency and counterdependency. *International Journal of Group Psychotherapy, 58,* 231–252. http://dx.doi.org/10.1521/ijgp.2008.58.2.231

Stacciarini, J.-M. R., O'Keeffe, M., & Mathews, M. (2007). Group therapy as treatment for depressed Latino women: A review of the literature. *Issues in Mental Health Nursing, 28,* 473–488. http://dx.doi.org/10.1080/01612840701344431

Sue, D. W. (2010). *Microaggressions in everyday life: Race, gender, and sexual orientation.* New York, NY: Wiley.

Sullivan, M., Deutsch, R. M., & Ward, P. (2016). Coparenting, parenting, and child-focused family interventions. In A. M. Judge & R. M. Deutsch (Eds.), *Overcoming parent–child contact problems: Family-based interventions for resistance, rejection, and alienation* (pp. 222–242). New York, NY: Oxford University Press.

Tasca, G. A., Flynn, C., & Bissada, H. (2002). Comparison of group climate in an eating disorders partial hospital group and a psychiatric partial hospital group. *International Journal of Group Psychotherapy, 52,* 409–417. http://dx.doi.org/10.1521/ijgp.52.3.409.45515

Taylor, R., Coombes, L., & Bartlett, H. (2002). The impact of a practice development project on the quality of in-patient small group therapy. *Journal of Psychiatric and Mental Health Nursing, 9,* 213–220. http://dx.doi.org/10.1046/j.1365-2850.2002.00478.x

Tchanturia, K. (Ed.). (2015). *Brief group psychotherapy for eating disorders: Inpatient protocols.* New York, NY: Routledge.

Thompson, L. W., Gallagher, D., Nies, G., & Epstein, D. (1983). Evaluation of the effectiveness of professionals and nonprofessionals as instructors of "coping with depression" classes for elders. *The Gerontologist, 23,* 390–396. http://dx.doi.org/10.1093/geront/23.4.390

Vannicelli, M. (2014). Supervising the beginning group leader in inpatient and partial hospital settings. *International Journal of Group Psychotherapy, 64,* 144–163. http://dx.doi.org/10.1521/ijgp.2014.64.2.144

von Maffei, C., Görges, F., Kissling, W., Schreiber, W., & Rummel-Kluge, C. (2015). Using films as a psychoeducation tool for patients with schizophrenia: A pilot study using a quasi-experimental pre–post design. *BMC Psychiatry, 15,* 93. http://dx.doi.org/10.1186/s12888-015-0481-2

Wheelan, S. A. (1997). Group development and the practice of group psychotherapy. *Group Dynamics: Theory, Research, and Practice, 1,* 288–293. http://dx.doi.org/10.1037/1089-2699.1.4.288

Yalom, I. (1983). *Inpatient group psychotherapy.* New York, NY: Basic Books.

Yanos, P. T., Roe, D., West, M. L., Smith, S. M., & Lysaker, P. H. (2012). Group-based treatment for internalized stigma among persons with severe mental illness: Findings from a randomized controlled trial. *Psychological Services, 9,* 248–258. http://dx.doi.org/10.1037/a0028048

Yeh, M., Tung, T., Horng, F., & Sung, S. (2017). Effectiveness of a psychoeducational programme in enhancing motivation to change alcohol-addictive behaviour. *Journal of Clinical Nursing, 26,* 3724–3733. http://dx.doi.org/10.1111/jocn.13744

3

THE INTERPERSONAL MODEL

The interpersonal model, one of the oldest approaches to group psycho-therapy, takes many different forms depending on the patient population and the setting in which it is applied. Yet, all applications emphasize the usefulness of interpersonal learning within the group. In the interpersonal approach, the group is seen as a social microcosm in which an individual's typical style of relating emerges (Yalom & Leszcz, 2005). Members have an opportunity in the here and now of the group to observe themselves and learn about others' reactions to their behavior. Increasingly, members have a realization of both their responsibility for their interactions with others and their power to alter them. This realization, when accompanied by a greater knowledge of their maladaptive patterns of behavior, creates an impetus to attempt new and more positive behaviors within the group and eventually in their lives outside of the therapy. Common to all versions of the interpersonal model is the notion that for the model to be effective, members must be both affectively and cognitively engaged in interpersonal learning.

http://dx.doi.org/10.1037/0000113-004
Group Psychotherapy in Inpatient, Partial Hospital, and Residential Care Settings, by V. Brabender and A. Fallon

This chapter focuses on four versions of the interpersonal model. The first version involves the application of the Sullivanian principles of social learning in a group session with a minimally structured format. This format continues to be used, particularly in partial hospital and residential settings. The second and third were developed by Yalom (1983) to address patients' decreasing number of days in the inpatient setting: The interactional agenda model was devised for group members who have a capacity to use exploratory and supportive interventions and have some minimal ability to tolerate anxiety, and the focus group model was created for group members who require exclusively supportive techniques. The fourth version, interpersonal psychotherapy–group (IPT-G), is different from the aforementioned types in that Klerman, Weissman, Rounsaville, and Chevron (1984) established it for the individual therapy situation and later extended it to group psychotherapy. This chapter contrasts these four types of interpersonal group therapy. The first three approaches are interpersonal because of their emphasis on here-and-now interaction, whereas the latter is defined by the interpersonal problems on which the approach focuses.

The influence of the interpersonal approach is so far-reaching that most likely every model in this book incorporates some element of it. Sometimes these connections are made explicitly but more often implicitly. The interpersonal model is a lens through which professionals, group psychotherapists and non–group psychotherapists alike, view group psychotherapy. That is why we begin with this orientation.

THEORETICAL UNDERPINNINGS

Harry Stack Sullivan's influence on the interpersonal approach to group psychotherapy is inestimable (Leszcz & Malat, 2012). His core notion was that psychopathology is at root interpersonal pathology. Sullivan (1940, 1953) saw personality as developing through the interplay of two opposing forces: the pursuit of satisfaction and the avoidance of insecurity. Psychopathology is the result of *parataxic distortion*, a maladaptive means of negotiating this conflict. A parataxic distortion is an unconscious misperception of another's response, a misreading based on early life experience and current need states. The parataxic distortion is gradually embedded in the complex network of perceptions, images, and fantasies about the self (or, in Sullivan's language, the *self-system*) to secure a particular satisfaction and enable the avoidance or lessening of anxiety. However, the distortion has little adaptive value because it is not tailored to contemporary reality and often begets the very reaction it is designed to avoid.

Other important contributors to the interpersonal approach were those theoreticians whose pioneering work brought recognition of the power of the here and now (i.e., the focus on members' contemporaneous interactions with one another). Prominent among these theoreticians are Moreno and Lewin. Moreno (1934)—who coined the term *here and now*—invited group members to bring family conflicts into the present through the enactment of psychodramas. Situating these experiences into the present proved to be an extraordinarily powerful technique in resolving longstanding conflicts. Lewin and his coworkers Benne, Bradford, and Lippitt (see Benne, 1964) observed T-groups designed to effect positive change among coworkers in an organization. Their observations led them to appreciate the change that individuals can undergo if they are provided with an opportunity to learn how others see them within their immediate context.

Irvin Yalom, perhaps the best-known American writer and thinker on group psychotherapy, is the originator and primary expostulator of the interpersonal approach to group psychotherapy. Yalom's approach is based on Sullivan's interpersonal theory and a here-and-now methodology. Yalom first proposed his interpersonal approach in his classic text, *The Theory and Practice of Group Psychotherapy*, published in 1970. Through all of the editions, including the most recent (Yalom & Leszcz, 2005), he has made the point that within the group forum, the exploration of genetic or early familial factors that produce psychopathology may not be as important, powerful, or effective as is interpersonal learning within the group. Although Yalom outlined a variety of mechanisms that can be used in the group to further the well-being of its members, the primary therapeutic factor is interpersonal learning within the here and now.

Interpersonal learning consists of a two-stage process. The first stage entails members plunging into a richly affective expression of their immediate reactions to one another. To achieve such an exploration, the therapist must possess a facility in "activating" the here and now. That is, the therapist must redirect members' focus from events that may be historical and out of the room to their present transactions with one another:

> Miguel, who had been describing to the group his rage at his neighbors' loud playing of their stereo, was questioned by the therapist as to whether any members were playing their music too loudly in the group. Miguel then spoke of his irritation toward Lan, who had dominated the prior week's session talking about her distress over her perception that her family placed too many demands on her. Other members then expressed their annoyance toward Lan, who reciprocated the expression of hostility.

If members were permitted to remain in this stage of affective expression, they might have obtained some temporary catharsis from the session but would have achieved little that could be transferred to interpersonal situations in their lives outside the group.

The second stage involves the analysis of the affective expressions:

Lan was asked to share perceptions she had of Miguel during the prior week. She said that he had appeared bored and indifferent. She noticed that he was the only member of the group who had nothing to say regarding her disclosures. Miguel then offered that he was waiting for her to finish because he, too, had something important to share with the group. The therapist asked the group whether anyone was able to detect that Miguel had something to share. Other members responded that Miguel seemed somewhat uninterested, as if nothing was or even could be of importance in the group. The therapist went on to help Miguel explore and test out some of his fantasies about what would have happened had he spoken up. The therapist also pointed out that Miguel was being much more active and direct during the present session and encouraged him to note members' reactions to this altered mode of relating.

Miguel learned that when he wants attention that others are receiving, he responds in a behaviorally passive way (i.e., by withdrawing). He saw the negative effect that his withdrawal had on others (they saw him as uncaring) and himself (he continued to be frustrated). He also experimented with a new mode of communication and tested in reality any fears that he attached to its adoption.

Frank (1963), describing inpatient groups in a state hospital setting, anticipated some of the elements (e.g., working within the here and now) that ultimately became central to the interpersonal approach. In the 1970s and the early 1980s, some inpatient group therapists (e.g., Beard & Scott, 1975), influenced by Yalom's work, conducted inpatient groups in pursuit of the interpersonal goal of helping members develop more effective ways of relating to others. These practitioners used the interpersonal methodology of focusing on members' here-and-now experiences in the context of an unstructured session in which members could reveal spontaneously their characteristic ways of interacting with others. Elements of insight were often incorporated into the treatment in consonance with the Sullivanian conflict-based premise that the perceptual distortions that give rise to maladaptive social behaviors are unconscious and are associated with hidden affects, impulses, and fantasies. In partial hospital programs (PHPs), Yalom's interpersonal approach tended to be less popular than the far more structured social skills training (e.g., Bellack, Turner, Hersen, & Luber, 1984), which we describe in Chapter 9 of this volume. However, this latter model has elements of the interpersonal approach, such as encouraging members to obtain feedback from other members on their behaviors in the group. Residential treatment centers (RTCs) during this period focused on either parent groups or parent–child groups that had a strong psychoeducational focus. Such groups continue to be popular in RTCs but exist alongside other group formats, which more explicitly engage interpersonal elements.

In 1983, Yalom published *Inpatient Group Psychotherapy*, a text that describes two models for using the interpersonal approach in an inpatient setting. The interactional agenda model was developed for relatively high-functioning inpatients and the focus group model for lower functioning inpatients. Although incorporating interpersonal goals and methods, they are modified in consideration of the special features of the inpatient environment—the brevity of members' tenures in the group, members' degrees of pathology, and the fact that the group takes place on a treatment unit. The agenda and focus group formats were based on Yalom's own experience in leading daily inpatient groups, his observation of groups in 25 inpatient settings (most of which were training settings with abundant resources), and his own research studies.

These two formats differ from the earlier applications of the interpersonal model in three ways. First, the agenda and focus group models are more structured than the original interpersonal approach, which involved relatively unstructured sessions in which members spontaneously produced material; the agenda and focus group models both have a highly articulated format. Second, the goals of the unstructured and structured applications are somewhat different. Although all versions of the interpersonal approach endorse the goal of helping members acquire more interpersonally effective behaviors, the unstructured versions appear to have remained truer to their Sullivanian origins. That is, they are consistent with Sullivan's conflict model of psychopathology wherein maladaptive social behavior is seen as serving a defensive function for the person. The modification of behavior does not entail simply the recognition of problem behaviors and their impact on others but also the development of insight into the impulses and feelings that have sustained the maladaptive behaviors. As we discuss later, Yalom (1983) saw the fostering of insight as having limited utility in the inpatient group. Third, the leader in the later models is more active than in the prior applications of the interpersonal approach. Given members' brief tenures in the group, the therapist must be more directive in helping members move toward their goals.

Although Yalom (1983) highlighted inpatient hospital programs (IHPs) in presenting his models, they have also been used in PHPs and RTCs. For example, Ferencik (1989) described the use of the interactional agenda approach in a group of substance abusers being treated in a PHP. Likewise, Kleiger and Helmig (1999) described an adolescent interactional group involving the setting of agendas in an RTC.

GOALS OF TREATMENT

A central goal of the interpersonal model is to foster members' development of effective social behaviors that will enable them to achieve more intimate, gratifying interpersonal relationships. This goal is derived from the

Sullivanian position that all psychological problems (no matter how individually centered they may seem) have a social undergirding. For example, although an individual's symptoms of depression might seem to reside in the person rather than in his or her relationships, an investigation will inevitably reveal interpersonal elements that sustain the symptoms. The individual might be depressed because of isolation from others, a perception that others have a negative valuation of him or her, or guilt about negative feelings toward others.

Although the traditional goal of the interpersonal model might be quite appropriate in PHP and RTC settings in which members remain in the group over weeks and months, it might be less so in the IHP group in which attendance of a single session or two is the duration of a member's participation. With extremely brief tenures of participation, the notion that members can modify features of their interpersonal styles is likely unrealistic. However, other interpersonally oriented goals can be pursued within an extremely brief time frame. One important interpersonal goal is the patient's increased openness to relationships within the milieu, with a lessening in the negativity attached to such relationships. At the time of their hospitalization, many patients exhibit a high level of withdrawal. This stance must be overcome for the patient to benefit from the modalities and interventions present within the setting, most of which have a social component. Even the dispensation of medication is a social transaction. In an interpersonally oriented group, members have an opportunity to explore their fantasies concerning the catastrophic consequences of relating to others. A group member who assumes that others are secretly laughing at her stammer may discover that although members do notice the stammer, they place little weight on it. She learns that members place much more weight on her forthrightness, a quality they value highly. This member's enhanced awareness that she has something to offer others is likely to enlarge her availability to others not only in the group but also in the milieu.

The interpersonal model is geared to accomplish the goal of increasing members' motivation and readiness for outpatient psychotherapy (particularly interpersonally oriented therapy). In fact, the primary goal of Yalom's (1983) agenda and focus group formats is to provide participants with a positive experience in therapy so they will wish to continue treatment after they are discharged. Within a motivational interviewing framework, we might think of the group as moving members from the Contemplation to the Preparation and Action stages of change (Prochaska & Norcross, 2001). The cultivation of their preparation and motivation for outpatient therapy has several dimensions. Within the interpersonal approach, members come to recognize their responsibilities for their difficulties. With this sense of responsibility comes an accompanying hopefulness of attenuating their problems.

The interpersonal approach also heightens members' awareness of the close tie between their interpersonal difficulties and their symptoms. In this way, members are led to see the usefulness of carrying on interpersonal exploration in their post-discharge psychotherapy. Yalom (1983) emphasized what he called the *problem-spotting function* of the IHP group (members' delineation of those interpersonal difficulties that can be addressed in a future, more long-term context). Finally, group members achieve an awareness of some of the common processes within an interpersonally oriented group. For example, Bryant, Kelly, and Zegarra (2010) described an interpersonal group for elderly individuals in an acute IHP. They noted that elderly individuals, in particular, are not likely to obtain feedback in their everyday lives. One of the positive outcomes of the group is simply to familiarize members with feedback and enable them to catch a glimpse of its potential usefulness.

TECHNICAL CONSIDERATIONS

Role of the Leader

Yalom's (1983) description of the leadership behaviors associated with the IHP version of his model is extensive. Some of his comments are pertinent to therapists using an interpersonal model in any setting, and others describe good leader behaviors in virtually any model. In this section, we focus on those aspects of leader behavior that are specific to the interpersonal model in an IHP.

The leader of the interpersonally oriented IHP group assumes a highly active posture (Hajek, 2010). This posture is required by the here-and-now focus of the group. Group members do not naturally focus on their immediate experience and often avoid it studiously. Instead, members are likely to dwell on other topics, such as the circumstances that precipitated their hospitalization. A newly formed group, in particular, requires therapist vigilance to ensure that members center themselves within the here and now. A high level of therapist activity is also required to achieve the appropriate balance between affect and cognition, a fundamental technical requirement of the interpersonal approach (Yalom & Leszcz, 2005).

In an IHP, a more vigorous intervention style is needed than in outpatient settings and long-term PHP and RTC settings. The IHP group therapist must be active in a number of respects (Yalom, 1983). The brevity of members' stays requires that the therapist be active in creating a highly structured session that enables each member to engage in significant interpersonal learning in every session. To stave off regression and diminish members' nonproductive anxiety, the therapist must provide an abundance of support. The interpersonal therapist must be efficient and strongly directive in managing the crises that frequently occur in IHP groups, such as when a member makes a threatening statement to another.

Therapist's Style of Relating

The therapist of the interpersonal group must cultivate an interactive style that is strong, authoritative, and yet egalitarian (Yalom, 1983). The authoritative aspect is important because a highly confident therapist is better able to assuage members' unproductive anxiety. Moreover, the therapist's confidence enhances members' willingness to participate in a process that, at the outset of treatment, might lack credibility as a means of addressing the difficulties precipitating members' hospitalizations. The therapist's egalitarianism is necessitated by the requirement of the interpersonal approach that the group members take considerable responsibility for self-disclosing and providing feedback to other members. A therapist who is either autocratic or unresponsive fosters infantile behaviors in members who are inspired to lay in continual wait for the therapist's dispensation of cures. A key means for the therapist to achieve an egalitarian relationship with members is to engage in the very activities in which members are encouraged to engage. For example, just as members are expected to give and receive feedback, so too should the therapist contribute his or her observations of the members and show a willingness to receive members' comments on his or her behavior.

Within the interpersonal approach, group psychotherapists show a fairly high degree of transparency, especially relative to other IHP models. Group psychotherapists are called on to be transparent particularly about their reactions to the group itself or specific events within the group, a type of sharing that Kiesler (1996) described as "therapeutic meta-communication" or "communicating about communication" (Leszcz & Malat, 2012, p. 53). Consider the following two examples of therapist transparency:

- A therapist may express to the group that she feels moved by members' courage in giving one another honest feedback.
- A therapist acknowledges feeling torn between allowing the group to continue focusing on an obviously distressed but inconsolable member and urging the group to move on to others who may be suffering, albeit less conspicuously so.

In the second example, the therapist's admission of having an internal struggle permits an explicit recognition of all members' needs and paves the way for the group to broaden its focus. In both these examples, the therapist's motivation in self-disclosing is to facilitate members' expressions of their feelings and observations. Within the interpersonal model (as in most models), the therapist must be sufficiently self-aware to know when a potential self-disclosure is in the service of the group's needs versus his or her own to ensure that only the former cross the behavioral threshold (Leszcz, 2008). However, Yalom (1983) pointed out that often the failure to be transparent is motivated by the therapist's wish to protect him- or herself.

Conflict in the Interpersonal Therapy Group

Anger commonly arises in the inpatient group and has many sources. Hospitalization itself evokes anger: Members are often angry because of their need for hospitalization as well as the inconveniences and annoyances of residing in a confined setting (e.g., loss of privacy, regimentation, frequent intrusions, exposure to more disturbed patients). These latter factors also attach to varying degrees to RTCs but less so to PHPs. Another source of anger concerns the group itself: the demand implicitly made on members to share the therapist, a feature of group life across all its applications. Particularly in the IHP group, the typically brief tenure of members in the group and the pressure they feel to change during this interval contribute to frustration with the group and a concomitant intensification of irritation. In PHPs and RTCs, members' relationships with one another are more longstanding. Any negativity that characterizes these relationships in the milieu or in other groups can easily enter the psychotherapy group.

In the interpersonally oriented group, members are invited to share openly their reactions to other members. It is natural that along with the positive feelings that members express toward one another, negative feelings of various sorts are present: irritation, hostility, impatience, exasperation, and so on. The interpersonal group therapist is faced with somewhat of a dilemma in helping the group to respond to the emergence of these feelings. Although it is essential that members learn to communicate their negative feelings effectively, such reactions have the power to produce further disorganization in the sender and the receiver (and even sideline observers) of such messages.

Interpersonal therapists differ in the ways they have responded to this challenge. In some interpersonally oriented groups (e.g., Beutler, Frank, Schieber, Calvert, & Gaines, 1984), the exploration of members' negative feelings is made a centerpiece of the group. The processing of affects such as anger and their multiple manifestations allows for the correction of internalized schemes—typically formed in childhood—about the interpersonal catastrophes that are likely to ensue following the communication of negatively toned feelings (e.g., "If I let her know she angered me, the relationship will be over"). It also allows members to broaden their repertoires in how they express negative feelings to strengthen relationships ("When I get angry, I need not explode; rather, I can verbalize my feelings"). In those RTCs and PHPs in which members are present for longer than a brief stay (i.e., weeks rather than days), members' opportunities to express and explore anger within the group can be extremely useful. However, Yalom (1983) believed that "the inpatient group is not the place for confrontation, criticism, or the expression and examination of anger" (p. 125). He saw an open, intense, or prolonged manifestation of conflict as destructive to the IHP group because it feeds members' fearfulness of group involvement. He argued that a conflict-ridden, hostile group subverts what for him is the cardinal goal of an IHP group: to develop members' perception of group psychotherapy as a supportive setting in which a high level of comfort with others and understanding of self and others is achievable.

Regardless of setting—IHP, PHP, or RTC—members' levels of hostility toward one another must be modulated for the group to be regarded by its members as a place of safety. Yalom (1983) identified a set of therapist techniques to achieve such a modulation. For example, the therapist might encourage the angry member to direct his or her hostility toward an abstract issue rather than toward the member associated with the issue. The therapist can offer him- or herself as the target of the anger (e.g., "You are saying that Jorges is taking up too much of the group's time, but perhaps you are feeling upset that I haven't intervened to provide you and others more of an opportunity to talk"). The therapist can also encourage a member who gets explosively angry to express hostility when it is in its more nascent form (or *young anger*, as Yalom [p. 148] called it). The common denominator of these and other techniques is that the therapist permits a limited discharge of anger to prevent its full flowering. Eventually, members might express irritation toward one another, but the therapist must ensure that it is done constructively and must attend carefully to how it is experienced by its recipient.

Use of the Here and Now

Although many applications of the interpersonal approach can be found in IHPs, PHPs, and RTCs, a core feature of all of them is the fostering of interpersonal learning through the use of the here and now. As we discussed earlier, the use of the here and now is predicated on the position of Sullivan (1953) and, later, Yalom (1985; Yalom & Leszcz, 2005) that most, if not all, psychological problems have an interpersonal aspect that can be explored within the immediacy of a relationship or, as in the case of a group, a set of relationships. A key technical consideration of all interpersonal group therapists is how to use the here and now most effectively. From Yalom's (1983; Yalom & Leszcz, 2005) standpoint, such effective use entails the two-step process that was outlined briefly earlier in this chapter and that we now describe in greater detail. The first step, the activation of the here and now, involves the delineation of those immediate elements that require the group's attention. Although, in a mature outpatient group, the group members themselves might identify those events or aspects of the group in need of exploration, in most other instances, the therapist must perform this task. Consider the following example of the therapist's activation of the here and now in a PHP group:

> Helen, a member of the group, spoke in a whining tone about her husband's failure to attend to her emotional needs. The therapist observed that she did not look at the other members while she delivered her narrative. When she was finished, members responded minimally to her. The therapist asked the group members whether they had noticed anything about how Helen related to them while she was talking about her husband. One member said that Helen had not looked at them, and others nodded (activation of the here and now). The therapist wondered aloud whether members had a reaction to Helen's lack of eye contact. (Here, the therapist was keying in on the affective layer of the group, a layer that often emerges vividly during this step.) Several group members declined the therapist's invitation by responding intellectually. They said they had inferred that Helen did not want to be interrupted, that she was invested in simply telling her story. However, one member, Mary, who had formed a strong relationship with Helen outside the group, indicated that she felt slightly annoyed and even a little hurt that Helen was not curious about how she might be responding. Other members then followed Mary's lead. One member said she was bored by Helen's monologue. Still another said she felt rejected by Helen in the latter's evident lack of interest in her opinion. Helen expressed some dismay and shock over both members' perception of her indifference and the feelings in them that these perceptions elicited.

Once members had put forth their feelings toward Helen and Helen responded by sharing feelings of her own, the group was in a position to understand the various reactions that the activation of the here and now had precipitated, a step Yalom and Leszcz (2005) described as the *illumination* of the here and now:

> The therapist then encouraged Helen to talk about the expectation she had about how the group members would receive her disclosures. Helen responded that she had expected exactly what she got: nothing. The therapist wondered aloud whether, as Helen spoke, the members did have thoughts they might have shared with her but did not. Again, Mary took a leadership role in indicating that she had many reactions that she wanted to share with Helen, and several other members revealed that they, too, had thoughts and feelings about her disclosure. The therapist commented, "Helen, your expectations about how members would respond led you to discourage them from responding. Because you assumed that the other

members don't care, you didn't give them an opportunity to show their caring for you." The therapist then showed the other group members that their behavior was much like Helen's. They assumed that Helen was indifferent to them and thereby denied her the feedback she craved. Helen, realizing the genuineness of members' interest in her, spontaneously expressed affection for the other members.

We can see that the therapist moved the group to a cognitive analysis of the raw reactions group events evoked in members. Throughout the process, however, affective and cognitive elements were present.

In this sequence, the members of the group were given a framework by which their present affective reactions and those of others could be seen as coherent. Although an element of confrontation underlay the interaction between Helen and the other group members, a high degree of support was present as well. If the group had merely brainstormed ways in which Helen could maneuver her husband into being more forthcoming, she would have failed to experience this support so directly. So, too, would she have neglected to recognize her responsibility in evoking others' seeming disattunement to her. Were the group to have taken this alternate direction (toward the there and then rather than here and now), members would have experienced the session as much less vibrant and compelling. More important, the proceedings would have been perceived as having relevance for only those members whose external situations closely resembled Helen's.

Content of the Session

In all applications of the interpersonal model in IHP, PHP, and RTC groups, the content of the session consists of the group's examination of their relationships with one another within the group. The conversation may be extended to an exploration of their relationship in the milieu. In less structured versions of the interpersonal model, members are encouraged to bring up material spontaneously. Often, members center on topics that, at least on the surface, are unrelated to their relationships with other members. The therapist uses this material to direct their attention to the immediate aspects of their experience. The therapist guides members in proceeding through the two-stage process just delineated. This format wherein the therapist is primarily reactive to members' offerings characterizes most of the session. In some cases, the therapist may elect, at the outset of the session, to introduce the goals and methods of the group—a feature included in recognition of the fact that, particularly in the inpatient environment, preparation for group participation might not be feasible before a member's first session.

Alternatively, the therapist can structure a sequence of events within the session. Such structure ensures a focused pursuit of goals in a way that enables them to be fulfilled given the group's limited period in which to work and many members' compromised resources for working (Yalom, 1983). However, the development of such a format requires that the group be relatively homogeneous regarding level of functioning. In 1976, Leopold formalized the notion of creating groups for members who occupied the same broad area of functioning. Here *level of functioning* refers to the patients' behaviors within groups and capacities to use different types of intervention. Although this concept is obviously related to diagnosis and level of adaptation in the extra hospital environment, it is nonetheless separate from both of these constructs. Patients are considered to be low functioning when their capacity to relate to others is enhanced by interventions of a primarily supportive, nonexploratory nature (i.e., those designed to effect an immediate lessening in the member's degree of anxiety or other disturbing affects). Patients are viewed as high functioning when they benefit not only from the aforementioned class of interventions but also from interventions designed to enhance their awareness of patterns of behavior and the impact of these behaviors on the social environment.

A *levels* approach entails the creation of separate groups and different session formats for high- and low-functioning members. Yalom (1983) proposed the agenda group for high-functioning patients and the focus group for low-functioning patients. Although these models are presented in a highly detailed way, they are not intended as exact blueprints of how other therapists should conduct their groups, in that all models should take into account the particulars of the group's context. In the sections that follow, we describe differences among interpersonal approaches; however, Table 3.1 describes their common features.

INTERPERSONAL APPROACHES

Interactional Agenda Group

A five-step process informs agenda group sessions.

Orientation and Preparation

In the first step, orientation and preparation, the therapist provides members with information about the structural features of the group (e.g., length of sessions, frequency of meetings, presence of observers), its purpose, and its mechanics. Group members are informed that the group is designed specifically to assist members in their interpersonal relationships. The therapist also explains the notion that by working on their relationships with one another, members can improve their relationships outside the group. Yalom (1983) saw this orientation as extremely important given the research evidence that members'

TABLE 3.1
Interpersonal Approach

Elements of the model	Characteristics of the model
View of psychological problems	Most human difficulties, including a wide range of symptom patterns, are due to a person's difficulty in relating to others.
Goals of model	Enhance an individual's capacity to relate positively to others.
Methods of action	Interpersonal learning involving activation of affect and cognitive framing.
Therapeutic techniques	• Fostering group cohesion • Focusing on the here and now • Supporting the exchange of feedback
Adaptation of the model to a brief time frame	When the member's typical tenure is brief (1–2 sessions), emphasis is placed on (a) fostering a positive attitude toward group psychotherapy, (b) helping the member to achieve familiarity with therapeutic processes, and (c) increasing openness to interactions and therapeutic interventions throughout the program.
Use of group process	Members focus almost entirely on their interactions with one another, learning how others experience their interpersonal behaviors. Members use the group as a laboratory to attempt new and potentially more effective ways of relating.

knowledge of the goals and working procedures of their groups enhances their performance within the group (e.g., Heitler, 1974; Houlihan, 1977).

Agenda Go-Around

The second step requires each member to identify some area on which he or she can work during this specific session. For example, a member might say, "Yesterday, I thought that all of you were secretly laughing at me when I shared my feelings with the group. Today I want to find out if you actually were." Yalom (1983) pointed out that the advantages of the go-around include enabling the therapist to identify the points of greatest tension with the group so the therapist can recognize problem areas that members can address in concert with one another and support patients in adopting an active participatory stance in the sessions.

In initiating the go-around, the therapist provides members with some instruction on what constitutes an appropriate agenda by allowing the more senior members to formulate their agendas first. Even with such an allowance, it is almost certain that some members will have difficulty creating their agendas. In such cases, the therapist must help members isolate problem areas, translate problems into interpersonal terms, and develop the problem formulations in such a way that they can be addressed within the here-and-now context of the group that day.

An example of the agenda-sculpting process is one wherein a group member offers as her agenda, "I'm sick of feeling worthless." The therapist (in some instances assisted by other group members) would engage in a discussion with the member leading to the development of an agenda that is realistic, interpersonal, and here-and-now focused. The member's problem may be rendered less abstract and more interpersonal through the following translation: "I want to value myself as much as I value others." Its contextualization within the group may be, "I want to speak up more today and not always defer to others who are also trying to speak." The formulation of agendas is envisioned to be a step that has therapeutic value in multiple respects (Yalom, 1983). Clearly, it accomplishes the problem-spotting function of the group and requires that members take control of their therapy (Leszcz, 1986). Moreover, to the extent that members can see themselves as having specific interpersonal problems that can be addressed in the group, their motivation to continue group therapy following discharge is enhanced. Finally, members typically perceive their formulation of agendas as successes, and this positive experience increases their attraction to the group.

Agenda Fulfillment

Either group members or the therapist may initiate the process of agenda fulfillment. However, what is important is that the therapist remains alert to the possibility of integrating as many agendas as possible into the field of action. For example, one member may have established as her agenda learning to focus on other members rather than on herself, and another member may have announced his wish to be more open in disclosing to the group his sense of humiliation about his stammer. The therapist might encourage the former to "draw out" the latter. Although most agendas are filled within the session, the therapist may give a member a "homework assignment" to complete on the unit between sessions. For example, if a given member wishes to practice taking the initiative in relationships, the therapist may suggest that the member initiates conversations on the unit with another group member who is striving to overcome his withdrawal. Alternatively, homework might involve staff members. For example, a group member lacking self-assertion skills might ask one of the staff for a desired privilege.

Wrap-Up—Part 1

The wrap-up consists of a two-part retrospective analysis of the session. In the first part of this step, the therapist and any other individuals who have observed the session provide an analysis of it. The inclusion of observers in IHP, PHP, and RTC settings is not uncommon because they all frequently serve as training venues. In the literature (e.g., Oldham, 1982), observers are typically portrayed in passive roles while the group is in session. The passivity and inscrutability of the observers can easily leave members feeling exploited and fearful about the preservation of confidentiality (Yalom, 1983). Yalom suggested an active role for the observers so that (a) the aforementioned negative effects of observers can be obviated, (b) the clinical and training functions of having observers can be preserved, and (c) the observers can actively advance the goals of the group. The observers' activity takes the form of sharing their observations about the group with the group members in the initial segment of the wrap-up period. Although the observers strive to be candid, they withhold any perceptions that might be narcissistically damaging or anxiety arousing to members. For effective participation in this nuanced fashion, observers must be carefully prepared for their roles.

The therapist's role in this discussion is to consider each member's progress in the session and to provide patients with additional support and attunement for unresolved issues and areas of future work. The therapist should be open to feedback from the members and acknowledge when a therapist behavior may have created an unintended consequence. This therapist behavior provides a model of openness. However, such admissions should be wrought with sensitivity and avoid those that may be disorganizing or distressing to members. If a cotherapy team conducts the group, discussion of the relationship between cotherapists also demonstrates for members constructive interpersonal exploration.

Wrap-Up—Part 2

In the second part of the wrap-up, group members bring the meeting to an end. Final events might include a discussion of their reactions to the observers' feedback or the therapist's analysis, the further processing of an unresolved issue from an earlier point in the session, or a focus on those members who have not had an opportunity to speak earlier. Group members are permitted to determine which direction to pursue because such an allowance fosters responsibility taking. At the same time, the therapist must seek opportunities to use this final period to support a self-review process in which members come to recognize more clearly what is effective work in psychotherapy. For example, the therapist may explicitly state that a given session was an especially valuable one because of members' obvious willingness to offer one another honest feedback (see Yalom, 1983, for a complete description of this model and a detailed clinical example).

Focus Group

The focus group model was designed for lower functioning group members who are sufficiently organized to sit in a group with others but whose ego functions are too disrupted by their symptoms to be able to profit from the more demanding agenda group. Although the activities of the focus group are quite different from those of the agenda group, they are nonetheless consistent with the general goals and principles of the interpersonal orientation. The group is directed toward constructively exploring members' interactions in the group to foster (a) their willingness to continue with therapy after discharge, (b) their recognition of the helpfulness both of talking and of concretely identifying problems, and (c) their capacity to engage with others both on the unit and outside the hospital (Yalom, 1983).

The particular activities of the focus group are designed with an awareness of the special limitations of these members. Because many individuals in this group will have exceedingly brief attention spans, activities are pursued for brief periods. Members' capacities for further decompensation necessitate that the exploration of conflictual areas is avoided assiduously. Given members' vulnerabilities to extraordinarily high levels of anxiety, specific exercises such as muscle relaxation are used to enable members to feel safer and more comfortable. Because members are likely to feel threatened specifically by being in a group, the therapist must create ways in which the members can experience success in the group instantly to diminish that threat. That is, the therapist must be attuned to, and poised to emphasize, all positive aspects of members' behavior, including their courage in simply attending the group. Although Yalom designed this format for IHPs, it is also particularly suited to application in day care PHPs (see Chapter 1).

Segment 1

Each session in the focus group is organized into four segments. The first segment, orientation and preparation, is essentially the same in content as that of the agenda group. Information about the time, place, goals, and methods of the group is shared. Even if there are no new members in a particular session, the therapist must never bypass this step given members' likely high levels of confusion.

Segment 2

The second segment, the warm-up, involves members' engagement in brief exercises that ease them into positive interaction with one another. Examples of such exercises are a ball toss, a go-around in which members describe a positive or negative feeling they experienced that day, or a go-around in which each member makes observations of another member of the group. It is important that the therapist ascertain the mood of the group in selecting a particular exercise.

Segment 3

The third segment consists of a set of structured exercises, each of which lasts from 5 to 15 minutes. Again, the particular exercise chosen (as well as its duration) is determined by the therapist's perceptions of the special needs and level of task endurance of each group. Yalom (1983) provided examples of various exercises and games in each category. Some exercises have a strong interpersonal focus (e.g., exercises that develop members' capacities for relating to others), whereas others do not (e.g., a psychoeducational discussion about a shared problem). The exercise can be tailored to enable members to process some event on the unit that may have upset them.

Segment 4

The fourth and final segment involves a review of the session. Given the difficulty these members have in organizing their experience, they are likely to profit from the opportunity to recollect the sequence of events that constituted the sessions. Following this memory exercise, the group then conducts an exploration of its reactions to the events of the session, much as is done by the agenda group. Observers are not involved because their mere presence might exacerbate members' inevitable difficulties with trust. For a complete description of this model with clinical examples, see Yalom (1983) and Vinogradov and Yalom (1989).

Interpersonal Psychotherapy–Group

Interpersonal psychotherapy (IPT; Klerman et al., 1984), like all interpersonal models, rests on the Sullivanian assumption that symptoms are highly connected to a person's difficulties in interpersonal functioning. Originally, the focus of IPT was on the treatment of depression. However, Wilfley and colleagues (Wilfley et al., 1993; Wilfley, Frank, Welch, Spurrell, & Rounsaville, 1998) saw the potential for adapting IPT for the treatment of individuals with binge eating disorders in a group format (IPT-G). In 2000, Wilfley, MacKenzie, Welch, Ayres, and Weissman published a manual that provides considerable helpful detail on conducting IPT groups. Because Wilfley and colleagues have developed the IPT-G format as a time-limited medium, it is particularly suitable for the three types of treatment environments described in this text but, most particularly, PHPs and RTCs. The therapist deliberately uses members' knowledge of the time limit to motivate them in engaging fully with the group.

Treatment Goal

The goal of treatment within IPT-G is to identify interpersonal problems that are attached to a set of symptoms and to provide the group experiences enabling the modification of those problems. The interpersonal problems connected to symptoms might be either precipitants of the symptoms or factors that maintain symptoms (Wilfley et al., 1998). For example, a group member might have become depressed because of unresolved grief over the death of a spouse, but the isolation caused by the death might maintain the depression. It is important to note that the interpersonal problems of interest are those emerging outside the group, a feature that distinguishes IPT-G from the other interpersonal models described in this chapter. IPT practitioners see this approach as focusing on the here and now. However, they use this term to describe current relationships in the individual's life, rather than historical relationships (e.g., the relationship an adult had with his parent when he was a child; Swartz, 1999).

Problem Areas

IPT-G addresses four problem areas. *Grief* refers specifically to a person's dysfunctional reaction to the death of a significant person in an individual's life. Other kinds of losses are not part of this category. *Interpersonal disputes* concern asymmetrical expectations in interpersonal situations. The following are some examples of interpersonal disputes:

- A parent of an adult child expects the latter to visit her weekly.
- An associate in a law firm feels he is inappropriately passed by for partner status.
- A man in a long-term relationship wants a commitment from his partner that is not forthcoming.

Human misery, in each instance, is instigated by different parties' beliefs or longings that conflict. *Role transition* relates to any major change in a person's life such as moving, ending a relationship, or beginning a new relationship. *Interpersonal deficits* describe individuals' long-term failure to establish or maintain fulfilling relationships, typically due to a lack of basic skills or ability to use them in an effective, coordinated way. Particular types of problem areas might be more common in particular patient groups (Wilfley, Stein, & Welch, 2005). For example, persons with binge-eating disorder and anorexia are likely to show interpersonal deficits more than other problem areas.

Group Development

Like all time-limited treatments, IPT-G consists of distinct beginning, middle, and end phases. However, the developers of IPT-G recognized that a psychotherapy group is constituted of different developmental phases that can either harmonize or work at odds with the goals of the model. The model developers have designed this approach to take advantage of the developmental opportunities presented over the group's life. In doing so, they use MacKenzie's (1997) stage model.

In MacKenzie's (1997) approach, the initial sessions revolve around members' engagement with one another, the therapist, and the group as a whole. The therapist assists members in building a cohesive group with the norms that will support members' goals. As members experience themselves as coming together, they are likely to have an increase in the hope that fuels work in later stages. They begin to recognize that though they have many similarities to one another, they also differ in important ways. They frequently express displeasure with aspects of the group, the therapist, or one another. This phase of differentiation is crucial to members seeing each other and themselves more fully, a capacity necessary for in-depth psychological work. Therefore, the therapist welcomes members' expressions and contextualizes them by helping members to see that addressing differences can be a sticking point in relationships outside the group (Wilfley et al., 2000). During the work phase of group life, which corresponds to the intermediate phase of group life, members delve into their highly individual social difficulties and practice skills enabling these difficulties to be ameliorated or overcome. The therapist helps members stay within the here and now, as this model defines it, and to refrain from becoming so immersed in their relationships with one another that the precipitating locus of the problem—their lives outside the group—is ignored. The therapist cultivates members' curiosity about how members are faring in coping with these problems outside the group. The fourth stage, termination, coincides with the last sessions of the group and offers members an opportunity to address what set of feelings is stimulated by the loss of the group, to look prospectively at challenges that lie ahead, and recognize the skills that have been developed to meet those challenges.

Assessment and Preparation

In this approach, the assessment is extremely important in that the information gleaned from this step frames the treatment. Whereas in other applications of the interpersonal approach, a formal diagnosis might not figure saliently in the treatment planning process, in IPT it does. This approach links the diagnosis to the individual's interpersonal problems. Hence, in the assessment interview, sufficient information must be obtained so that establishing an accurate diagnosis is achieved. A positive effect of diagnosis, IPT thinking holds, is that the prospective group member can embrace the sick role, thereby justifying obtaining care and gaining relief from everyday responsibilities (Wilfley et al., 2000).

During the assessment, the therapist interviews the patient about past and current relationships. However, enhancing interview data is the therapist's use of assessment tools. Particularly important are tools that reflect the individual's interpersonal functioning, such as the Inventory of Interpersonal Problems (Alden, Wiggins, & Pincus, 1990) and the Social Adjustment Scale (Weissman & Bothwell, 1976). The unfolding material is considered through the lens of the four problem areas described previously: grief, interpersonal role disputes, role transitions, and interpersonal deficits. From all the data the clinician has amassed, it might become clear that the patient has a plethora of problems in relating to others. In a time-limited group, only a few can be addressed. Therefore, one of the tasks during this assessment and preparatory stage is to whittle down the array to those that are most highly connected to the individual's current symptom pattern (Swartz, 1999). On the basis of the patient's most concerning current interpersonal problems, patient and therapist collaboratively establish goals.

In the sections that follow, we describe the format of the sessions once the group itself commences. We refer the reader to Wilfley et al. (2000) for a more extensive description and actual language that the therapist might use in delivering specific interventions. Moreover, our characterization is broadbrush. For example, whereas we characterize the initial phase as a whole, Wilfley et al. talked about each session in specific terms. Over the course of the group, the therapist provides each member with several individual sessions as a way of ensuring that that member's problem areas are being addressed adequately. This feature emerged from the research showing that IPT-G is most potent when it is also combined with some individual work. The extensive assessment and preparation further strengthen the focus on the individual member.

Initial Phase

Within a 15-session time frame, this phase would correspond roughly to the first five sessions. We previously described the importance of the therapist's building a group culture in which significant work can be done. In addition, however, these initial sessions are designed to help members appreciate that the symptoms they have are not unusual and can be treated and help them learn about how IPT-G specifically seeks to treat them. Each member of the group receives the group's attention by way of a consideration of that member's interpersonal inventory. This process consummates in the drawing up of a treatment contract with each member.

At the conclusion of each of the sessions, the therapist allocates time for a wrap-up. Often, emotions are stimulated by the sessions, and members benefit from having the opportunity to gain perspective on them before departing. It also provides some material for the framing of the subsequent session. As members proceed through these initial sessions, the building group cohesion and their greater levels of individual comfort lead them to be progressively more disclosing about their interpersonal struggles.

Intermediate Phase

The intermediate phase is when the lion's share of the work is done. The specific strategies the therapist uses depends on the area in which the member's problem resides. For example, suppose a member's difficulty was associated with the area of grief. In that case, the therapist would help that member identify the particular issue that hindered the individual from managing grief reactions in a way that is not immobilizing.

Suppose Nancy, a young adult, never mourned the death of her mother but nonetheless spent years barely functioning. During the assessment and preparatory phase, it might become clear to Nancy and the therapist that her family never allowed her to mourn the death of her mother. After her mother's death, the father insisted that they cease talking about her, and Nancy was discouraged from attending her mother's funeral because of the notion that it would be "too much for her." In the initial phase of the group, Nancy might feel the support of the group—support she lacked from her family—to garner the courage to be able to approach grief reactions. In the intermediate stage, she would unpack her relationship with her mother, both the positive and negative aspects. Action elements might be introduced, such as having her write a eulogy for her mother or take a mental journey through her mother's funeral. In the process of Nancy's hearing from other members how they connected with her experiences, she would be opening herself up to new relationships, a task for those attempting to move beyond the kind of grief that impairs everyday functioning. In this example, Nancy and the members readily took up the task of examining her grief. However, had she or others been reluctant, it would have been the therapist's responsibility to make sure she addressed the problem (MacKenzie & Grabovac, 2001).

As another example, some patients might require considerable attention in the area of interpersonal role disputes. Amira and her husband had been trying to conceive a child for many years. It became clear that an alternate way of building a family would have to be embraced, but her husband was steadfastly against doing so. Amira was committed to both the relationship and the goal of having children. When she entered treatment, she was experiencing considerable misery at the prospect of either leaving her husband or abandoning her long-held wish to have a child. The therapist had to help Amira to assess whether the conflict was in the renegotiation stage such that her investment in her relationship with her husband continued or whether they were at an impasse wherein no tolerable resolution was possible within the confines of the relationship. If Amira decided that living a life without having a child was unacceptable to her, she might be assisted in proceeding to the dissolution stage. The latter entails managing the loss and the need to rebuild her life.

Final Stage

The final stage, termination, occurs as the group nears its end, with only five sessions remaining. For all patients, but particularly those who struggle with depression, the end phase represents an opportunity to address reactions to loss, with loss being a key precipitating factor in depression. Some patients are likely to experience a range of painful feelings, and the therapist should encourage their expression. Such facilitation can take the form of the therapist's recognizing the group's ending as a loss for members and explicitly stating that it might evoke difficult reactions, which can be shared in the remaining sessions. In addition, the therapist should be sensitive to when members are indirectly talking about the ending of the group by focusing on other parallel events in their lives. The therapist can help them see that what they are describing about an event or transition external to the group also has immediate relevance.

Other tasks are important during this termination phase (Wilfley et al., 2000). An important activity for each member is taking stock of progress made over the course of the group. The therapists and the other group members share their observations of the gains each member has made, and each member forms his or her self-observations, based not only on changes manifested in the group but also in the patient's everyday environment. For patients in a PHP, this focus on external relationships is augmented by the member's immersion in these relationships outside program hours. Inpatient programs and RTCs provide more limited opportunities for members to work on external relationships. In this process of noting changes, it is not unusual for members to attempt to minimize progress or attribute gains to factors other than their exertions. The therapists have to be alert to this possibility and to counter this dismissal. Doing so enhances members' motivation to continue to strive to apply the learning obtained in the group.

The group is also forward looking in anticipating those circumstances that are likely to be challenging for members (Wilfley et al., 2000). For example, a member might recognize that when tension increases in his marriage, he is likely to engage in risky sexual behavior outside his marriage. Identifying alternate strategies for responding to the tension is of critical importance, and one strategy that is likely to have an important place in the mix is seeking additional therapy. Often, it can be helpful if significant others in the individual's life provide assistance. For example, a bipolar patient might be encouraged to enlist family members in identifying when he is showing the irritability that might be a harbinger of an incipient episode and in recognizing what other helpful steps might be taken.

Following the ending of the group, members are encouraged to have an individual follow-up visit with one or both of the therapists 4 to 6 months following treatment (Wilfley et al., 2000). Knowledge of the follow-up serves as an incentive for members to persist in their efforts to consolidate and expand on their gains. It also offers an opportunity to the treatment team to make an intervention if the client foundered following termination from the group. For example, the individual might be referred to another group or perhaps individual treatment.

CLINICAL ILLUSTRATION[1] OF AN INTERPERSONAL APPROACH

The vignette presented in this chapter features an unstructured version of the interpersonal approach. We are showing this type of interpersonal approach because, to varying extent, the other more structured approaches derive from this format. The group in this vignette was composed of relatively high-functioning members. In this session, the therapist had already oriented the members to the group with the help of the more senior members. Although this PHP group consisted of eight members, for ease of exposition, we describe only five.

Group Members

Marv, a middle-aged man, had been in the PHP for 3 weeks following a week of inpatient hospitalization after his revelation to his outpatient therapist that he had a suicidal plan that the therapist deemed serious. He entered the program in a mournful mood but in the past week appeared filled with bombast. Outside the group, he zealously attempted to help all who encountered him, staff and patients alike, and did so in a way that was so intrusive and condescending that others were avoiding him steadfastly. He had been in the group for four sessions.

Hazel, an elderly group member, was participating in her second group session. In the previous day's session, members commented that although they found her to be amiable, they noticed that when several members had made complaints about their life, Hazel attempted to minimize their concerns. At the end of that session, Hazel congratulated members on having been so perceptive of her during the prior session because her inability to acknowledge to herself or express to others any negative reactions had much to do with her unhappiness in her marriage and her need for admittance to the PHP. With the therapist's help, she formulated a plan that when she experienced even minor dissatisfaction in the group, she would speak up.

---

[1]This clinical illustration and all of the illustrations in this text are fictional accounts.

Gabe was a young man who had been in the PHP for a week. He was preoccupied with perverse, harm-wishing thoughts toward other people, and because of his fearfulness that others might somehow become aware of them, he had progressively isolated himself from his family and friends. Despite an initial refusal to join the group, he became more and more comfortable as he experienced himself being helpful to others. In the previous day's session, he had surprised other members of the group by disclosing his fears of rejection. He articulated a goal to test in the group the legitimacy of these fears.

Sally, an extremely sociable young woman, revealed in her 2 weeks of being in the group an ease in connecting with others. She was a highly liked and admired member of the group, and members frequently commented that she seemed more like a staff member than a patient. Members did not understand why she was attending the program and assumed it had resulted from a practitioner's misjudgment.

The Session

The therapist conducted a brief orientation about the nature and scope of the group.

<dl>
<dt>Sally:</dt>
<dd>What's wrong with you?</dd>

<dt>Marv:</dt>
<dd>Nothing.</dd>

<dt>Sally:</dt>
<dd>Well, something's wrong . . . I don't know . . . you seem miserable today.</dd>

<dt>Marv:</dt>
<dd>Okay, I guess I have to level with you: I've been feeling down—I just feel that I'm not connecting with anyone here, and it was so different when I first came. I felt that everyone here was my friend. But now, no one is. I mean, if I talk to people, they cut me off or look not that interested. I know I'm dense sometimes, but I'm picking up a negative vibe everywhere.</dd>

<dt>Therapist:</dt>
<dd>You said that people in the program seemed to be pulling away from you, but it would be important for us to know if you feel the same thing is going on in here.

[In this comment, the therapist is placing Marv's complaint within the here and now, encouraging him to take responsibility for his behavior and bolstering him in that effort.]</dd>

<dt>Marv:</dt>
<dd>Out there, it's a jungle . . . in here people seem nicer, but there is something that makes me suspicious. Yesterday when I was asking Hazel some questions, Sally said, "Stop badgering her." Now maybe you were kidding, but you used to have lunch with me, and you don't anymore.</dd>
</dl>

Therapist: So you're wondering what is going on?

Marv: I suppose.

[*Sally does not respond immediately, but as she sees members staring expectantly at her, she responds in a perfunctory tone.*]

Sally: I know you were trying to help and, in fact, I think you were doing a good job.

Gabe: But you did say, "Stop badgering her."

Sally: Well . . . maybe . . . I just wondered if you weren't coming across a little too strongly. After all, it was Hazel's first session.

Hazel: [*Giggles with embarrassment*] Don't worry about me, dear.

Therapist: It looks like we have a nice opportunity here because Marv wanted to get feedback on whether there was anything he was doing to alienate others in the group or make you feel less close to him. [*To Hazel*] Sally thought maybe Marv had scared you, but we really don't know unless you tell us how you felt toward Marv. And, Hazel, you did say that one of your goals was to be more open with the group members about your feelings, particularly, your negative feelings.

[*Here, the therapist is attempting to mesh the therapeutic needs of group members.*]

Hazel: Well, Marv asked me a lot of questions. I know he was just trying to be helpful . . . and he was . . . he was very helpful.

Gabe: But remember that you said last night that you had a headache when you left here.

Hazel: [*Giggles*] The session sort of left my head buzzing.

Therapist: Hazel, Marv is really eager to find out if there is something he did to make you feel that way.

Hazel: Nothing in particular.

Sally: Oh, come on, Hazel.

Hazel: Well, like I said . . . all the questions.

Sally: [*To Hazel*] But, Hazel, you're not saying how you reacted to his questions.

Hazel: I guess I felt a bit overwhelmed. I can't say I was annoyed at Marv. He was trying to help me, that's all.

Therapist: You said you felt overwhelmed by Marv's rapid-fire questioning. What would have been more helpful to you?

[Hazel had identified for Marv a behavior that induced in her a negative reaction. Here, the therapist is encouraging Hazel to identify a positive behavior in which Marv might engage both to assist his interpersonal experimentation within the group and to avoid the pain that might be attached to a more prolonged focus on negative behaviors.]

Hazel: I really don't know . . . well, I think I would feel more at ease if Marv would let me recover a little bit from one question before he asks me another one. Sometimes I need a time-out.

Marv: Now, why is that the first time that someone around here has said that to me?

Therapist: So let me just check out, Marv, what you think Hazel is asking of you. What change is Hazel asking you to make in how you help her?

[Having Marv paraphrase the feedback helps Marv to conceptualize it in terms coherent to him and provides him with additional opportunities to correct any misimpressions of what others are attempting to communicate to him.]

Marv: She says she would feel more comfortable if I would ask her something, let her answer, and maybe move onto someone else for awhile and then maybe get back to her later.

Sally: *[To Hazel]* Is that right?

Hazel: Pretty much. I didn't mean you could ask me only one question. It's just that as soon as I finish answering one, you have another one. You don't even act as though I answered the first question. It's just that as soon as I finish answering one, you have another one . . . it's like my husband . . . he always wants more than I can give him.

Therapist: *[To Hazel]* With Marv, you didn't realize that you can let him know when he's asking too much.

Hazel: I don't know if he'd accept it like Marv did.

Gabe: You might as well give it a try!

Therapist: *[To Marv]* So maybe it's not just the number of questions. Sounds that when Hazel gives you an answer to a question, she wants something more from you than another question.

Marv: That's cool. I didn't even realize I was shooting one question after another at her . . . like I'm the prosecuting attorney, and I have her on the stand. *[With an exaggerated voice of authority]* "Where were you the night he was shot?" *[laughs]*.

Hazel:	That's exactly how I felt—like I was on the stand!
Therapist:	Marv, you did something today that I haven't seen you do before. You took the lead in asking for feedback from another member, and then you really listened when it was given to you. I think that Hazel was able to put her finger on something that you can continue to work on even after you leave the hospital: recognizing when your own beliefs about what's best for another person get in the way of being sensitive to what that person actually needs. And Hazel, you, too, took an extraordinary step in clarifying for yourself what you need from Marv.
Sally:	Yea, Hazel. Way to go!
Therapist:	Another step was that you let Marv know about what you need and don't need from him.
	[This intervention was directed to support members' engagement in risk taking. Within this approach, the therapist necessarily takes a highly active role in establishing the norms of the group and educating patients on what constitutes work in the group.]
Therapist:	But there were other members, who, like Hazel, wanted to work on being more fully open with the group.
	[This intervention supports members' ability to learn vicariously.]

Comment on the Session

At the beginning of the session, members appear to be well socialized in the norms of a process-oriented group, as is seen in Marv's amenability to exploring parallels in the group with his problems within the program at large. Of course, in many cases, the therapist will be presented with the task of helping a patient like Marv to formulate what he expressed spontaneously. For example, had Marv merely indicated that he felt "crummy," it would have been incumbent on the therapist to shape this complaint into a concern that could be addressed directly within the group. The therapist might have wondered aloud whether something in either the program or the group provoked in Marv this unpleasant feeling.

After helping Marv create a meaningful here-and-now focus, the therapist's next intervention involved providing encouragement to Hazel to give feedback to Marv. This intervention was an effort to weave together the therapeutic needs of different members, in this case, Marv and Hazel. The therapist also underlined the value of direct communication among members by implying that only Hazel (not Sally) could accurately report on how Hazel reacted to Marv. When Hazel spoke in general terms about Marv's behavior toward her, the therapist helped her to articulate her perceptions in a more specific way. This greater specificity on Hazel's part was necessary for Marv to acknowledge particular behaviors that he could attempt to modify. Later, the therapist encouraged Hazel to reframe her response to Marv in positive rather than negative terms (a behavior that he could do rather than attempt not to do). The motive for this intervention was to assist Marv's interpersonal experimentation with the group and to protect him from the pain that might be attached to a more prolonged focus on negatively perceived behaviors.

Once Hazel and Marv had finished their exchange, the therapist reminded other members that some members among them had expressed having a difficulty in communicating openly that was similar to Hazel's. Through this intervention, the therapist facilitated members' further sharing and fostered a process of vicarious learning. This therapeutic factor (Yalom & Leszcz, 2005) is a mechanism that enhances the extent to which members can profit from participation in a group, including those in short-term or brief settings. If a member does not have an opportunity to address a particular problem within a given session, he or she can be helped by identifying with the work of a member who was more behaviorally active during that session. Although this process often occurs spontaneously, the therapist's invitation to members to identify with one another ensures and intensifies its occurrence.

STATUS OF THE RESEARCH

Research on the interpersonal approach specifically in IHPs, PHPs, and RTCs has accrued slowly. In those studies that have been conducted in the last few decades, ascertaining the effects of interpersonal group therapy has been difficult. Often, the interpersonal model is combined with another model or type of intervention. For example, Schramm et al. (2007) conducted a study on acute inpatients who were randomly assigned to pharmacologic treatment versus interpersonal group and individual therapy, and pharmacologic treatment alone. The group receiving the interpersonal therapy exhibited less depression at the end of treatment and at the 3-month and 12-month follow-up. Notably, they also exhibited higher levels of social functioning at both follow-ups, an important finding given that the interpersonal model targets interpersonal change. However, the contributions of group versus individual therapy could not be disentangled. The elimination of the effects due to medication is not so important given that a high percentage of inpatients are placed on medication, thereby giving the findings some ecological validity. Because this type of study is characteristic of what can be found in the literature, we lack information on the usefulness of this approach when it is applied in a nonhybrid or pure form.

Outcome Findings

The small group of IHP, PHP, or RTC studies that have been done on the interpersonal or interactional approach have generally supported its effectiveness. To identify this group of studies, we considered not merely how the authors identified the theoretical approach but also the way in which they described the group process. We culled those studies that emphasized interpersonal learning within the here and now and that compared the interpersonal/interactional format with some other group intervention.

Unstructured Interpersonal Approach

One of the earliest and methodologically strongest studies was Beutler et al.'s (1984) study of the interpersonal inpatient group pitted against emotional/expressive, behavioral, or no-group conditions. Participants were randomly assigned to conditions. Only the interpersonal group entailed the exploration of members' here-and-now experience with the goal of delineating each member's role within the group. The research team found that the interpersonal group exhibited the greatest degree of symptomatic change, and this change had sustained itself at a 13-month follow-up. The investigators also found that participants in the emotional/expressive group, which strongly emphasized the affective rather than cognitive aspects of experience, showed a worsening of symptoms. This finding supports Yalom's (1983) view of the importance of keeping cognitive and affective elements in balance in inpatient groups.

Coché, Cooper, and Petermann (1984) compared problem-solving group therapy with interactional group therapy over the course of an eight-session inpatient group. Although diagnostically heterogeneous, most members had some type of affective disorder diagnosis. The two forms of therapy were equivalent overall. However, problem-solving therapy was more helpful in alleviating subjective distress and the manifestations of thought disorder. Interactional therapy was more successful in raising members' levels of social adjustment. Overall, men gained more from problem-solving therapy, and women from interactional therapy.

Interactional Agenda Model

Pollack, Harvin, and Cramer (2000) compared self-management and interactional group psychotherapy with inpatients diagnosed with bipolar disorder. This study is important because the authors followed closely the format of Yalom's (1983) interactional agenda model. On average, individuals received four sessions of group psychotherapy, although some members were present for only a single session. Participants' symptomatic status was assessed at the beginning of group participation, before discharge, and 3 months after discharge. The interactional group exhibited significantly less symptomatic behavior and higher functioning relative to their pre-group assessment; the self-management group did not show this favorable pattern. The groups did not exhibit a change in coping resources across the three measurements. The investigators found that member satisfaction decreased for the interactional agenda group members from their assessment at discharge to that 3 months later but remained stable for the members of the self-management group.

Interpersonal Psychotherapy–Group

The original study on IPT-G entailed the comparison of IPT-G with group cognitive behavioral treatment for a group of women with bulimic eating disorder (BED; Wilfley et al., 1993). The participants were randomly assigned to IPT-G, group cognitive behavior therapy, or a wait list control group. The treatment groups lasted for 16 sessions. The investigators found that the two treatments effected a lessening of binge eating, unlike the wait list control group. As promising as these findings were, they were not as favorable as those of other studies at the 6-month and 1-year follow-up (Wilfley et al., 2000).

In a subsequent study, Wilfley et al. (2002) fine-tuned IPT-G, in part by adding several individual sessions. A randomized trial of IPT-G compared this treatment with group cognitive behavioral treatment for BED. Twenty 90-minute group sessions and three individual sessions took place. Both treatments were successful in decreasing the number of binge days for participants during treatments, and relative to pretreatment levels, binge eating continued to be less at the 1-year follow-up. Improvements in psychosocial functioning were also observed in both conditions, and gains in this area continued to be made posttreatment. The treatments appeared to be comparably effective in addressing BED, with the one exception that the cognitive behavioral group produced a more rapid acquisition of dietary restraint.

A pilot study (Schaal, Elbert, & Neuner, 2009) seeking to assess the utility of IPT with children compared IPT-G with narrative exposure therapy (NET) in a group of Rwandan genocide orphans, all of whom lived in orphanages or child-headed houses. Both interventions were designed to assist participants with alleviation of grief-based reactions. Whereas the IPT was delivered in group sessions, the NET entailed individual sessions involving the recounting of traumatic experiences. Both interventions produced a reduction in depressive symptoms, guilt cognitions, and posttraumatic stress disorder symptoms at the end of treatment and at a 6-month follow-up. However, at the 6-month follow-up, those receiving NET were considerably improved over the IPT-G participants. The fact that a modality difference existed alongside a model difference creates ambiguity in the interpretation of the results.

In a larger randomized trial, IPT-G was compared with creative playgroups and a wait list control group in its usefulness to depressed youths (ages 14–17) in internally displaced persons camps in Northern Uganda. Participants identified all four areas of IPT as relevant to them. For example, social deficiencies were associated with having spent much of their young lives in the bush and having developed few linguistic skills to communicate with others. All three groups showed a reduction in depression scores, but IPT-G participation produced a greater reduction. Neither treatment led to a reduction in anxiety symptoms or conduct problems or a gain in functioning. Although neither of these studies took place in IHP, PHP, or RTC settings, they did involve treatment of individuals living in a collective situation.

Therapeutic Factors

The greatest concentration of studies on the interpersonal approach has been on the mechanisms of change in group therapy, or therapeutic factors. Corsini and Rosenberg (1955) initially devised this system, which Yalom (1970), who developed a system of 12 factors, later refined. Therapeutic factor research can in one respect address the usefulness of the interpersonal model. One of the goals of this model is to develop members' awareness of the importance of interpersonal exploration. The presumption is that members recognizing the usefulness of the kinds of therapeutic processes that emerge in an interpersonally oriented group will increase the likelihood of their continuing such an involvement on an outpatient basis. Of course, this latter expectation would have to be tested separately. However, at least while the patient is in the IHP, PHP, or RTC, therapeutic factor research can provide information on whether terminating members see factors that are more interpersonally oriented (e.g., learning from interpersonal actions) as being more integral to their progress than individually oriented factors (e.g., self-understanding).

Most studies on inpatient groups have suggested that members do value interpersonal factors. Across various types of interpersonal inpatient groups from structured (Leszcz, Yalom, & Norden, 1985; Mushet, Whalan, & Power, 1989) to relatively unstructured (Brabender, Albrecht, Sillitti, Cooper, & Kramer, 1983), certain therapeutic factors emerge as relatively important to members. These include interpersonal learning, vicarious learning, and universality. These factors all pertain to the relationships between or among members. However, research findings are not wholly consistent. De Chávez, Gutierrez, Ducaju, and Fraile (2000) conducted a study comparing schizophrenic inpatients and outpatients. For the inpatients, the most important factors were instillation of hope, self-understanding, and universality. Of course, this study would benefit from replication, but in the meantime, the findings point to level of functioning as a potentially relevant variable. Perhaps the capacity to see interpersonal factors as having greater worth than others requires a certain level of ego functioning.

Sayin et al. (2008) investigated the ratings of therapeutic factors of 60 Turkish/Muslim inpatients at the time of discharge. These patients rated the existential factor (referring to the affirmation of the realities of the human condition such as personal responsibility and death), hope, and self-understanding as most key to their progress in an interpersonal group. The authors noted that the finding is curious in that the culture itself is collectivist and the factors the clients endorsed were individualistic. Group psychotherapy might stand to make its biggest contribution when it operates outside the client's paradigm. In any case, the study points to the limits of the generalizability of findings from one culture to another and, hence, the need for cross-cultural research.

DEMANDS OF THE MODEL

Clinical Mission

The interpersonal approach requires a relatively high level of support from the unit or program staff. For any particular version of the interpersonal model to be effective, the members of the treatment team must embrace its goals and understand the methods by which it enables their achievement. This support is seen to be essential for several reasons. First, the boundary separating the interpersonal group from the unit is a fluid one. Interactions with members and other staff outside the group may be brought within the group and vice versa. To avoid undermining such explorations, staff must see the value in them. Second, the members of the group might be given interpersonal homework assignments that include staff members. Third, in the case of the agenda group, members of the treatment team could observe the group; if so, they must have a willingness to assume an active role during the review phase of the session. Although the interpersonal approach requires staff support, it does not demand staff members' detailed technical knowledge about the workings of the model.

Temporal Variables

The interpersonal approach is extremely flexible regarding the time frame it can accommodate. Some versions have been designed for a group lasting only a single session, such as the interactional agenda group and the focus group (Yalom, 1983), and others for groups with a stable membership over far longer periods, such as the IPT-G. For example, Griffin-Shelley and Wendel (1988) described an inpatient interpersonal group in which members remained in the group for 5 to 6 months. The frequency of the meeting is also not a limiting factor. Yalom believed that the group should meet as frequently as possible, preferably daily. Yet, less frequent meetings do not preclude the use of the interpersonal model. A short-term interpersonal inpatient group meeting only twice weekly produced positive symptomatic changes, which were maintained 13 months later (Beutler et al., 1984).

A temporal factor that is likely to be more constraining is the length of the session, particularly for the structured models. The agenda model requires that each member develop an agenda. In an average-sized group (6–10 patients), a session of at least 75 to 90 minutes is necessary to accommodate this requirement. As Froberg and Slife (1987) noted, some settings are not able to guarantee a session of this length because of scheduling conflicts with other activities. Having members take turns in crafting agendas from session to session is a potential modification of this model. Alternatively, the different stages of the model could be spread over successive sessions (Taylor, Coombes, & Bartlett, 2002).

IPT-G requires a close-ended structure wherein members begin and end the group together. It also requires a sufficient number of sessions so that the group proceeds to the work phase of development. Twelve to 15 sessions are characteristic of this format. However, Wilfley et al. (2000) indicated that the model could be adapted to a shorter term time frame in an open membership format. It would require limiting the number of problems members could address and placing greater weight on vicarious learning. That is, while the therapists worked with a given member, other members could observe the process and derive benefit from it. This modification could make this model appropriate for IHPs and PHPs with brief lengths of stay.

Size of the Group

The agenda model has a low ceiling on the number of members it can accommodate. If the group were to go beyond 10 members, even in a 90-minute session, the therapist might find it impossible to proceed through all the designated stages of the group. In fact, even 10 might be too many, and eight is likely to be a more comfortable number. However, a small number of members (e.g., three) does not preclude the model's use (Yalom, 1983). The less-structured versions of the interpersonal approach enable the inclusion of a larger number of members. However, any version requires that all members participate in active ways (e.g., giving feedback) such that the therapist must exercise good judgment on what the maximum number should be.

Composition of the Group

Unstructured applications of the interpersonal approach have been developed for depressed patients (Coché, Cooper, & Petermann, 1984), chronic regressed patients (Beard & Scott, 1975), diagnostically mixed patients (Beutler et al., 1984; Garrick & Ewashen, 2001), patients with schizophrenia (Kanas, 1991; Yehoshua, Kellermann, Calev, & Dasberg, 1985), and individuals with borderline personality disorder (Marziali & Munroe-Blum, 1994), alexithymia (Spitzer, Siebel-Jürges, Barnow, Grabe, & Freyberger, 2005), and extreme levels of perfectionism (Hewitt et al., 2015). Delmonico, Hanley-Peterson, and Englander (1998) developed a version of the interpersonal approach for persons with traumatic brain injury who experience frustration and substance abuse. Beutler et al. (1984) found that the efficacy of an interpersonal approach is not dependent on diagnostic category or degree of psychological disturbance. In general, then, it appears that the unstructured version of the interpersonal approach is somewhat protean in its ability to accommodate different types of patients.

The agenda and focus group versions are more stringent in their composition requirements. Probably the most fundamental requirement is that potential group members be subdivided according to level of functioning. Some settings (e.g., a psychiatric unit of a general hospital) may have so few patients that a critical mass at the level of functioning suitable for either the agenda or focus group model is not present. The agenda and focus group versions of the interpersonal model seem to be effective when members have a wide range of diagnoses and symptom patterns. Particularly for the agenda group, diversity in symptoms might be useful.

Even more important than diagnostic or symptomatic variability is diversity in the interpersonal styles present in the group. Such diversity facilitates the interlocking of members' stated or unstated agendas that is so vital for efficient work within all groups but especially those with a limited time frame. In the clinical vignette presented earlier, Marv, who was working on asking questions in a more sensitive way, could be encouraged to interact with Sally, the surrogate staff member, who wanted to be more receptive to others' helping efforts. Most applications of the interpersonal model have been with adult patients, although some attempts have been made to use the agenda model in the treatment of adolescents. We suspect that an adolescent population, in particular, would find the agenda model to be appealing given that the process of peer validation is very much alive with this age group. From their review of the empirical literature, Burlingame, McClendon, and Alonso (2011) concluded that across theoretical orientations, a focus on member-to-member interaction, emphasized by the interpersonal approach, leads to increases in cohesion. Further, adolescent and young adult populations show especially large gains in outcome when cohesion is present. In a geriatric population, a sense of isolation is an extremely common problem to which group psychotherapy can be an antidote (Husaini et al., 2004). Inpatients with organic brain syndromes might be especially helped by the format of the focus group. The systematic review, held at the end of the session, is specifically designed to reduce confusion. Hence, the interpersonal approach appears to have sufficient flexibility to accommodate all age groups from adolescence onward.

Cultural diversity is likely to be of benefit to all applications of the interpersonal approach in two important respects. First, it makes the group a better microcosm. Members are likely to encounter others with a range of cultural identities in their world outside the group. Interactions within the group ready them for this eventuality. Second, individuals from different cultural backgrounds provide different perspectives on others' social behaviors. For example, whereas individuals from more individualistic cultures might emphasize the extent to which a person's communications convey that person's views, persons from collectivistic cultures might recognize when an individual's actions in the group evoke discomfort in other group members.

IPT-G has been used primarily with members who share particular psychological problems, particularly eating disorders and depression. This homogeneity supports the group's rapid development of cohesion. Nonetheless, the workings of the group would not seem to preclude diagnostic heterogeneity among group members.

Therapist Variables

All versions of the interpersonal model require that the therapist be skilled in helping members to relate to one another. This competency is unique to group psychotherapy and requires an investment in training and supervised practice. It entails helping the group to focus on and explore the here and now and to be attuned to process rather than content. The therapist must have a comfort with self-disclosure alongside an awareness of what self-disclosures will benefit the group.

The interpersonal group can be led either by a cotherapy team or by a single therapist. Cotherapy can be useful in enabling the therapists to perform competently the many tasks associated with the agenda group. In the focus group model, cotherapy may be helpful in monitoring individual members' anxiety levels to ensure that each member experiences the group as supportive rather than threatening or disorganizing. When the group is designed as a single session, sessions can be held with alternate therapists, which allows for greater staffing flexibility, and to be held on weekends, when IHPs and RTCs have few active treatments.

The inclusion of staff and students into the treatment model and therapist level of disclosure and the interactional approach supported by this model is an especially good choice for diverse cultural groups who value an initial personal and relational approach to the therapeutic work (Aguilera, Bruehlman-Senecal, Liu, & Bravin, 2018) and respect for the collective wisdom of the group (*simpatia*).

SUMMARY

The interpersonal orientation has led to the development of a set of approaches that embraces the Sullivanian position that psychological problems are, in essence, problems in relationships. To further the well-being of the individual, it is necessary to alter, in a positive direction, an individual's way of relating to others. In psychotherapy, such alteration can most readily be achieved, so the interpersonal approach holds if the individual works on his or her immediate experiences with others.

Existing versions of the interpersonal model differ from one another in the degree of structure. Before the 1980s, those inpatient group psychotherapists who applied the interpersonal orientation to their group work did so in a fairly loose fashion. Although these practitioners emphasized the interpersonal domain within the here-and-now context of the group, they did not use a highly structured session. Today, those IHP, PHP, and RTC settings with these same time frames permit a less-structured application of the interpersonal approach. However, the short-term time frames of many PHP, RTC, and most IHP groups require a higher level of structure. To satisfy this need, Yalom (1983) devised two formats for interpersonally oriented groups, each of which is characterized by a high level of structure, particularly concerning the format of the session. The agenda group for high-functioning inpatients is designed to foster a positive attitude toward therapy, to enable members to appreciate that engaging in exchanges with other members is beneficial to their well-being, to isolate problems that might be addressed in long-term therapy, and to relieve that anxiety generated by the treatment situation itself. The focus group, designed for low-functioning inpatients, embraces the need to help members socialize in a nonthreatening way and to bolster their orientation to reality. Group psychotherapists (e.g., Hajek, 2010; Taylor et al., 2002) have modified particular features to accommodate the demands of their treatment contexts. The IPT-G model was developed out of the individual IPT approach to depression. IPT-G treatment entails a close-ended group preceded by a careful assessment and preparation and focuses on four types of interpersonal problems: grief, interpersonal role disputes, role transitions, or interpersonal deficits. The close-ended aspect of the group requires the therapist's attendance to, and therapeutic use of, group developmental issues. Individual therapy sessions run along IPT lines often accompany the group treatment. These groups have usually been run with diagnostically homogeneous members.

We said over 20 years ago that "the outcome data on the interpersonal model are rather thin" (Brabender & Fallon, 1993, p. 171). Despite the accrual of data on many other models, the empirical evaluation of the interpersonal model languishes. Still, what studies have been published support the effectiveness of the structured and unstructured application of the interpersonal approach.

REFERENCES

Aguilera, A., Bruehlman-Senecal, E., Liu, N., & Bravin, J. (2018). Implementing group CBT for depression among Latinos in a primary care clinic. *Cognitive and Behavioral Practice, 25*, 135–144. http://dx.doi.org/10.1016/j.cbpra.2017.03.002

Alden, L. E., Wiggins, J. S., & Pincus, A. L. (1990). Construction of circumplex scales for the Inventory of Interpersonal Problems. *Journal of Personality Assessment, 55*, 521–536. http://dx.doi.org/10.1080/00223891.1990.9674088

Beard, M. T., & Scott, P. Y. (1975). The efficacy of group therapy by nurses for hospitalized patients. *Nursing Research, 24*, 120–124. http://dx.doi.org/10.1097/00006199-197503000-00010

Bellack, A. S., Turner, S. M., Hersen, M., & Luber, R. F. (1984). An examination of the efficacy of social skills training for chronic schizophrenic patients. *Psychiatric Services, 35*, 1023–1028. http://dx.doi.org/10.1176/ps.35.10.1023

Benne, K. D. (1964). From polarization to paradox. In L. P. Bradford, J. R. Gibb, & K. D. Benne (Eds.), *T-Group theory and laboratory method: Innovation in re-education* (pp. 216–247). New York, NY: Wiley.

Beutler, L. E., Frank, M., Schieber, S. C., Calvert, S., & Gaines, J. (1984). Comparative effects of group psychotherapies in a short-term inpatient setting: An experience with deterioration effects. *Psychiatry, 47*, 66–76. http://dx.doi.org/10.1080/00332747.1984.11024227

Brabender, V., Albrecht, E., Sillitti, J., Cooper, J., & Kramer, E. (1983). A study of curative factors in short-term group psychotherapy. *Hospital & Community Psychiatry, 34*, 643–644.

Brabender, V., & Fallon, A. (1993). *Models of inpatient group psychotherapy.* Washington, DC: American Psychological Association. http://dx.doi.org/10.1037/10121-000

Bryant, J., Kelly, V., & Zegarra, A. (2010). Developing and delivering a psychotherapeutic group on an acute psychiatric ward. *PSIGE Newsletter, 11*, 32–37. Retrieved from http://www.psige.org/public/files/newsletters/PSIGE_111_web.pdf

Burlingame, G. M., McClendon, D. T., & Alonso, J. (2011). Cohesion in group therapy. In J. C. Norcross (Ed.), *Psychotherapy relationships that work: Evidence-*

based therapy relationships (pp. 11–12). New York, NY: Oxford. http://dx.doi.org/10.1093/acprof:oso/9780199737208.003.0005

Coché, E., Cooper, J. B., & Petermann, K. J. (1984). Differential outcomes of cognitive and interactional group therapies. *Small Group Research, 15*, 497–509. http://dx.doi.org/10.1177/104649648401500404

Corsini, R. J., & Rosenberg, B. (1955). Mechanisms of group psychotherapy: Processes and dynamics. *The Journal of Abnormal and Social Psychology, 51*, 406–411. http://dx.doi.org/10.1037/h0048439

De Chávez, M. G., Gutierrez, M., Ducaju, M., & Fraile, J. C. (2000). Comparative study of the therapeutic factors of group therapy in schizophrenic inpatients and outpatients. *Group Analysis, 33*, 251–264. http://dx.doi.org/10.1177/0533316400332006

Delmonico, R. L., Hanley-Peterson, P., & Englander, J. (1998). Group psychotherapy for persons with traumatic brain injury: Management of frustration and substance abuse. *The Journal of Head Trauma Rehabilitation, 13*, 10–22. http://dx.doi.org/10.1097/00001199-199812000-00004

Ferencik, B. M. (1989). Cognitive and affective patterns of alcoholics: Implications for group therapy. *Group, 13*, 31–41. http://dx.doi.org/10.1007/BF01456550

Frank, J. D. (1963). Group therapy in the mental hospital. In M. Rosenbaum & M. Berger (Eds.), *Group psychotherapy and group functions* (pp. 453–468). New York, NY: Basic Books.

Froberg, W., & Slife, B. D. (1987). Overcoming obstacles to the implementation of Yalom's model of inpatient group psychotherapy. *International Journal of Group Psychotherapy, 37*, 371–388. http://dx.doi.org/10.1080/00207284.1987.11491056

Garrick, D., & Ewashen, C. (2001). An integrated model for adolescent inpatient group therapy. *Journal of Psychiatric and Mental Health Nursing, 8*, 165–171. http://dx.doi.org/10.1046/j.1365-2850.2001.00374.x

Griffin-Shelley, E., & Wendel, S. (1988). Group psychotherapy with long-term inpatients: Application of a model. *Small Group Behavior, 19*, 379–385. http://dx.doi.org/10.1177/104649648801900306

Hajek, K. (2010). Interpersonal group therapy on an acute inpatient ward based on Yalom's model. In J. Radcliffe, K. Hajek, J. Carson, & O. Manor (Eds.), *Psychological groupwork with acute psychiatric inpatients* (pp. 156–174). London, England: Whiting & Birch.

Heitler, J. B. (1974). Clinical impressions of an experimental attempt to prepare lower-class patients for expressive group psychotherapy. *International Journal of Group Psychotherapy, 24*, 308–322. http://dx.doi.org/10.1080/00207284.1974.11491833

Hewitt, P. L., Mikail, S. F., Flett, G. L., Tasca, G. A., Flynn, C. A., Deng, X., . . . Chen, C. (2015). Psychodynamic/interpersonal group psychotherapy for perfectionism: Evaluating the effectiveness of a short-term treatment. *Psychotherapy, 52*, 205–217.

Houlihan, J. P. (1977). Contribution of an intake group to psychiatric inpatient milieu therapy. *International Journal of Group Psychotherapy, 27*, 215–223. http://dx.doi.org/10.1080/00207284.1977.11492294

Husaini, B. A., Cummings, S., Kilbourne, B., Roback, H., Sherkat, D., Levine, R., & Cain, V. A. (2004). Group therapy for depressed elderly women. *International Journal of Group Psychotherapy, 54*, 295–319.

Kanas, N. (1991). Group therapy with schizophrenic patients: A short-term, homogeneous approach. *International Journal of Group Psychotherapy, 41*, 33–48. http://dx.doi.org/10.1080/00207284.1991.11490631

Kiesler, D. J. (1996). *Contemporary interpersonal theory and research.* New York, NY: Wiley.

Kleiger, J. H., & Helmig, L. (1999). Evolution of a group therapy model for adolescent residential treatment. *Journal of Child and Adolescent Group Therapy, 9*, 187–197.

Klerman, G. L., Weissman, M. M., Rounsaville, B. J., & Chevron, E. S. (1984). *Interpersonal psychotherapy of depression.* New York, NY: Basic Books.

Leopold, H. S. (1976). Selective group approaches with psychotic patients in hospital settings. *American Journal of Psychotherapy, 30*, 95–102.

Leszcz, M. (1986). Interactional group psychotherapy with nonpsychotic inpatients. *Group, 10*, 13–20. http://dx.doi.org/10.1007/BF01469737

Leszcz, M. (2008). The interpersonal approach to group psychotherapy. In G. M. Saiger, S. Rubenfeld, & M. D. Dluhy (Eds.), *Windows into today's group psychotherapy* (pp. 129–149). New York, NY: Routledge.

Leszcz, M., & Malat, J. (2012). The interpersonal model of group psychotherapy. In J. L. Kleinberg (Ed.), *The Wiley Blackwell handbook of group psychotherapy* (pp. 33–58). New York, NY: Wiley.

Leszcz, M., Yalom, I. D., & Norden, M. (1985). The value of inpatient group psychotherapy: Patients' perceptions. *International Journal of Group Psychotherapy, 35*, 411–433. http://dx.doi.org/10.1080/00207284.1985.11491425

MacKenzie, K. R. (1997). *Time-managed group psychotherapy: Effective clinical applications.* Washington, DC: American Psychiatric Association.

MacKenzie, K. R., & Grabovac, A. D. (2001). Interpersonal psychotherapy group (IPT-G) for depression. *Journal of Psychotherapy Practice & Research, 10*, 46–51.

Marziali, E., & Munroe-Blum, H. (1994). *Interpersonal group psychotherapy for borderline personality disorder.* New York, NY: Basic Books.

Moreno, J. L. (1934). *Who shall survive? A new approach to the problem of human interrelations.* Washington, DC: Nervous and Mental Disease Publishing.

Mushet, G. L., Whalan, G. S., & Power, R. (1989). In-patients' views of the helpful aspects of group psychotherapy: Impact of therapeutic style and treatment setting. *British Journal of Medical Psychology, 62*, 135–141. http://dx.doi.org/10.1111/j.2044-8341.1989.tb02820.x

Oldham, J. M. (1982). The use of silent observers as an adjunct to short-term inpatient group psychotherapy. *International Journal of Group Psychotherapy, 32,* 469–480. http://dx.doi.org/10.1080/00207284.1982.11492365

Pollack, L. E., Harvin, S., & Cramer, R. D. (2000). Coping resources of African-American and white patients hospitalized for bipolar disorder. *Psychiatric Services, 51,* 1310–1312. http://dx.doi.org/10.1176/appi.ps.51.10.1310

Prochaska, J. O., & Norcross, J. C. (2001). Stages of change. *Psychotherapy: Theory, Research, Practice, Training, 38,* 443–448. http://dx.doi.org/10.1037/0033-3204.38.4.443

Sayin, A., Karslioglu, E. H., Sürgit, A., Sahin, S., Arslan, T., & Candansayar, S. (2008). Brief report: Perceptions of Turkish psychiatric inpatients about therapeutic factors of group psychotherapy. *International Journal of Group Psychotherapy, 58,* 253–263. http://dx.doi.org/10.1521/ijgp.2008.58.2.253

Schaal, S., Elbert, T., & Neuner, F. (2009). Narrative exposure therapy versus interpersonal psychotherapy. *Psychotherapy and psychosomatics, 78,* 298–306. http://dx.doi.org/10.1159/000229768

Schramm, E., van Calker, D., Dykierek, P., Lieb, K., Kech, S., Zobel, I., . . . Berger, M. (2007). An intensive treatment program of interpersonal psychotherapy plus pharmacotherapy for depressed inpatients: Acute and long-term results. *American Journal of Psychiatry, 164,* 768–777.

Spitzer, C., Siebel-Jürges, U., Barnow, S., Grabe, H. J., & Freyberger, H. J. (2005). Alexithymia and interpersonal problems. *Psychotherapy and Psychosomatics, 74,* 240–246. http://dx.doi.org/10.1159/000085148

Sullivan, H. S. (1940). *Conceptions of modern psychiatry.* New York, NY: Norton.

Sullivan, H. S. (1953). *The interpersonal theory of psychiatry.* New York, NY: Norton.

Swartz, H. A. (1999). Interpersonal psychotherapy. In M. Hersen & A. S. Bellak (Eds.), *Handbook of comparative interventions for adult disorders* (pp. 139–155). New York, NY: Wiley.

Taylor, R., Coombes, L., & Bartlett, H. (2002). The impact of a practice development project on the quality of in-patient small group therapy. *Journal of Psychiatric and Mental Health Nursing, 9,* 213–220. http://dx.doi.org/10.1046/j.1365-2850.2002.00478.x

Vinogradov, S., & Yalom, I. D. (1989). *Concise guide to group psychotherapy.* Washington, DC: American Psychiatric Association.

Weissman, M. M., & Bothwell, S. (1976). Assessment of social adjustment by patient self-report. *Archives of General Psychiatry, 33,* 1111–1115. http://dx.doi.org/10.1001/archpsyc.1976.01770090101010

Wilfley, D. E., Agras, W. S., Telch, C. F., Rossiter, E. M., Schneider, J. A., Cole, A. G., . . . Raeburn, S. D. (1993). Group cognitive-behavioral therapy and group interpersonal psychotherapy for the nonpurging bulimic individual: A controlled comparison. *Journal of Consulting and Clinical Psychology, 61,* 296–305. http://dx.doi.org/10.1037/0022-006X.61.2.296

Wilfley, D. E., Frank, M. A., Welch, R., Spurrell, E. B., & Rounsaville, B. J. (1998). Adapting interpersonal psychotherapy to a group format (IPT-G) for binge eating disorder: Toward a model for adapting empirically supported treatments. *Psychotherapy Research, 8,* 379–391. http://dx.doi.org/10.1080/10503309812331332477

Wilfley, D. E., MacKenzie, K. R., Welch, R. R., Ayes, V. E., & Weissman, M. M. (2000). *Interpersonal psychotherapy for group.* New York, NY: Basic Books.

Wilfley, D. E., Stein, R., & Welch, R. (2005). Interpersonal psychotherapy. In J. Treasure, U. Schmidt, & E. van Furth (Eds.), *The essential handbook of eating disorders* (pp. 137–154). West Sussex, England: Wiley.

Wilfley, D. E., Welch, R. R., Stein, R. I., Spurrell, E. B., Cohen, L. R., Saelens, B. E., . . . Matt, G. E. (2002). A randomized comparison of group cognitive-behavioral therapy and group interpersonal psychotherapy for the treatment of overweight individuals with binge-eating disorder. *Archives of General Psychiatry, 59,* 713–721. http://dx.doi.org/10.1001/archpsyc.59.8.713

Yalom, I. (1970). *The theory and practice of group therapy.* New York, NY: Basic Books.

Yalom, I. (1983). *Inpatient group psychotherapy.* New York, NY: Basic Books.

Yalom, I. (1985). *The theory and practice of group psychotherapy* (3rd ed.). New York, NY: Basic Books.

Yalom, I., & Leszcz, M. (2005). *The theory and practice of group psychotherapy* (5th ed.). New York, NY: Basic Books.

Yehoshua, R., Kellermann, P. F., Calev, A., & Dasberg, H. (1985). Group psychotherapy with inpatient chronic schizophrenics. *Israel Journal of Psychiatry and Related Sciences, 22,* 185–190.

4

PSYCHODYNAMIC FAMILY OF MODELS

Psychodynamic psychotherapy group approaches have a long history of application to inpatient settings. In fact, some of the major psychodynamic concepts in relation to group psychotherapy at large were derived from observations of inpatient groups. During World War II, military personnel experiencing symptoms associated with trauma (called, at that time, *battle fatigue*) received group psychotherapy as an efficient mode of treatment during psychiatric hospitalization (Brabender, Fallon, & Smolar, 2004). Seminal thinkers such as Wilfred Bion (1959) identified phenomena such as the basic assumption and work groups that have informed major contemporary approaches.

This chapter attempts to capture some of the richness of psychodynamic approaches designed for the three types of settings by presenting three different models, followed by their integration in a case illustration toward the end of the chapter: the basic model, the object relations/systems (OR/S) model, and the mentalization model. First, we begin with core principles that are common to the psychodynamic approaches.

http://dx.doi.org/10.1037/0000113-005
Group Psychotherapy in Inpatient, Partial Hospital, and Residential Care Settings, by V. Brabender and A. Fallon

CENTRAL CONCEPTS

Central to all applications of psychodynamic psychotherapy—group and individual, inpatient, and outpatient—are the concepts of psychic determinism and the dynamic unconscious. In relation to the concept of psychic determinism, Sigmund Freud (1914/1965) posited that all experiences and behaviors, no matter how seemingly trivial or random, serve at least one of the twin goals of any human being, which are to pursue pleasure and avoid pain. To appreciate why we often are unable to see the purposes underlying our experiences and behaviors, it is necessary to recognize that only part of what resides within the self is accessible to the person. Many emotions, thoughts, urges, and fantasies are outside awareness—that is, unconscious. Moreover, these elements have a role in shaping experiences and behaviors, as do conscious elements. The *dynamic* aspect of the unconscious refers to the fact that various elements, conscious and unconscious, can come into conflict with one another. For example, unconsciously, an individual might have the urge to express aggression, yet this urge might be objectionable to the person's conscious self. Conflict between elements creates tension, the alleviation of which comes through various means. One of these means is the use of a defense mechanism by which the individual denies the direct and full expression of one of these elements. Defense mechanisms can be adaptive or maladaptive. Individuals with particular personality styles and types of psychopathology will be likely to emphasize certain defense mechanisms over others (Horowitz, 1974/1996).

Associated with these central concepts of psychodynamic psychotherapy are seven characteristic elements that Blagys and Hilsenroth (2000) identified by examining the process and technique of group psychodynamic and cognitive behavior therapies, as described in studies comparing manualized applications. We consider here each of these elements and briefly discuss its ramifications for psychodynamic inpatient group psychotherapy. The first two principles concern feelings, with the first notion being that psychodynamic psychotherapy, including group applications, supports the awareness and expression of emotions and affects. In group psychotherapy, the awareness of feeling that is cultivated is not only of one's own but also that of other members of the group. The second principle is that psychodynamic psychotherapy helps members recognize those defenses they erect against the awareness and expression of feelings. These first two principles go hand in hand because, without reckoning with the defenses, it may be difficult or impossible to become aware of the feelings. Although relative to other therapies, the psychodynamic approach places emphasis on emotions, cognitions are also the object of exploration. For example, early on in the life of the group, a member might think, "If I express hostility toward the therapist, she may retaliate." This content has both an affective component (probably fear) and also a cognitive component (the belief about the likely relationship between the member's and therapist's actions).

Principle 3 involves recognizing and exploring recurring themes. In psychodynamic group psychotherapy relative to individual treatment, this thematic focus typically pertains to those ideas or concerns that emerge across members. In some cases, the theme results from each member's being affected by other members' communications. As each member speaks, others consciously or unconsciously ask themselves what they might identify with in another member's expression. From a series of communications with each member identifying with others, a theme emerges. However, themes also result from members' reactivity to common developmental issues. As noted in Chapter 2, a group proceeds through stages of development. During a given stage, members are faced with a common set of conflicts, the expression of which will have a thematic character. Finally, in inpatient hospital program (IHP), partial hospital program (PHP), or residential treatment center (RTC) groups, members' issues are stimulated by events occurring in the broader treatment environment. For example, the loss of a popular staff member might lead to the emergence of a theme of abandonment.

Principles 4, 5, and 6 are best considered together in their application to group psychotherapy. Principle 4 concerns the relevance of early experiences to the patient's current difficulties. In fact, these early experiences account for the thematic elements described in Principle 3. Principle 5 refers to psychodynamic psychotherapy's focus on interpersonal relations. In group psychotherapy, the relationships within the room are a primary focus. Indeed, seeing what issues and difficulties arise among members allows for a reckoning with early life problems without discussing them directly. As was discussed for the interpersonal approach (Yalom & Leszcz, 2005), the there and then comes alive in the here and now. Principle 6 speaks to the importance of the therapeutic relationship. In group psychotherapy, not only is rapport and trust crucial in terms of each member's relationship with the therapist, but members' relationship with the therapist is also a valuable area of exploration. For example, it is not uncommon for members to feel disappointed in the therapist and his or her limitations. This reaction provides a springboard for examining feelings of dependency on authority figures. The reactions of members are not restricted to the other members or the therapist. At times, one or more members may have a response to the group as a whole (Kauff, 2012), as when, for example, members declare that they can be understood only in the present group and nowhere else.

Principle 6 recognizes the usefulness of exploring the patient's fantasies and longings, a process that can be achieved only if the patient has sufficient leeway in the session to be able to speak freely. Often, to fully understand affects (Principle 1), it is necessary to recognize the wishes to which they are attached. For example, patients might feel disappointment in the therapist because of a wish that the therapist will meet their every need. Yet, if the session is so highly structured that members are given little space to talk about their feelings toward the therapist, such a connection is unlikely to be made. Therefore, as in psychodynamic individual therapy, in psychodynamic group therapy, even with structure, group members are given the opportunity to speak spontaneously, to say what comes to mind. This flow of associations among members is termed the group process and is akin to free association in individual psychodynamic psychotherapy (Kauff, 2012).

A variety of group formats have been developed for IHPs, PHPs, and RTCs that adhere to the core principles we outlined. Existing models differ from one another in a range of respects, including the degree of structure of the session and the specificity of focus.

BASIC MODEL

This model is termed *basic* because it has a generic character. It incorporates the lowest degree of session structure, thereby providing the greatest latitude for the emergence of the members' associations and the most general guidelines for the therapist's mode of intervention within the group. This latter feature accords the group the potential to be maximally responsive to members' individual needs. At the same time, it may hinder the group from pursuing any one particular goal with maximum efficiency. Our presentation of the basic model draws from Rice and Rutan (1987), Radcliffe and Diamond (2007), and others. However, the term *basic* is ours, and we use it primarily to distinguish it from the other models we present in this chapter.

Goals of Treatment

From the outset of treatment, individuals harbor feelings that are unacceptable to them. Being unwanted and often unrecognized, these feelings possess the power to hinder the individual's functioning and induce suffering. The goal of treatment is to enable the group member to acknowledge them fully and accept them. This broad goal necessitates the pursuit of other more specific goals. Those defenses by which the individuals spare themselves the full realization of feelings must be relaxed, a goal often achieved through their identification. The recognition of other intrapsychic elements, such as wishes and cognitions, associated with particular emotions also support the overarching goal of increased emotional awareness and tolerance. For example, a member may discover a long-held belief that the expression of anger leads to rejection by others. An additional goal is for members to learn about the interpersonal effects of their emotions and impulses, as well as the mechanisms that members use to defend against the emotions, wishes, and impulses (Radcliffe & Diamond, 2007).

For example, an individual might discover that he listens with minimal attentiveness to other members speak because he is afraid of what they might evoke in him. Members misconstrue his spotty attentiveness as mere indifference, a perception that evokes frustration and irritation. This individual can come to appreciate that his effort to limit his self-awareness has a negative social consequence. This goal of learning the effects of one's behaviors on others is not the exclusive province of the psychodynamic model. In fact, it is central to the interpersonal approach described in Chapter 3. The difference is one of emphasis. Whereas the psychodynamic approach places stress on the member's gaining access to those intrapsychic elements that are linked, directly or indirectly, to maladaptive social behaviors, the interpersonal approach places a more pronounced and sustained focus on the latter. However, because of the overlap in goals, the two models are highly compatible and lend themselves to integration with one another (e.g., Callahan, Price, & Hilsenroth, 2004; Wells, Glickauf-Hughes, & Buzzell, 1990).

Intervention Style

Several features characterize the activity of the psychodynamic group psychotherapist: building a growth-fostering group, establishing a contract consistent with the goals of a psychodynamic group, intervening at multiple levels, conceptualizing group process developmentally, and monitoring his or her reactions.

Boundary Setting and Maintenance

A primary function of the therapist is to create an environment conducive to the group's accomplishing its goals. Prominent among the tasks the therapist performs is to establish consistent, predictable group boundaries, the presence of which creates a sense of safety (Rice & Rutan, 1987). Although boundary maintenance is important for most inpatient groups, it is particularly essential to the success of a psychodynamic group because the emergence of a spontaneous group process requires that members feel reasonably safe. For many inpatients, the prospect of being in a group psychotherapy session is anxiety arousing. However, when the prospective member can rely on the experience unfolding in a particular way, anxiety is lessened. Among the boundaries that are particularly salient to members are those concerning time, place, and membership. Temporal boundaries pertain to the therapist's efforts to begin and end the group at the agreed-on time, a challenging task in IHPs, PHPs, and RTCs, where a variety of factors might affect the members' timely appearance for group. The latter includes a member's resistance. The therapist might establish a policy wherein once the group begins, late members cannot enter that session. A constant meeting place is also important, and once again, unlike most outpatient groups, the group therapist may find that other activities intrude on the group's access to its regular room. Both time and place boundaries require that the therapist be an advocate for the group with the other staff of the unit. The therapist is most likely to be successful in performing this function if he or she assists others in understanding the reasons why these sources of consistency are so important to the functioning of the group.

Preparation and Contracting

Often in inpatient and day hospital settings, it is not possible to offer members a preparatory session. It nonetheless is important for the therapist to establish with members the goals for their group participation, a contracting process that typically takes place at the beginning of the session. Members need to know what they are working on, how they are accomplishing this work, and what behaviors will help or hinder their progress (Kauff, 2012). As a prelude to their group work, members benefit from understanding that feelings, thoughts, and urges that may not be in their full awareness can limit their effectiveness in being with others, engaging in work, and finding fulfillment in life. Members are then encouraged to pursue greater awareness of their internal lives by speaking as spontaneously as possible within the session, with particular attention to any feelings or thoughts about other members or the therapists. Like the interpersonal group, the psychodynamic group focuses on the here and now, where the power of the group is seen as residing. Through such instruction, the therapist catalyzes the group process. Giving emphasis to the importance of expressing impulses and affects in words rather than actions supports the development of healthy norms in the group that will also support the group's work.

Multilevel Interventions

A distinctive feature is that the psychodynamic group psychotherapist directs his or her interventions to different levels of group activity: individual, dyadic, subgroup, and group as a whole. From the standpoint of general systems theory (von Bertalanffy, 1950, 1966), a framework commonly used by psychodynamic group psychotherapists, each of these units can be seen as subsystems of a progressively larger system, existing within a hierarchy of systems. Because these systems have boundaries that are porous, that is, for import and export information, a change in any one unit reverberates throughout the systems in the hierarchy (Agazarian, 2001). For example, a change in an individual member results in changes of the same character in that member's subgroup and, ultimately, the group as a whole. For this reason, psychodynamic psychotherapists do not confine their interventions to a single level but rather direct interventions to that social unit most likely to be receptive to it.

A Developmental Focus

The psychodynamic group psychotherapist has a cognizance that group process does not emerge randomly but does so in an orderly fashion. As is the case with individual human beings, groups show a consistent pattern of development wherein a series of stages emerges (Bakali, Wilberg, Klungsøyr, & Lorentzen, 2013; Brabender & Fallon, 2009). Completion of the developmental tasks of one stage ushers in the next stage with its unique challenges. The developmental stages through which the group proceeds provide members with the opportunity to address the relational difficulties that members bring to group psychotherapy. For example, Stage 1 activates issues related to trust and attachment. Those members who experience attachment anxiety or avoidance in their individual lives are prone to experience such difficulties in the group as well (Marmarosh & Markin, 2007). Early in the group's life, members are likely to show these dysfunctional responses with particular clarity. However, it is not only the individual members who struggle with attachment insecurities but also the group as a whole. A basic tension exists in the group at large as to whether it is worth coming together and facing the perils that attend human contact (e.g., rejection) or stay safely apart. In an inpatient group, the fear of joining with others is often seen in more dramatic ways than in outpatient groups. Rice and Rutan (1987) described the patient who stood outside the door of the group session before summoning the courage to enter the room. Typically, members will subgroup according to their position on their stances on the conflict confronting the group (Agazarian, 2001). For example, those seeking to avoid contact will tend to affiliate with one another, and the therapist can support this subgroup process by identifying similarities in members' positions. In the safety of their subgroup, members can begin to confront their fears of connection and the costs of acceding to them.

In Stage 2, members confront their medley of reactions to the authority figure in the room, the therapist. On the one hand, members long to have all their needs met by the therapist in the way the mother does for the infant, and on the other, they fear that demanding that such needs be met and expressing frustration and anger with the therapist might induce some retaliatory or rejecting response from the therapist. Members, to varying degrees, experience the acknowledgment of dependency on the therapist as a challenge to their autonomy. Although the conflicts of this stage are universal, for the members of IHPs, PHPs, and RTCs, the fairly common difficulties with respect to early attachments make this stage a highly laden and hence potentially productive one. From it, members can gain greater access to the various elements underlying their struggles with authority figures and find means to harmonize these elements with one another.

Stage 3 is a brief stage of euphoria following the group's successful challenge of the therapist's authority. This stage affords members the opportunity to make deeper self-disclosures, and the positive aura gives members an experience of deep acceptance in relation to these communications. In the meantime, members use their newfound greater perceptiveness of one another to begin the process of offering feedback. The emotional tone of this stage all but ensures that it will be positive and bolstering, important characteristics that inoculate members against some of the stress of having close observations made of their persons. A major responsibility on therapists in this stage is to reinforce boundaries, which may be challenged as members feel the impulse to merge and blend with one another as fully as possible. Members' increasing discomfort with and mistrust of the Stage 3 longing for total intimacy usher in Stage 4. In Stage 4, members struggle to balance the need to retain their individual selves with the yearning to have intimate ties. No longer operating under the sway of an idealized view of one another, members can recognize not only one another's strengths but also their weaknesses. This period is when the important work is done on helping members see their dysfunctional social behaviors but, as important, the intrapsychic elements underlying these behaviors. The therapist's interventions during this period cover a range from the behavioral level of helping members to offer feedback that is operational, precise, and balanced to making those observations, clarifications, and interpretations that will enhance members' awareness levels of the conscious and unconscious elements attached to their behaviors.

The last stage of development, Stage 5, involves members' termination from the group. This period in group life most clearly achieves the status of a stage when all members terminate together. The potential of this era in group life is especially important for individuals in IHPs, PHPs, and RTCs because it is precisely the inability to tolerate loss that precipitates a breakdown in functioning necessitating a high level of care. The loss of the group frequently activates feelings associated with prior losses members have experienced in their lives. To avoid the discomfort associated with current and past losses, members resort to defensive maneuvers that prevent them from fully grappling with the loss in a way that would support their receptivity to new relationships. The therapist plays an important role in identifying both the defense and the feelings, impulses, and fantasies that evoke its use:

> Justin, who had developed strong connections in the group, said during the last session that he was glad the group was ending because it was beginning to be an unwanted burden. Several members expressed hurt over Justin's cavalier attitude toward losing the group. The therapist wondered aloud whether Justin and others might find it easier to see the group as having little value and, hence, as being dispensable than to feel sad that something of worth was coming to an end.

With this intervention, we see the therapist identifying the defense of devaluation, which is commonly used at the group's termination. The therapist universalizes Justin's reaction by making it clear that others may share it, a tack that is likely to reduce Justin's defensiveness. In making this interpretation, the therapist should also maintain empathy for Justin's identity status. The therapist might wonder whether cultural prescriptions for how to cope with loss might inform his response. A benefit of the group-as-a-whole interpretation is that it provides the individual some greater latitude to continue to use modes of responding that, though defensive, might be helpful and culturally consistent for the person. At the same time, the individual is assisted in joining with others in recognizing feelings that might be difficult to process were they to be faced alone.

Each ensuing stage provides an opportunity to explore a new aspect of human relating and more fully develop a healthier internal working model of relationships from which fulfillment and adjustment flow. The psychodynamic group psychotherapist thinks and intervenes developmentally by assisting members in recognizing the key developmental conflict at hand and how individual members, and subgroups of members, relate to it. Observations, clarifications, and interpretations are all deployed in the service of helping the group as a whole and the members in it to advance to the next developmental stage.

Monitoring Countertransference

Freud (1912/1958) identified a phenomenon wherein the patient transfers feelings that originate in his or her relationship with other people onto the therapist. This exploration of *transference* within treatment is a primary means by which psychodynamic psychotherapists help patients understand their internal working models of self and others. In group work, the therapist's interventions are predicated on the notion that aspects of the member's responses are derived from internal working models of self and others originating in early relationships. In other words, many responses group members have toward one another are transference-based responses.

Serving as a counterpart to transference is *countertransference*, a term capturing the therapist's reactivity to the patient. Although Freud and his successors saw countertransference as rooted in the therapist's issues, a more relational understanding of treatment emphasizes that countertransference is co-constructed within the therapeutic relationship. Because the patient participates in the instigation of countertransference, this set of therapist reactions can be mined for their ability to point back to features of the patient's own psychological life and especially that life as the person interacts with others. This reformulation of countertransference encourages the therapist to use his or her reactions to recognize facets of the patient's inner world that otherwise might be hidden. For example, countertransference responses can cue the therapist into a transition from one stage to another:

> Dr. Vick had been leading a new group in an RTC that had been meeting for three sessions. In the first three sessions, he had been pleased with the group's progress. It appeared that members were connecting with one another in positive ways. No one appeared to be excluded. In the fourth session, he noticed himself feeling irritated with the members, even though ostensibly, members' behavior appeared unchanged. Observing these behaviors more closely, he realized that members were showing minor acts of disattunement—one member looking at her watch, another sighing loudly as another member spoke at length, another looking longingly at her cell phone. He contemplated that these minor signs were perhaps not minor at all. They signified to Dr. Vick that the sense of unity existing at the end of Stage 1 might have transitioned into the fractiousness of early Stage 2. He observed the group for additional evidence of the accuracy of this hypothesis.

In short-term psychodynamic group work, time must be used efficiently. Doing so requires that the therapist tap into all the sources of information available. For Dr. Vick, early detection of Stage 2 could enable him to intervene in a fashion that allows members to approach more expeditiously their displeasure with the group, the therapist, and one another. For example, Dr. Vick could facilitate members with a common complaint in identifying with one another by using an intervention such as,

> Jorges, your concern that the group is spending too long talking about Mark's problem is similar to Mildred's worry that Ellen is not receiving the support she needs. For you, and maybe others, doubt seems to exist as to whether the group is doing what it ought for everyone.

By identifying a subgroup of members sharing what is often a difficult reaction to share, dissatisfaction with the therapist, Dr. Vick has reduced the risk for individual members in delving into this affective domain (see Agazarian, 2001, for further discussion of functional subgrouping). However, note that these technical maneuvers originally emanated from Dr. Vick's sensitivity to his own reactions and the group member behaviors tied to these reactions.

KIBEL'S OBJECT RELATIONS/SYSTEMS MODEL

The OR/S model is a psychodynamic approach to inpatient group psychotherapy that was first proposed by Howard Kibel in the late 1970s and has been of interest in the United States but, more especially, in Western Europe (Heinskou, 2010; J. Radcliffe, personal communication, December 15, 2015), where this format has been termed a *Kibel group*. A central tenet of Kibel's (1986, 1990, 1992) approach is that the tenor of members' interactions with one another on the hospital unit and in the psychotherapy group is reflective of the organization of their internal lives. According to this model, because a person's intrapsychic organization determines the quality of his or her relationships, it is this organization—not symptoms or social behaviors—that is the primary target of change.

Theoretical Underpinnings

Kibel's approach integrates two theoretical motifs, each of which we discuss in turn: object relations theory and general systems theory.

Object Relations Theory

Object relations theory has its roots in the work of Klein (1952) and other writers in the British school of psychoanalysis. *Object relations* refer to the complex interrelationships between the self or images of the self and others or images of others. An *object* can be either a real person or the image of a person. Central to object relations theory is the notion that individuals form internal schemata of their experiences with others, a process termed *internalization*. These templates shape the individual's future social experiences, determining their quality and tenor. Although changes in an individual's templates can occur through life, and certainly as a function of psychotherapy, those experiences that are most formative occur in the first few years of life in relation to primary caregivers. Object relations theorists in describing the vicissitudes of the infant's mental life have emphasized the criticalness of two developmental processes—splitting and projective identification—in accounting for the organization in the infant's experiences with her or his mother. The understanding of the unfolding of these processes in development is necessary to appreciate how they are disrupted in people who require care in hospital or residential facilities.

Normal Development

The earliest representations of experience occur when the infant lacks the capacity to discern where she begins and the mother ends. Hence, the initial schemata are not representations of a distinct self and a distinct mother but rather, of a self–mother unit. During this period from 1 month to 6 to 8 months, the distinction the infant is able to make is between what is pleasurable and what is painful. This period ends when the infant reliably differentiates self from mother. Another important achievement is the infant's gradual construction of associative networks of positive and negative self–mother representations. For example, the infant may associate the mother's gentle touch with her soothing voice and all other pleasure-evoking aspects of her person. The increased ability of the infant to synthesize various images of mother and self creates a potential crisis for the infant. If the infant were to associate positive and negative images of the mother with one another, the infant would be at risk of losing his or her sense of a positive tie with the mother. The developing constellation of positive representations is highly fragile. Were negative representations to be integrated with the positive, the infant would experience the positive representation network as under attack by her aggression. Later on, as this positive associative network achieves greater prominence and strength in the infant's intrapsychic life, the infant is able to experience continuity in the existence of this network despite being the object of the infant's aggression. To protect the positive self–mother images, the infant uses the mechanism of *splitting*, a defensive but developmentally needed operation wherein opposite-valenced representations are actively kept apart while the positive representational network develops.

The integration of positive self–mother representations is the foundation of the good ego core, which includes both the individual's emerging positive sense of self as well as her ability to adapt to the environment. As the constellation of positive representations acquires a more focal position in the infant's intrapsychic world, the negative representations, through the infant's use of splitting, are experienced as more peripheral to the self.

The second class of mechanisms, projection and projective identification, enables the infant to give unwanted elements of experience a less central place in the representation of self and other. Their use during this period rests on both the infant's burgeoning ability to distinguish internal from external and self from other, as well as the partial accomplishment of these discriminations. Both of these mechanisms involve the placement of some unwanted aspect of the self on another or, more accurately, on one's representation of another. An example of simple *projection* occurs when a person finds her envy to be unacceptable, projects it onto others, and sees a particular individual or group of individuals as being envious of her. *Projective identification* involves extruding some loathed part of the self, unconsciously acting in a coercive way to elicit an internal and behavioral response from another person. It is because of this second step that projective identification is a mechanism that connects the intrapsychic with the interpersonal (Ogden, 1979). The third step involves a continued identification with the projected-on object. If that person can manifest a tolerant attitude toward the expelled element, the projecting individual—whether an infant or adult—can incorporate into the self some element of this tolerance. For the infant at this stage, the perception of being at once one and not one with the mother makes the latter the quintessential object of projection. This act of projection serves a valuable function for the infant: In seeing the mother as having these unwanted feelings, the infant spares him- or herself the full force of their burden. The mother serves as a container for the infant's disturbing feelings until the infant can accept these feelings as her or his own. Moreover, the mother's capacity to show tolerance of the feelings the infant is projecting on her provides the foundation for the infant's development of acceptance of negatively toned feelings and impulses.

At approximately 6 to 8 months, the infant begins to accomplish the integration of the good and bad images of the mother and the good and bad images of self. Once this task is completed, the child realizes that the image of the loathed mother and the loved mother are one and the same mother. This realization requires the child's abandonment of the idealized (all-good) mother, and with this abandonment comes a sense of responsibility for having brought about her demise. It is this sense of responsibility that gives rise to feelings of remorse, shame, and guilt (Klein, 1952). Still, the child's ability to integrate positive and negative aspects of self and others is important because it renders the child's perception of self and others more stable and more realistic given that neither the self nor others are all good or all bad. Through this process, the child also acquires a more robust self-concept, capable of remaining stable in the midst of affirming and disconfirming external events.

Development of Psychotic and Borderline Organizations

The Kibel approach draws on a developmental characterization of individuals with borderline personality disorder[1] and individuals with psychosis during their premorbid states versus regressive episodes. Individuals with premorbid borderline personality disorder are persons who have failed the integration stage of object relations development previously described.

---

[1]Here, *borderline* refers to a level of personality organization described by various psychodynamic writers including Kernberg (1975a). It is used in contrast to the symptom-based diagnostic term used in the *Diagnostic and Statistical Manual of Mental Disorders* (fifth ed.; American Psychiatric Association, 2013).

Individuals so organized maintain an internal equilibrium and adapt to the environment through the use of splitting. For these individuals, decompensation (or the inability to perform everyday tasks) is the failure of splitting. With decompensation comes erosion in the capacity to distinguish self from others and of separations between benevolently and malevolently toned representations. The associative networks developed deteriorate so that the individual's perceptions of self and others become highly fragmented.

In contrast to the individual with borderline personality disorder, the person with premorbid psychosis is unable to distinguish between self and other, thoughts and their referents, and internal and external events. However, like the infant, the individual with psychosis can make a rudimentary differentiation between positive and negative representations. Through this differentiating process, the person with psychosis can achieve some modicum of inner harmony. For the person with psychosis as for the patient with borderline personality disorder, regression involves the loss of ability to organize representations according to their affective valence. The unavailability of the defense of splitting places the individual in great peril in responding to the demands of the environment. As was previously described, the ego's ability to function is based on the coalescence of positive and the extrusion of negative representations. It is precisely because the ego has been immobilized that the structured setting of the program becomes essential, performing for individuals that which they cannot perform for themselves. If regression involves the deterioration of the organizational aspects of the ego—the loss of those defenses on which the individual customarily relies—treatment must be directed toward their reconstitution. However, the particulars of how this goal might be accomplished require knowledge of the inpatient environment and of how the environment is likely to interact with the patient's pathology.

General Systems Theory and the Treatment Environment

General systems theory, described earlier in this chapter, has been applied over the past 20 years to long-term outpatient psychotherapy groups (e.g., Agazarian & Peters, 1981; Durkin, 1972), PHP groups (e.g., Greene, Rosenkrantz, & Muth, 1985) and long-term and short-term IHP groups (e.g., Brabender, 1988; Rice & Rutan, 1987). General systems theory is particularly appropriate for IHPs, PHPs, and RTCs because it provides a language to describe the reality that none of these groups stand alone. Rather, they are embedded in a series of hierarchically and dynamically related systems. These groups are subsystems of the hierarchy of systems (e.g., the unit, the hospital) in which they are nested. Because the boundaries of all of the systems and subsystems in a hierarchy are porous, happenings at one level affect all other levels. If, for example, at the level of the suprasystem of the hospital, a conflict exists among key administrators concerning treatment philosophy, this conflict will appear in some fashion in all subsystems embedded in this suprasystem, including the psychotherapy group. Although the notion of a hierarchy of systems possesses some descriptive value, as Kernberg (1975b) pointed out, the concept is limited. A more realistic model, Kernberg suggested, is a concatenation of systems with any one subsystem belonging to multiple supersystems. Each supersystem might bear down on a given subsystem at any time. For example, the supersystem that might reflect the humanistic values of the organization could exert itself more or less strongly as could the supersystem that is responsive to financial pressures.

It stands to reason that although all systems in a hierarchy (or concatenation of hierarchies) influence and are influenced by one another, those systems and subsystems that are contiguous to one another show the most dramatic influences. The psychotherapy group is most likely to be affected by the immediate environment in which it is embedded. One way in which the group is related to the unit is in composition. Typically, all the group members are residents of the program. Frequently, the therapists are members of the treatment team. The tenor of members' relationships with one another as well as the issues that emerge in their relationships cannot help but be carried into the group. Another related aspect of the group and unit or program is the high level of information exchange between the two. Conversations on the unit continue into the group, happenings in the group are reported at staff meetings, affective states stimulated in one venue are carried into another. Because of their interrelatedness, it is impossible to think about the dynamics of the psychotherapy group independently of those of the larger program.

Integration of Object Relations and Systems Theory

Both object relations and systems theory, examined in concert with one another, provide an understanding of the challenges the group presents and the opportunities the psychotherapy group offers in relation to these challenges.

The Inpatient Unit

The reconstitutive aspects of inpatient psychiatric hospitalization are well known (Rice & Rutan, 1987), and many of these features apply to PHP and RTC settings as well. The unit offers sanctuary from everyday stressors, relief from decision making, and diminished requirements to attend to the responsibilities of everyday life. Those inpatients bereft of social supports outside the hospital or the program find them in greater abundance in their new setting. The institution of a medication regimen frequently reduces the intensity of symptoms. All these forces are aimed at helping patients regain their premorbid levels of functioning.

Another set of forces not only fails to support reconstitution but also induces deeper levels of regression (Kibel, 1978). The inpatient unit is a large group in which the members have multiple roles in relation to one another. Any given patient encounters others who are seeking to rid themselves of their negative affects and impulses via projection and projective identification. For example, Stan, who is trying to rid himself of anger, encounters Barry, who is doing the same and will do so by perceiving Stan as the bearer of hostility. In fact, Barry will endeavor to provoke Stan into feeling and behaving with hostility. Moreover, the inpatient unit typically has clear authority figures that evoke transferential responses related to early parental figures (Kibel, 1981). With all these factors at play, the inpatient unit can readily become a toxic environment for individuals seeking sanctuary and restoration. It is here that the psychotherapy group can play an important role in lessening the corrosive and strengthening the supportive influences.

The Psychotherapy Group

The restitutive and regressive forces in the larger program are also contained within the psychotherapy group. However, within the group relative to the program, these forces are more identifiable and, as such, more amenable to exploration and alteration (Kibel, 1981). Members' reactions achieve clarity in the group because the group is seen as providing a strong safety net, which facilitates the less disguised appearance of regressive reactions. In contrast, in individual therapy, the patient is unable to express fully angry feelings toward the therapist because such expressions induce concern for the power of such expressions to obliterate the therapist. Patients in the midst of their self-perceived helplessness cannot, they believe, afford such obliteration. In the psychotherapy group, members can express negative feelings toward the therapist and still retain a positive tie to the group as a whole (Kibel, 1987a). In addition, the group is conducive to the full-blown manifestation of conflict because it encourages the verbal expression of affect and thereby renders the extent and nature of the affect clearer to all (Kibel, 1987b). Whereas the program is large and diffuse with many different interactions occurring simultaneously, the group is small, focused, and contained. These latter qualities create an inescapability wherein members are forced to respond to feelings in a more direct fashion. Finally, while functioning in the confines of the group, staff members are relieved of other burdens, thereby facilitating their assumption of an exploratory attitude toward patients' communications and abetting their capacity to serve as healthy repositories for members' projections.

Because the psychotherapy group symbolically contains the issues experienced by the larger program, it is a place in which important work can be done with effects on all systemic levels. Through the group's analysis of members' reactions to the regression-promoting stimuli on the unit, the restitution-fostering features of the patient's stay can be actualized most completely.

Goals of Treatment

Kibel's model seeks to promote the necessary intrapsychic change to enable members to return to their premorbid level of functioning. This model views the primary impediment to members' reattainment of their former healthier level of level of functioning to be their inability to use splitting. In the absence of splitting, infusion of the central ego core with aggression occurs, leading both the self and others to be experienced as toxic. The goal of this model is to neutralize and circumscribe group members' aggression. As the use of splitting is restored, and as aggressive images of self and others become less consuming, the individuals' capacities to summon positively toned representations are enhanced. The developmental task of moving beyond splitting is left to long-term outpatient treatment.

The intrapsychic change sought by this model begets external change. Members' experiences of others and members' social behaviors move from the toxic to the benign. Members become more capable of adapting to their environments and coping with the stressors of everyday life, including those of the larger program in which they participate. The individual member also would be expected to show greater willingness to participate in outpatient group psychotherapy. The restitution of the good ego core enables the use of those processes such as self-reflection that were casualties of regression. Such a function as self-reflection is critical not only for the patient's participation in exploratory psychotherapy but also for his or her awareness of the value of such an exploration.

The Change Process

The interventions of Kibel's approach are targeted toward (a) segregating and reducing the intensity of the members' negative images of self and other and (b) bolstering the good ego core, which is the organized totality of the positive images of self and others. A primary strategy to accomplish the first goal is to help members establish linkages between present emotional reactions and recent events, particularly events related to the experience of being hospitalized:

> Members of a group on an adolescent unit became quite irritated with Dr. Pell for "invading their space." "Why did Dr. Pell need to ask such personal questions," they wondered. Dr. Pell found this to be a curious criticism in that he had not asked any questions in that session. He had made a few reflective comments that went a little further than what

members had said themselves. However, in thinking about one member's use of the term *invade*, the therapist related members' irritation to a recent drug screen that had taken place for all adolescents on the unit due to staff suspicions that some were "using." Dr. Pell shared this connection with members and commented that anger in response to feeling invaded was quite understandable. After members decried the staff for this action, they expressed fears about being found the culprit whether they had used illicit drugs or not. Members who were surprised that others feared being deemed guilty despite innocence laughed and developed a fantasy of the patients on the unit taking the same action on the staff.

The therapist identifying parallels between members' experiences in the group and precipitating events in the larger program helped members recognize that their emotional reactions were comprehensible rather than confusing or bizarre. It also validated members' reactions by claiming that their irritation, given the situation, was not unreasonable. This validation removed other painful affects such as shame and guilt from the anger and thereby diminished the intensity of the latter. Such an intervention altered in a positive way the members' representational world because it harnessed and at least partially neutralized those aggressive introjects that had invaded the good ego core.

Splitting is reinstated not only by diminishing the bad but also by bolstering the good. Members in the group are given an opportunity to respond to one another in a nurturing fashion. Such displays of caretaking of others enhance self-esteem and strengthen the individual's self-perception of being good. Members' identifications with one another also fortified their positive representations. When a group becomes cohesive through these identifications, the self-images of the members coalesce into a collective group ego (Kibel, 1987a) that is better able than that of any one individual to ward off aggressive urges. The inter-member binding of positive and negative representations enables the group to accomplish externally the splitting that is so crucial for the members' returns to their premorbid states.

Technical Considerations of the Object Relations Model

Beyond those features that were ascribed to the therapist role in the psychodynamic psychotherapy group, particular aspects of the therapist's functioning in Kibel's approach are important.

Boundary Management

The therapist maintains an optimal level of permeability of the boundary between the group and the unit. Information must flow from the psychotherapy group to the treatment team because the group therapists are in a position to get important information about patients from the standpoints of diagnosis, dynamics, and progress in treatment (Kibel, 1987b). Heinskou (2010) described how information from a Kibel group could be used to establish the focus of monthly staff meetings. This contribution advantages patients and staff and develops in the latter a positive attitude toward the group. The therapist must also receive information from the unit staff to understand the dynamics of the group fully. For example, learning that an angry exchange occurred in the middle of the night between two roommates and awakened others on the hall might be important in understanding tensions within the current session. The therapist must also regularly offer staff information about the group's work that might enhance their grasp of individual member or group dynamics.

Supportive Interventions

Relative to the long-term outpatient therapist, the therapist using a Kibel approach is active in involving the members of the group. To stimulate discussion, the therapist may ask questions, seek clarifications, or even address a unit-related topic. An important supportive activity is to help members bond with one another through recognition of commonalities in one another's experiences. For example, if a new member expresses anxiety about entering the group, the therapist might remind other members that they had a similar feeling in the days prior. The therapist thereby facilitates the establishment of a bridge between new and old members. The therapist also offers support by exhibiting and fostering in others a nonjudgmental attitude toward members' contributions (Kibel, 1987b).

Clarifying Interpretations

Here, the therapist assists the group in seeing how members' communications in the group are reflective of reactions (often overreactions) to the broader therapeutic milieu. An example of this process was given in the preceding section in which the therapist decoded for members the symbolism in their irritation over his putatively probing questions. In encouraging members to ventilate their anger, the therapist offered himself as an object for this displaced anger. This displacement occurred readily because the therapist was, as is typically the case, seen as a representative of the treatment team and the larger psychiatric system. The therapist was then able to "contain" (Bion, 1962) the aggression for the members. That is, the therapist demonstrated a capacity to tolerate being the target of such feelings. When members use projective identification vis-à-vis the therapist and see that the therapist does not respond with vengeance, they are then able to take in a diluted, less frightening form of anger.

By directing anger toward the therapist, members can test out their concerns about the consequences of being angry and expressing it in a real context. For example, members may come to see that the manifestation of anger does not necessarily lead to retaliation or abandonment. This process of testing is important because members' concerns about the catastrophic consequences of expressing anger are a major factor in causing their aggressive impulses to be so intolerable to them. In this model, the therapist takes an active role in helping members articulate and test their fears. In some cases, it may be beneficial for the therapist to reassure members that certain negative anticipations will not be met. For example, the therapist may make it clear to members that he or she will not delay their discharge from the treatment program simply because they express anger toward him or her.

Content of the Session

The Kibel approach entails an unstructured session in which members bring up material spontaneously. Early on in the session, the therapist uses a variety of interventions to get members to respond to and establish identifications with one another. Throughout the session, the therapist fosters a here-and-now focus by encouraging members to talk about immediate reactions. In this context, *immediate* refers to reactions occurring on the unit or in the group. If a member describes a reaction in the there and then, the therapist might seek a parallel between that reaction and one in the present context, "You say you have been angry at your boss, but as the session ended yesterday, you talked about a similar feeling toward Dr. Suds." Thus, the therapist makes linkages between immediate reactions and events in the larger treatment community.

Typically, the reason the group has warded off recognition of its emotional reaction in relation to an event on the unit or an aspect of hospital life is the fear that acknowledging the connection will bring about something untoward. The working through of a group-as-a-whole interpretation involves some attention to the fears that members have about the awareness of particular feelings and the events that provoked them. Members should be encouraged to test their fearful anticipations of what the consequences of such expressions would be inside or outside the group. Particularly common are fears of retaliation by the person to whom a certain feeling is expressed. Table 4.1 summarizes characteristics of the OR/S model.

MENTALIZATION GROUPS

A group approach that has more recently come onto the practice landscape is the mentalization (or mentalizing) group, which is based on the work of Bateman and Fonagy (2001). The concepts proposed by mentalization

TABLE 4.1
Object Relations/Systems Model

Elements of the model	Characteristics of the model
View of psychological problems	Psychological problems are due to the failure in the integration of different experience of self and other and to the use of relationship-undermining defenses in the effort to avoid integration.
Goals of model	To help members achieve access to the defenses used premorbidly so that they can return to a long-term treatment situation in which integration can be pursued.
Methods of action Intervention techniques	Detoxification of negative self and other experiences • Use of group-as-a-whole comments to help members identify with one another's experiences. • Identification of the precipitants of negative experiences, thereby assisting members in recognizing the reasonableness of their reactions. Precipitants include in-group and in-program events.
Adaptation of the model to a brief time frame	Establishing the goal of the restoration of premorbid defenses is a significant adaptation of the model, which would ordinarily posit integration as a goal.
Use of group process	Group process is a major focus as members explore the relationship of their shared affects and impulses as they relate to precipitants in the group and on the unit or program.

theory are particularly, although not exclusively, conducive to application in IHPs, PHPs, and RTCs because this treatment was developed for persons who function at a borderline level as defined by the *Psychodynamic Diagnostic Manual* (2nd ed.; Lingiardi & McWilliams, 2017). As noted previously, this patient population predominates in these three settings. Although this approach was proposed in the early 1990s, in the last 15 years, its prominence and popularity have rapidly grown, as has its application to a broader range of treatment settings and modalities. Indeed, in the last decade, considerable attention has been paid to the use of mentalization approaches in psychotherapy groups (e.g., see Karterud & Bateman, 2012) because the group setting provides an especially rich environment for individuals to strengthen their mentalizing abilities (Haslam-Hopwood, Allen, Stein, & Bleiberg, 2006).

Mentalization is the capacity of a person to be mindful of his or her intentions, desires, and goals, which might inform that person's experiences and behaviors, and to recognize the same elements in others, particularly as they shape others' behaviors (Coates, 2006). It entails realizing that one has a mind and so do others (Bateman & Fonagy, 2006). For example, mentalization is in evidence when one group member says to another, "I think you are looking at the clock so much today because you want the group to end before someone confronts you about your hurtful comment yesterday." Mentalizing also occurs when the member says about herself, "I think I made that hurtful comment to you because I am envious of you." Bateman and Fonagy (2006) noted that such acts of mentalization require imagination in that one, strictly speaking, can never know what is occurring within another person. It is also primarily preconscious. Although, for example, the comments made by the group members involved conscious acts of mentalizing, typically, individuals continually engage in this activity automatically, outside the bounds of consciousness.

Mentalization theory has its roots in the discoveries over the past 2½ decades concerning the attachment process and the developmental benefits that accrue from a young child's success in establishing a secure attachment to a caregiver, typically the mother. John Bowlby saw psychoanalysis as placing excessive emphasis on the fantasy life of the infant, independent of the infant's actual experiences in his or her interpersonal world, particularly those with his or her primary caregiver, usually the mother (Bretherton, 2006). Initially, Bowlby homed in on the consequences of the separation of the infant and her mother, a separation created, for example, by the child's hospitalization. He and his colleagues documented the extreme psychological and physical toll these separations took on the child. His work, in collaboration with Mary Ainsworth, established the criticalness of the mother's presence to offer security to the child and attunement to assist the child in managing physical and emotional discomfort. Through the "secure base" the mother establishes for the child, the latter can develop healthy internal working models of self and other, which in turn fuel the child's interest in and willingness to explore her or his inner and outer world (Ainsworth, Blehar, Waters, & Wall, 1978/2015).

Fonagy, Gergely, Jurist, and Target (2002) described how in the infant's first 5 months of life, he or she engages in face-to-face interaction with the mother in which the latter functions as a *pedagogue*, teaching the infant that he has a mind. The instrument of her teaching is contingent, marked, and ostensive mirroring, a type of instructive communication for which the infant is biologically primed (Choi-Kain & Gunderson, 2008). *Contingent mirroring* involves the mother's matching the infant's internal state in her expressions. *Marked mirroring* occurs when the mother conveys to the infant that she grasps the state of his or her mind. The marking takes the form of exaggerating her expression of a state so that the infant can see that she is referring to his or her mind and not her own. *Ostensive mirroring* taps into a biological readiness on the part of the infant for particular cues that evoke a receptive, student-like attitude toward the interaction. These cues are the mother's eye-to-eye contact with the infant and particular intonational patterns that elicit what Gergely (2007) called "a specific receptive and interpretative attitude (the 'pedagogical stance')" (p. 57).

Through this carefully choreographed but nonetheless spontaneous dance, the mother conveys to the infant a grasp of the infant's intentions, even before such time that the infant is aware of having intentions, enabling the infant to take baby steps toward achieving the realization that he or she and others have a mind.

At about 6 months, due both to maturation and the consistency of the mother–infant interaction, the infant begins to engage in *teleological thinking*, which is the capacity to see behavior as leading to a future state or goal, an achievement that is a mentalization forerunner. As mother–infant interactions continue, ever so gradually, the infant develops the ability to realize that the mother has various thoughts, feelings, and impulses to which her behaviors are connected—in other words, something underpins what the infant can directly touch, see, and hear. Infants' experiences help them grasp the presence of their minds. Infants sense wanting things—that is, having goals such as wanting to nurse at the mother's breast. The immediate context provides a particular array of opportunities for achieving this goal. The infant could cry, or merely yell. If he or she is close to mother, the infant could bob up and down, giving a kind of postural communication. The infant's burgeoning capability to sense goals versus the acts needed to achieve them contributes to the infant's nascent sense that he or she has an internal life. Somewhere around the age of 2, and of course, it varies from infant to infant, the child appreciates that like him or her, other people have goals and intentions. With the dual realization of the other and the self as having an interior, the child has achieved both a rudimentary capacity to mentalize and a primitive theory of mind.

Characterizing this early stage of mentalization are three ways by which the child represents his or her affects and those of others—psychic equivalent, pretend, and teleological (Fonagy et al., 2002). These modes are key to grasping the mental lives of individuals who populate inpatient groups. The *psychic equivalent mode* entails seeing an internal content as directly and precisely reflecting external reality. The *pretend mode* is, as it sounds, imagining. It is the creation of an internal reality that the child knows explicitly to be at odds with external reality. In fact, in the pretend mode, the child steadfastly avoids what might seem to bear a resemblance to external reality because doing so would activate psychic equivalence. For example, the wicked witch is acceptable only as long as she is imagined as quite distinct from any women in the child's life. The pretend mode provides the child with a space to play with possibilities and to make strides in developing a representational system. The *teleological mode* entails acknowledging an inner state only when it has an external correspondent (e.g., "You don't love me unless you give me flowers"; Fonagy et al., 2017).

At about the age of 4, these activities merge, leading the child to the crowning achievement of full-fledged mentalization. This transition is in part fostered by the parent who engages in imaginary play with the child while affirming the boundary between the representational and outside world (Fonagy et al., 2002). What the child comes to know through this developmental work is that the internal representation of the outside world is just that, that it need not be perfectly aligned with outside reality and that others may have different representations of the same reality. Mentalization entails forming secondary representations of one's emotional states. These secondary representations serve as the basis for the child's capacity to engage in self-regulation. Rather than affects directly driving behavior, the child can now contain the affects through use of the secondary representations, which can then serve as mediators of social interaction. Mentalization also is key to the formation of a sense of self. Once a child can grasp that he or she has a representation of the external world that is his or her own, that quality of "mindness," the establishment of the self begins. As representations develop and interconnect, the sense of self correspondingly becomes more palpable and coherent.

The developmental theory of mentalization provides assistance in understanding the central issues of persons who commonly present for treatment in IHPs, PHP, and RTCs—that is, individuals with borderline pathology. As noted previously, here, borderline pathology is not the personality disorder identified in descriptive psychiatry systems such as the *Diagnostic and Statistical Manual of Mental Disorders* (fifth ed.; American Psychiatric Association, 2013) but, rather, a level of functioning characterized by massive ego weakness and propensity for severe disorganization. Borderline pathology originates in the child's lack of a secure attachment to the mother. The young child with a disorganized attachment avoids grappling with the parent's threatening internal states. It is the child's penetration of the parent's internal world that teaches that child about his or her own. In avoiding the parent's internal world, the child is deprived of achieving awareness of his or her mental states. Insofar as these internal states constitute a self, the child is hindered in achieving awareness of it. Alternately, the parent's responses to the child, rather than accurately capturing the child's self-state, might have been "off"—an insufficiently close reflection of the child's current inner state. This circumstance leads the child to develop secondary representations of his or her emotional states that are slightly at odds or removed from the states themselves, somewhat like labeling an experience with a word that is almost apt. Although the child's mentalizing capacity will not be absent, it will be compromised.

The borderline individuals who commonly present in IHPs, PHPs, and RTCs are distinguished by particular difficulties in mentalizing, difficulties that impinge on other crucial areas such as affect and impulse regulation. Although such individuals can mentalize, they are unable to do so consistently, especially when affect surfaces (Fonagy & Bateman, 2008).[2] Bateman and Fonagy (2010) posited that constitutional factors and trauma could be restraining forces against the development of mentalizing capacities and particularly exert their effects when a child receives noncongruent mirroring from a caregiver. They hold, too, that the lack of adequate mirroring results in an extremely reactive attachment system. Finally, the aforementioned steps deprive the person of the ability to direct attention and to represent one's own and others' affect, particularly when emotional distress is evoked in relation to a loss. The incapacity of symbolically representing feelings is associated with affective dysregulation. Incongruent mirroring also deprives the person of enjoying continuity in the sense of self in that the cognizance of an "I" proceeds from discerning the operation of a mind that controls behavior. Without a palpable mind, no "I" exists (Bateman & Fonagy, 2006).

In the context of a secure attachment, the mentalizing approach to group psychotherapy strengthens members' abilities to attend to and represent their own and others' emotional reactions, even during conditions of affective stimulation. Mentalization that is both enriched and stable provides the means wherein an individual can gain control of his internal life and behavior. Such greater control lessens the person's suicidal tendencies, strengthens the positive tenor in his or her relationships with others, and provides a fortified sense of self.

Goals of the Treatment

Although writers on mentalization-based therapy frequently mention the utility of a group format, Sigmund Karterud (2015; Karterud & Bateman, 2012) and Fonagy, Campbell, and Bateman (2017) have provided the most extensive coverage of group therapy centered on mentalization. Karterud and Bateman (2012) distinguished between mentalization-based treatment and mentalization-informed group therapy. The former is a conjoint treatment in which patients receive both individual and group psychotherapy, each driven by mentalization theory. Mentalization-informed group therapy involves using this theoretical approach in a stand-alone treatment. Both of these applications have relevance to IHPs, PHPs, and RTCs.

In Karterud's (2015) text, he described the flexibility of the mentalization-based model in accommodating different temporal frames, but he emphasized that the goal must be adjusted to meet the time frame. In the case of short-term treatments, the goal is psychoeducational: Members become acquainted

---

[2]For more information about the development of borderline pathology within a mentalization framework, the reader is urged to consult Fonagy and Bateman (2008).

with the concept of mentalization and acquire the rudiments of applying it to events in their lives, particularly those involving close relationships. As the time frame expands, the expectation also increases that members will be able to undergo an intrapsychic shift in which mentalization regularly and automatically occurs as an individual's response to interpersonal events in his or her life.

In longer term experiences (e.g., 12 sessions), members' mentalization is enhanced by their acquisition of four basic mentalizing competencies (Fonagy, Luyten, & Bateman, 2015). Each competency represents the achievement of balance on a continuum that is anchored by contrasting processes or foci. The first continuum is the automatic versus controlled polarity. It reflects the extent to which the individual's mentalization is uncontrolled, spontaneous, and unconscious as opposed to conscious, verbally articulated, and deliberative. For example,

> Dhanya said to the new member, Roscoe, that she knew they would not get along. The therapist wondered why Dhanya was so sure, and the latter responded that she simply was. On being pressed further, she claimed that she was "picking up a hostile vibe" from Roscoe.

Dhanya formed a quick, intuitive judgment about the new member. In fact, her identification of the hostility was not initially accessible until the therapist urged her to engage in some additional processing. If we follow this interaction further, we see another dimension emerge:

> The therapist wondered what it was that Roscoe had done to make Dhanya think he had hostile feelings for her. She said that while Roscoe is speaking in the group, he occasionally looks at her and scowls.

Dhanya is, at least according to her report, relying on external cues such as facial expressions to make a judgment about the mind of another member. If her comment were representative of her usual way of seeing others, she could be regarded as at the end of the continuum from externality to internality in her engagement in mentalizing. The goal of the therapist would be to move her more toward the center of the continuum by helping her to recognize that Roscoe's external manifestations could have a variety of internal roots:

> The therapist asked the other members whether they could think of other reasons why Roscoe scowls when he looks at Dhanya. One member said that Roscoe's scowl was simply a manifestation of his thinking about something. The scowling—he inferred—was a sign of concentration. Other members agreed and noted that he scowled at them, too, but they interpreted it differently. Dhanya then asserted that she had a talent for knowing who was hostile toward her and who was not, and it made her angry that the group could not trust her judgment.

Dhanya's response illustrates another continuum—that between affect and cognition. Rather than taking in the alternate interpretation from the group—a new cognitive framing of Roscoe's behavior—Dhanya reasserted her intuitive and emotional view of Roscoe's stance toward her. The goal for Dhanya would be to help her to shift to a position that integrated the two poles of affect and cognition.

At the same time that Dhanya is expressing the conviction that her view of Roscoe is accurate, she is ignoring any data that he might offer that could be helpful to her forming an accurate view of his internal experience. That is, on the polarity between self and other, Dhanya resides at the extreme self end of the continuum. In the group, the goal would be to help her situate herself between the self and other pole by encouraging her to focus on whatever pole is being neglected. In this case, the therapist might respond as follows:

> Although you are quite sure you know how Roscoe feels, Roscoe might have something to say about his feelings that would be important to consider. I know I am curious about what Roscoe would have to say given what you and others have said about him. Perhaps by asking him about his feelings toward you, you would be able to develop a fuller picture.

Here, the therapist is not only directing Dhanya's attention to the other but also nurturing her inquisitiveness about others in her interpersonal world, an inquisitiveness that will support her effort to represent others' inner states.

Process of the Group

To create an environment in which members can improve their mentalization skills, the group, like any treatment situation, must activate members' attachment systems. If members experience the group as a secure base, they can adopt the exploratory attitude that mentalization requires. As members pursue their exploratory work, they come to associate it with the secure base provided by the group, which only encourages further investigation of others' minds and their own (Bateman & Fonagy, 2004). To offer a secure base, the group psychotherapist must establish safety through the provision of a consistent workspace. The therapist must also offer mirroring for the group members and mark the mirroring in a way that the members understand that it is their own experiences the therapist is reflecting back and not the therapist's.

If the goal of mentalization-based group psychotherapy is to foster good mentalization by members' achievement of balance on each of these four continua, the therapist must foster those processes that support this goal. Early in treatment, the group psychotherapists work with members to help them restructure their understanding of their feelings, particularly those feelings that have a destabilizing effect on them. To gain access to affects, members describe events that stimulated those affects. The events should be those occurring in the group, in the treatment program, and outside the treatment environment. In some cases, members might not have mentalized at all and thereby have to engage in reflection that will make these feelings clearer to them. In other cases, members will be capable of identifying affect states but in a way that fails to do justice to the four polarities described previously. By drawing the member's attention to the neglected pole, the therapist can enable him or her to move in the direction of greater balance.

Technical Considerations of Mentalization Groups

The Role of the Therapist

The group therapist in mentalization-based group therapy has a complex set of tasks, not all of which are fully captured in this section (the reader is referred to Karterud, 2015, for a more elaborate exposition). For our purposes, what is important to recognize is that all the therapist's activities—both inside and outside the group—must be congruent with the ethos of this approach. That is, in how the therapist administers the group, reflects on the group, and conducts the group, the therapist must place mentalization at the heart of his or her activities.

Mentalization and the Therapist's Relational Stance

The therapist must establish the group as a kind of transitional space where members can safely explore emotions, thoughts, wishes, needs, and desires (Bateman & Fonagy, 2004). The therapist creates the transitional space through many means, not the least of which is the therapist's demonstrated comfort with the kinds of primitive prementalization activity in which members engage. Members' residency at a borderline level of functioning ensures that (a) seeing inner reality and outer reality as one and the same, (b) experiencing feelings as disconnected from other elements in the person's internal world, (c) symbolizing affects with difficulty, and (d) oscillating with stunning rapidity in their attitudes toward the therapist are routine (Bateman & Fonagy, 2004). The therapist must also maintain a poised and reflective stance toward the enactments that inevitably occur in a group of individuals who are at borderline level. The therapist's consistency as a mentalizing presence will serve to contain members' disturbing inner states and provide a model for members' mentalizing efforts. At times, the members will place parts of themselves onto the therapist. These parts constitute an alien self, whose continued presence within the self is a challenge to the person's self-cohesion. The task for the therapist is to reject this alien self but to allow its extrusion until such time that the member develops the mentalizing skills to assimilate it.

For mentalizing to occur, members have to operate from a secure base, the presence of which fuels their drives to explore their inner and outer lives. In doing so, the therapist helps members develop epistemic trust in all group members, including the therapist, meaning that the member has an openness to others' communications (Fonagy et al., 2017). Many of the therapist's interventions are designed to ensure that the group serves as this secure base. For example, the therapist manifests a caring attitude and encourages members to do the same toward one another. The therapist urges members to attach to the group.

Mentalization and Specific Interventions

In this approach, members are prepared carefully for the group experience. Fonagy et al. (2017) discussed the usefulness of presenting to members the concept of attachment styles and how these styles relate to the struggles members endure. In this preparation, the therapist nurtures a promentalization environment by letting members know that mentalizing is the goal of the group. Members are taught to distinguish between good and bad mentalizing and are told they will be assisted in achieving the former. At this time, the therapist cultivates norms that will support mentalizing during the sessions. Among these are members' bringing up events from their lives that can be mentalized, responding to one's events and others' in a mentalizing manner, and showing caring for other members (Karterud, 2015).

The therapist also attends to the phases. In this model, the group session is seen as organized in three phases. In the beginning phase, the therapist provides any updates since the last meeting. Information is provided about any members who are not in attendance. Members are invited to comment on these messages. The therapist offers a summary of the themes of the prior session both to reinforce mentalizing and also to foster group cohesion (Fonagy et al., 2017). The therapist then creates connections to the prior meeting by offering observations of the work done by members. Each member is mentioned. This sharing both sets the stage for the work in the current session and reveals to members that the therapist has kept the group in mind—a means of highlighting the importance of mentalizing and the need for its consistent application.

In the next phase, the therapist initiates a go-around. The therapist either establishes a direction (e.g., that one member will begin followed by another) or allows the members to do so, typically based on the themes that the therapist outlined in relation to the last session. As each member is sharing, the therapist encourages the others to listen and not interrupt (Fonagy et al., 2017). The therapist monitors the time and each member's participation. If any group member expresses intent to self-harm, that event should be given priority (Bateman & Fonagy, 2004). The therapist fosters a process in which members search for any stimulus within the group that might have given rise to self-harm ideation (Bateman & Fonagy, 2004).

Toward the end of the session, the therapist reminds the group of the passing time and engages the group in a decision-making process as to how the last portion of the session will be spent. In this way, the therapist enlists members' higher order cognitive processes in judging their own and one another's mental states in light of the reality-based time limitations of the session. Frequently, the therapist ends the group with a summary of key thematic elements in the present session to set the stage for future work (Fonagy et al., 2017).

The therapist's constant objective throughout all stages is to foster mentalization. The therapist punctuates the sessions with questions that serve as invitations to the members to activate their mentalizing resources:

> Why is the patient [member] saying this now? Why is the patient behaving like this? Why am I feeling as I do now? What has happened recently in the therapy or in our relationship that may justify the current state? (Fonagy et al., 2017, p. 204)

In group psychotherapy, the scope of the questions concerns not only the therapist but also the relationships among group members, the group as a whole, and staff in the treatment program. Although at any point in the group, the scenario discussed might belong only to a single member, the therapist engages all the members in its exploration. All members have the opportunity to practice mentalizing by, first of all, being encouraged to adopt a not-knowing posture (Karterud, 2015) and, then, by identifying questions that are relevant to pose about the scenario. Continually, the therapist models a not-knowing stance, which counteracts the dependent position members can readily assume.

As members engage in efforts at mentalizing, the therapist helps them recognize when their attempts constitute *good mentalization*, which has a number of qualities such as flexibility, integration of cognitive and affective aspects of self and others, openness to discovery, and recognition of the tentativeness of formulations, to name a few (Luyten, Fonagy, Lowyck, & Vermote, 2012). For example,

> Charlene reported that she had been sulking in the back seat of her friend's car. Her two friends in the front seat carried on a lively conversation. Charlene said they asked her a question, she responded monosyllabically, and then they continued talking to one another.

Charlene shared that she realized she was keeping herself out of the conversation lest she should make an effort and be rejected. She decided to ask the two a question and thereby declare herself a participant. The therapist said, "You gave yourself a mental space to realize that fear preceded your withdrawal, which in turn caused the very thing you didn't want. Your new thought led you to cope differently. How was it for you having this new perspective?"

As Karterud (2015) noted, the therapist's acknowledgment should engage the member in a here-and-now analysis of the event. Had Charlene exhibited a failure in mentalization, the therapist would have helped her see how her response might be enriched in a way that makes it a more effective instance of mentalization. For example, if Charlene had become stuck in her feeling that she was left out, she could have expanded her view to explore what she was feeling right before she had this "left-out" reaction. In addition, other members could be enlisted to share their perspectives.

> The therapist then turned to the group, "Others have heard Charlene talk about her experience of being the odd person out. In fact, others have shared the worry of being in that position. How were you affected by Charlene's sharing?"

Here, the therapist is ensuring that the session will not devolve into individual therapy in a group but will keep members engaged and aware that all that transpires is relevant to each of them.

The therapist in this approach also uses particular technical interventions to advance the group dialogue and each member's mentalizing work. For example, the intervention of *triangulation* can be summoned when two members establish a kind of cabal, resonating to each other's experiences while excluding other members. As Fonagy et al. (2017) explained, the therapist can enlist a third member who can either share reactions to the dyad's conversation or relate his or her experiences to it. In this way, the therapist interrupts what has devolved from a self–other interaction to a self–self interaction in which members regard each other as entities lacking distinctiveness vis-à-vis the self.

Content of the Session

Although we have discussed the mentalization session in its broad lines, the middle phase of the session warrants further consideration. In this middle phase, the group attends to a series of events presented by individual members. The therapist might invite members to propose an event to the group for mentalization. What constitutes an event is a happening either inside or outside the group that has an interpersonal aspect. Karterud (2015) noted that, typically, the events most productive for the group are those that generated some affect that was significant for the member. For example, Stacey might disclose that she argued with her mother the morning of the group session. Immediately, the therapist knows this event has the potential for a rich analysis given that the event was interpersonal and involved the generation of feeling. Stacey is then encouraged to delve into her inner world further. What was she feeling during the argument? Stacey indicates that she was feeling angry with her mother. On being asked what was driving her anger, Stacey responds that her mother's opening her mail provoked her. She goes on to state that preoccupation with the argument resulted in her attending minimally to work tasks. Stacey's exploration led her to identify an event (the argument) associated with affect (anger) and a consequence of the angry exchange (inattention at work). She thereby had achieved a coherent narrative and had mentalized the event.

Often, members struggle to mentalize their internal states. It is here that the therapist assists them in clarifying those states and connecting them to other states and behaviors, both through their questioning and through their encouragement of other members to investigate a given member's mind. For example, Stacey might have easily talked about her expressing her disagreement with her mother's behavior but not being able to acknowledge having angry feelings toward her mother. It is here—through the group's sensitive questioning—that Stacey is helped to achieve this realization. All group members who participate either through their questioning or their careful tracking of the discussion are receiving practice in the skill of mentalization. Those members who are addressing the protagonist's event are strengthening their capabilities in mind reading—sensing what is occurring internally with another person. The member whose event is being explored is acquiring greater competency in attending in productive ways to his or her mind. Both in reading their own and other members' minds, the members exhibit failures in mentalization. For example, when Stacey describes her mother's behavior, members might take her presentation of her mother as intrusive at face value. The therapist helps the group recognize the assumptions they are making and the need to gather more information to determine whether the assumptions are warranted.

No one protagonist is permitted to dominate the session. Rather, members take turns in presenting their events. The therapist monitors the time given to each event, recognizing that some events take longer than others to mentalize due to the characteristics of the event itself, those of the person relating the event, or the group climate at that time. The therapist, on discerning that a particular event has been sufficiently mentalized, encourages the member to stand back and take stock of the progress made. Doing so stimulates metacognition or cogitating about one's cognitive states, an

TABLE 4.2
Mentalization Model

Elements of the model	Characteristics of the model
View of psychological problems	Psychological problems are rooted in a failure to mentalize in the context of an attachment relationship.
Goals of model	The model seeks to support the development of healthy mentalization.
Methods of action	Members are engaged in mentalizing events within and outside the group as a means of gaining practice and feedback on mentalizing skills.
Intervention techniques	• Therapists encourage members to identify internal and external events, which they then mentalize. • Therapist takes care of group and members so that group becomes a secure base and members' attachment systems are activated. • Foster a not-knowing stance among members • Challenge pseudomentalizing • Regulate affect
Adaptation of the model to a brief time frame	Brief group experiences allow for psychoeducational training in mentalization sufficient to gain some understanding of the concept.
Use of group process	Group members use their interactions with one another to gain practice in mentalization in attachment relationships.

activity that strengthens the member's sense of self ("I am looking at my own thinking"). Table 4.2 summarizes the features of the mentalization model.

CLINICAL ILLUSTRATIONS OF THE PSYCHODYNAMIC FAMILY OF MODELS

We now illustrate the three approaches outlined in this chapter using three segments of a group. First, we illustrate the relatively unstructured psychodynamic approach. We proceed to the OR/S model, followed by a mentalization-informed therapy group. We use the same characters, all fictional, and each group scenario is a continuation of the prior one. This group took place within a PHP on the campus of a large psychiatric hospital. It contained seven members and two therapists.

Group Members

Darby, a woman in her late 20s, was placed on the inpatient unit after slashing her wrists and then was admitted to the PHP. Precipitating this suicide attempt was her discovery that her boyfriend of 3 months was having an affair. She had been in the PHP for 2 weeks.

Kathy, a woman in her mid-20s, entered the day treatment program directly after having sustained several weeks of vegetative symptoms of depression following the birth of her second child.

Ralph, a middle-aged retired marine, entered the hospital after being consumed by the unfounded belief that the FBI was investigating his military career. He conjectured that his neighbors were part of an FBI connection, and his repeated attempts to spy on their spying led to his commitment. He had been treated at a Veterans Affairs hospital, but when staff judged that the setting was exacerbating his fears, he was transferred to a private facility where he claimed to feel safe. He entered the PHP a week ago.

Delila, a 28-year-old transgender woman, entered the PHP after her employer's discovery of her gender identity led to her dismissal. Delila had made a serious suicide attempt. Delila was an assistant director at a social services agency that treated the elderly. She feared a future of unsuccessful attempts at gaining stable employment. This session is her first.

Frank, a highly obsessive middle-aged man, entered the hospital because the intensification of sexual preoccupations and his fear that others were aware of them prevented him from going to work. He had been in the day hospital program for 3 weeks and was being discharged in 2 weeks.

Serena, a woman in her early 30s, had attempted to kill herself and her baby by falling off of a bridge. Both were rescued. She claimed to have heard voices telling her to take this action. She had had a lengthy hospitalization, been transferred to the day treatment program, transferred back to the inpatient unit, and was now once again in the PHP.

Classic Model

This group format offers the group the greatest leeway of the three models to develop a train of associations, thereby permitting the emergence of unconscious elements. These, in turn, can be tied to members' conscious experiences and behaviors. In work with heretofore-hidden material, the therapist continually keeps in mind the group's stage of development.

The Session

One of the therapists opened the session by explaining that the purpose of the group was for members to learn about the thoughts and feelings that are attached to how they relate to one another. The therapist, Brenda, emphasized the importance of open, nonjudgmental communication and the willingness to give one another feedback on how they saw members relating to themselves and the other members. Then, the other therapist, Mike, asked each of the members to introduce themselves. The exchange presented next followed the introductions.

Frank: So, can you tell us a little bit about why you are here?

Delila: I lost my job, and it made me extremely sad and, actually, hopeless. There were complexities but let me just say that I was really good at what I did—I was an administrator . . . in an agency.

Ralph: Did you have problems with your supervisor? I know all about that!

Delila: I suppose you could say that. But as I said, it's complex, and I don't know if, at this point, I want to . . .

Frank: Don't feel as if you have to tell us everything about yourself. I never feel that I have to divulge everything in this group.

Darby: Frank, I don't see how you think we can help you and everybody if we aren't open with one another. [*She nods toward Brenda, the therapist.*] Brenda just said a few minutes ago that we should be open.

Serena: I don't think Brenda meant that we have to spill the beans in our first session here.

Darby: No, but I think pretty soon we all have to get to it. Otherwise, what's the point?

Frank: We can share some things without sharing everything.

Serena: I don't think that's how it works.

Therapist Brenda: Some members feel that it's important for a member to be willing to share everything that might be of concern, and others doubt whether it's necessary or even a good idea. Perhaps some of these concerns have to do with circumstances and situations outside the group. I'm wondering what it would be like to be open about the thoughts and feelings you are having to one another right within this room, right now.

[*Here, the therapist is attempting to help members identify their common positions and to establish the venue where work is most likely to be productive. A mature group eventually addresses the topic of personal secrets, but this group is not ready for such an undertaking, and the encouragement of members to disclose prematurely could adversely affect their continuing motivation to engage with the other members.]*

Delila: I feel I could do that—be open in that way.

Frank: Well, there again—I would think it would be smart for me to share some things but not everything. And that's exactly what I've done. I've told members things about them that irritated me and things that make me like them more, but I certainly haven't said everything that's gone through my mind.

Therapist Mike: When you [*looking around to all the members*] think of sharing everything that goes through your mind, do any feelings come up for you?

[*The therapist is helping members identify feelings that might restrain communications in the group.*]

Serena: Well, what goes through my mind in saying something that hurts someone's feelings and then I'm left with the guilt for the rest of the day, maybe longer.

Therapist Brenda: Who else can relate to Serena's worry?

Frank: Well, me, for sure. I've had things said to me from past groups, and they stung for a long time. I wouldn't want to do that to anyone else. I feel bad about myself most of the time, and I don't need any more ammunition.

Ralph: I would just worry about retaliation—I mean, you do something to someone, and what are they going to do? Sit around and take it? I don't think so.

Delila: I've never been in a group before, but it seems to me that if you say something with a good heart—really trying to give someone something they crave—then it's not going to be damaging. And, Ralph, if one of us senses that you are speaking for their benefit, I doubt if anyone would retaliate.

Ralph: I'm not so sure. You're too gentle to see the ugly side of folks.

Darby: In fact, I would appreciate hearing anything any of you have to say about me because, most of the time, it's just not possible to know what people are thinking about any of us . . . even if they're smiling and acting nice.

Serena: I agree with Darby. I really want to know what you all think about me.

Therapist Mike:	I'm hearing that group members have a couple of different feelings about sharing our impressions with one another. On the one hand, there is some fear about hurting another member and with it, concern about feeling guilty or worrying about retaliation. On the other hand, members are curious about others' impressions and see our group as a special place to learn about oneself. I suspect that the tension between wanting to share and fearing it is something that exists—perhaps in varying degrees—in each of us.

Comment on the Session

The therapist is helping members see the psychological forces that are linked to their behaviors in the group. Each member is seen as giving expression to an element that is likely present within the group as a whole. Because this is an early group—insofar as a new member is present—resistances to trust are likely to emerge prominently. Helping members to articulate them lays a foundation for greater openness among members.

Object Relations/Systems Group (Kibel Group)

This vignette illustrates a segment of a Kibel group with the same members as in the prior segment. However, in this group, members have been with one another for at least a week.

The Session

In the community meeting that preceded this meeting, a popular psychiatrist announced that he would be marrying a nurse on the upcoming weekend and would be vacationing with her in the Bahamas the subsequent week.

Kathy:	[To Serena] I heard you before the meeting say to the nurse that you wanted to be transferred back to the inpatient unit. I know why. There's that really good-looking resident you worked with while you were there.
Darby:	Yeah, we saw him come over here and visit you when you first arrived.
Ralph:	I remember that.
Serena:	[Looking at the therapist beseechingly] I really don't feel like being here today. [She rises to leave.]
Therapist Brenda:	Wait, Serena, I think perhaps you don't feel like being here because some things are upsetting you. In fact, I

think others in here may share your distress. It's important for you to stay here so we can explore them.

[*The departure of Serena from the group would not only intensify her sense of failure already stimulated by her need for first inpatient hospitalization and then day hospital treatment but would also make members more self-critical because they would have proof within the group that their show of aggression has destructive consequences.*]

Therapist Mike: The group has been focusing on Serena's visit from her psychiatric resident, but maybe something about this special visit is making the group feel a little nervous, maybe a little annoyed.

Darby: [*Rolls her eyes*] Can't you take anything at face value?

Kathy: [*To Darby*] Yeah, well, the real reason you mentioned the cute doctor is because you are feeling edgy since your own dream doctor told us he is getting married and leaving for the Bahamas. You were prickly during lunch. I think you're afraid that you will miss him.

Darby: I'm glad he's leaving because he's getting you-know-who out of my grill.

Frank: I've been in many programs like this over the last 20 years, and it's quite common for staff to marry one another. I've heard that 65% of all marriages are forged in the workplace.

Therapist Brenda: Maybe so, Frank, but it sounds like this particular marriage may be upsetting to group members.

Darby: I don't care who or what he marries . . . and just like I said, I'm glad he is giving me a break from her because she is annoying in the extreme with her constant checking.

Kathy: Amen to that.

Therapist Brenda: A lot of intrusions occur here, and there's nothing to like about them.

[*The therapist acknowledges the reality in relation to their feelings.*]

Darby: But the one thing I don't like is seeing him run off to the Bahamas when I have just one more week to spend in this place. If I have a setback, it will be on him.

Frank:	Be realistic. Do you expect him to make arrangements around your hospitalization? We'd all like that to happen, but it never will.
Darby:	I didn't say that I expected anything. I don't expect nothing!
Therapist Mike:	I'm sensing right now that there's a shared sense of abandonment here in the group and in the community with the departure of two staff members. And, understandably, some anger over being abandoned.
	[*The therapist does not pursue the notion that the reaction is an overreaction. In this model, what is important is acknowledging the feelings as coherent and understandable responses to the circumstance at hand.*]
Darby:	It's not that easy for me to open up to someone. Remember when I started here 2 weeks ago—it took me about four days before I even said one word. Then, I got to like . . . sort of trust this doctor and he just . . . evaporates! So, this morning, I started feeling sad, but then I said to myself, "You're just a hard luck case. You don't have anybody to care about you . . . no family or nothing . . . so you get upset about the doctor like he's family." Like someone said, "Therapy is like buying a friend."
Frank:	The saying is, "Therapy is the purchase of friendship," and it is (a) true and (b) very pathetic.
Delila:	I don't think it's pathetic at all—it's very natural to care about your therapist and to feel really annoyed when he's not there. I would feel the same way.
Serena:	I left my therapist and, still, I was annoyed with him that he couldn't follow me here. What Delila says is true—it's just human to feel that way.
Therapist Brenda:	[*Speaking broadly to the group*] It sounds as though Delila, Serena, and maybe others can relate to Darby's feelings of missing her therapist and anger that you've been placed in a position of missing your therapist. And, at the same time, there's a wish to protect yourself from such losses maybe by putting the relationship down, seeing it as something "pathetic."
	[*Here, the therapist is aiming to give expression to the two dominant forces in the group—the yearning for a connection with a caregiver and the countervailing wish to protect the self from that yearning, while also conveying once again the legitimacy of these reactions.*]

Comment on the Session

The therapist's first responsibility is maintaining the boundaries of the group, a task the therapist performed by getting all members to stay and translate feelings into words rather than actions. The therapist has an awareness of some of the current tensions in the unit, one of which is the departure of a popular psychiatrist. The fact that he is marrying a nurse is understandably evocative of envy on the part of program participants. The therapist opens a door for members to share feelings about this transition, and members walk through. Members share feelings not only about the departure but also an aspect of life in the community—loss of privacy. The therapist conveys that these reactions are perfectly understandable given the circumstances. As one or more members give voice to what might be disturbing content, the therapist attempts to convey that those members are not alone with that element. This kind of intervention—usually entailing a group-as-a-whole statement—creates safety for those members who have repudiated an element but are moving toward acknowledging it. It also helps those members giving expression to the element to feel less alone.

Mentalization Group

The Session

This vignette illustrating a mentalization approach finds our same members in a session of a group that has enjoyed a constant membership for 2 weeks. This was the group's 10th session. Darby, who thought she was leaving the program the prior week has been forced to stay after her suicidal ideation intensified following the departure of her psychiatrist.

The therapists begin the group by sharing with members their thoughts about the last session. Therapist Brenda posed to the group the question of whether the group should pick up on one of the threads from the last session or pursue a new event.

> *Delila:* I think we should get back to Ralph. [*Turning to him*] You said a little bit about what has been going on with you, but you were so tense, it seemed you could hardly talk. Then this morning, I heard you yelling about something.

> *Therapist Brenda:* [*To Delila*] It sounds as though you've been thinking about Ralph and maybe having some feelings about him, too.

> *Delila:* That's right. Fear is what I was feeling. And concern. Deep concern. Ralph, you seem desperate, and I'm worried you are going to do something desperate.

> [*Ralph is silent as he hangs his head.*]

Therapist Mike:	Ralph, are you having any reaction to what Delila is saying to you?
Frank:	C'mon, Buddy. Open up.
Ralph:	[*Smiles at Frank and then looks at Delila*] I feel comforted. [*To Delila*] I know that when you say something you mean it. I feel grateful that you would even think about me. I wish I had a friend like you on the outside, but I don't have any sort of friend on the outside. I have to worry about everybody. I learned this morning that I am going to be evicted from my apartment because of the disturbance I caused there when I accused my neighbors of being part of a spy ring.
Therapist Mike:	I think maybe we can be most helpful to you by looking at some reactions you have in here that might be similar. I remember that when you first came to the group, you said you were kind of suspicious of a few of us. But now?
	[*The therapist moves the issue into the here and now where it is more readily addressed and engages the other members more actively.*]
Ralph:	No, not so much.
Therapist Mike:	That's what I thought, but I needed to ask.
	[*The therapist models checking out assumptions about others' minds.*]
Therapist Brenda:	When we began, who in the group made you fearful?
Frank:	Me? Usually, it's me.
Kathy:	You can tell me if it's me. I'm okay with that.
Ralph:	Well, no. Three people in particular . . . Darby and you two [*indicating the two therapists*].
Therapist Mike:	And now? You said, "Not so much." It sounds as though sometimes you do become afraid.
Ralph:	Well, it's much better, but still you can and you *do* sometimes.
Darby:	Guess I'm in good company. But what is it that we do?
Therapist Brenda:	Good question, Darby.
	[*Therapist sees Darby obtaining information for her mentalizing efforts and reinforces this activity.*]

Ralph: You ask many questions. It gives that I'm-being-investigated feeling.

Delila: "Investigated" in a bad way? Like they're trying to get information about you to hurt you?

Ralph: Well, that's how it seems to me in the moment. Just like my neighbors. But in here, I'm off base. Out there, I'm not.

Kathy: So, you're saying you don't always feel the therapists and Darby are trying to hurt you?

Ralph: No, not most of the time. Most of the time, I feel you're [*speaking to Darby and the two therapists*] trying to help me by your questions. But, say, if Darby asks me questions rapidly—one after another—I say to myself "Who's she working for?"

Therapist Brenda: And then you feel . . .? I'm trying to put my finger on how that makes you react.

Ralph: Really scared. Trapped.

Therapist Mike: I like, Ralph, how you put together the connection of the pace with which Darby and maybe others ask you questions and the thoughts and feelings it evokes. When people ask you rapid-fire questions, you feel fear. I could imagine myself or, really, any of us responding in that way. Yeah, I think you have a handle on the pattern.

Darby: I ask questions quickly when I get really worried about someone, not because I'm working for the FBI or anything like that.

Serena: Darby, I feel glad when you ask me a lot of questions, like someone is finally paying attention.

Delila: I understand what Ralph is saying, though. I've had that—if I see someone staring at me, I get unnerved.

Ralph: Yeah, it's like "Why all of the interest?"

Delila: Exactly! But you know what? Sometimes it's nothing bad at all . . . that's what I've learned. Most of the time, it's okay. And I think you've learned that, too, from these three people. I don't think they've ever been menacing toward you.

Therapist Brenda: Does that seem on target, Ralph?

Ralph: For sure! It's just something that goes through my mind, but it's way off in this case, and I have to remind myself of that and try not to jump to any conclusions.

Therapist Mike: I have a sense we just accomplished a great deal. Ralph, it sounds like you're moving into a different frame of mind, one in which you can identify different explanations that might correspond to that thought you have that people might be after you. And once you have those explanations, you slow down and collect the evidence to see which idea fits what actually is happening. I'm wondering, Ralph, whether you and others feel we are ready to move on.

Comment on the Session

The members of this group demonstrated their developing mentalizing skills, borne out of the group's nine sessions of practice. The group dove into sharing events that would lend themselves to mentalizing activities. Delila realized that Ralph was struggling with an emotionally charged happening that could be explored to his benefit and relief. Ralph was easily able to access feelings within the group that paralleled those outside. However, he benefitted from guided questioning to identify what specifically evokes the fear. He furthered his mentalizing efforts by comparing his thoughts about other members' motives with how they actually behaved over time. He was thereby able to achieve an enhanced awareness that others might have motives other than what his quick inferences would suggest.

Comparison of the Three Models

One dimension on which these three models vary is structure. As we move from the classic to the Kibel to the mentalization-informed model, we see increased levels of structure. In the classic model, the therapist has knowledge of characteristic group dynamics and a readiness to tap them to aid members in pursuing their therapeutic goals. The therapist in the Kibel model also possesses and uses this knowledge but, in addition, is armed with a grasp of the events and dynamics of the larger treatment community. That therapist is vigilant to see what linkages might exist between the dysregulated feelings members are experiencing and the local events that might have precipitated them. In the mentalization approach, the therapist creates a structured session consisting of phases the therapist manages. In the opening phase of this vignette, we could see the cotherapy team helping members to mentalize about the prior session and then moving the group into addressing affect-laden events identified for individual members. The therapists would also assist the members in closing the session. For example, the therapists might direct the members' attention to any loose ends that had to be tied up.

The level of structure in the group is related to the variation in group goals among the models. In the classic model, the therapists are fostering a group process that will enable members to gain access to conflictual material and work toward a more integrative resolution to the conflicts. Better resolutions, it is postulated, give rise to stances that are less defensive vis-à-vis self and other, a state that also lessens vulnerability to symptoms. In the vignette, then, we saw therapists Mike and Brenda helping members address the issue of trust ("To what extent can I trust other members in the group?") via decision making in relation to self-disclosure. The therapists use interpretations as a vehicle for change. In contrast, the Kibel group is focused on the much shorter term goal of assisting members in becoming sufficiently affectively regulated to be able to leave their intensive treatment program. Whereas the classic model seeks to assist members in progressing to a higher developmental level, the Kibel model aims to fortify members' premorbid defenses so that they can move to a long-term treatment situation in which goals such as those posited by the classic model can be fruitfully pursued. In this process, they use largely clarifying comments as interventions. Group therapy focusing on mentalizing is at root a skills training approach. It homes in on the skill of mentalizing in interpersonal and affect-activating situations because this capacity consistently is associated with a variety of positive mental health outcomes. For some members, successful application of the model might help in the reacquisition of mentalizing skills. For others, the treatment might strengthen their capacities for mentalizing beyond what they had achieved on a premorbid basis.

The systems perspective that informs the conducting of a Kibel group requires that the therapist operate on the supposition that members are subject to the common forces of the broader dynamics of the treatment community. For this reason, the therapist can begin by addressing a single member's concern but then broaden the formulation to the group. Likewise, the therapist can make a reasonable assumption that members identify with one another's concerns, especially if they involve their life with others in the program. These assumptions enable the group to maintain an unstructured character even though the group has a distinct focus. In the mentalizing group, each member must have opportunities to practice the skill of mentalization. Although mentalization-oriented group therapists do assume that members engage in vicarious learning, the presumption is also that the individual member's work is important. Accordingly, the therapist in the mentalization group does more coordinating and directing, relative to other psychodynamic approaches, to ensure that all members have practice opportunities. Moreover, the therapist rarely uses the kinds of group-as-a-whole statements (Karterud & Bateman, 2012) commonly used in the OR/S approach.

All these models, but particularly the mentalizing approaches, require openness on the part of the therapist, a willingness to share his or her mentalizing activity with the group (Karterud & Bateman, 2012). Mentalizing approaches see the therapist's sharing of his or her mentalizing activity as stimulating the members' mentalizing processes.

STATUS OF THE RESEARCH

Outcome Findings

Studies testing the effectiveness of general psychodynamic approaches in group psychotherapy are almost nonexistent. Although some studies have been included as part of a larger meta-analysis (e.g., Leichsenring & Leibing, 2003; Leichsenring & Rabung, 2008), they did not form a sufficiently large subgroup to warrant a separate statistical analysis. One reason for the dearth of research is the tendency of psychodynamic group psychotherapists to focus on process rather than outcome (Kösters, Burlingame, Nachtigall, & Strauss, 2006). In some studies, process is examined in relation to outcome. For example, Dinger and Schauenburg (2010) investigated the relationship between members' individual perceptions of group cohesion and interpersonal style in their effects on outcome in 327 participants in 12-week inpatient group psychotherapy. The investigators reported significant symptomatic change with a .95 effect size (ES). They also found that the stronger the perception of cohesion, the greater the symptomatic improvement. Moreover, the investigators found an interaction between the group members' degree of affiliation and degree of perceived cohesion. Members low in affiliation had greater symptomatic improvement when cohesion increased over the course of the treatment; for members low in affiliation, a slight decrease in cohesion led to poorer outcomes. This study lacked a comparison group, most likely because (even though outcome data was collected) the outcome aspect of the study was not the emphasis. However, findings suggest that personality variables might be key in understanding what group atmosphere produces the most favorable outcomes in members.

Kirchmann et al. (2009) provided another example of a process study that had implications for outcome evaluation. A total of 289 inpatients received psychodynamic group psychotherapy at six different hospitals. The investigators explored the relationship between participants' attachment styles and the Dusseldorf therapeutic factors as they affected outcome. Overall, investigators found a large ES of .70 for an index of symptom severity and a moderate ES of .42 for change on interpersonal measures. More central to their aim was the finding that attachment characteristics of the members could affect group climate, which in turn affects outcome.

Explorations of psychodynamic groups that link process and outcome in IHPs and PHPs are extremely valuable. They help practitioners understand how groups can be run to produce optimal outcomes. For example, Kirchmann et al. (2009) suggested the importance of attending to members' attachment styles. An earlier study by Greene and Cole (1991) drew attention to the level of functioning of the group member as a determinant of the usefulness of the psychodynamic group. MacKenzie and Tschuschke (1993), studying long-term inpatient groups, demonstrated the importance of the member's relatedness or sense of connection to the group as a determinant of that member's success in reaching treatment goals. They demonstrated that when members do achieve positive change, they can sustain it for at least an 18-month period. Tschuschke, MacKenzie, Haaser, and Janke (1996) found that when in the life of a group (first, second, third, or fourth quartile) members do their most intensive work determines what they can derive from group participation. For example, in-depth work at the beginning of the group's life is associated with highly favorable outcomes at the 18-month follow-up. Such a finding suggests that the therapist must ensure that all members are fully engaged with the group from the beginning of its life. Although process–outcome studies are helpful, they do not provide the essential knowledge of how psychodynamic groups fare against other types of groups, knowledge that can be gleaned only from pitting psychodynamic groups against alternate models using a randomized design.

Object Relations/System Model

Our review of the literature failed to reveal any outcome studies in which a Kibel group was contrasted with either groups run according to alternate models or control groups. The research on this model might be especially sparse because the target of change is intrapsychic. Concepts such as "the detoxification of aggression" are not readily translated into operational terms. However, some of the theoretical postulates of this model have been investigated. One major supposition is that events, issues, and affective facets of the unit affect the process of the inpatient psychotherapy group. The findings of a series of classic studies (Astrachan, Harrow, & Flynn, 1968; Harrow, Astrachan, Becker, Miller, & Schwartz, 1967; Karterud, 1989) support this supposition.

Another distinctive feature of the OR/S model is the notion that processing negative feelings such as hostility—particularly toward members or aspects of the community—can be helpful to members. Koch (1983) directed his research team to tape sessions from a psychodynamically oriented group in a PHP and to analyze the degrees of different types of affects. He found that the greater the expressed hostility and affection, the better the outcomes as measured by increased self-esteem and diminished subjective anxiety. Karterud (1989) found that when members of inpatient groups were able to use splitting and projection to express anger toward staff, they also were able to participate in community life in positive ways. These findings suggest that the focus of the OR/S model of helping members to tolerate feelings of hostility is an appropriate one, given the abundance of aggression on an inpatient unit. Moreover, such work might enhance favorable outcomes.

Still, this model merits a rigorous empirical evaluation because it fills a niche. It is one of the few psychodynamic group models that can be used in extremely brief time frames. Moreover, this model warrants evaluation because it is used in Western Europe and, to a lesser extent, the United States. The approach can be used not only in the psychotherapy group but also in the community meeting (Kibel, 2003), thereby lending coherence to the overall therapeutic efforts in the IHP, PHP, or RTC. Research on this model must be directed toward assessing its success in achieving its specific goals—fostering the reacquisition of premorbid defenses, greater tolerance for negative affects, and diminished self-derogation because of negative affects. Because the model is aimed to alleviate group tensions, another relevant outcome might be the climate of the unit.

Mentalization Groups

Those models that have emerged since the blossoming of the evidence-based practice movement show a much stronger orientation toward a continual examination of the model's success in producing outcomes consistent with the model. The mentalization model is no exception to this trend: The effort to study the effectiveness of the mentalization model has gone hand-in-hand with its development. In 1999, Bateman and Fonagy reported on their landmark study based at a psychoanalytically oriented[3] PHP. The investigators randomly assigned 38 individuals, all of whom were diagnosed as having borderline personality disorders, to either a PHP or treatment as usual (TAU). In the PHP, over a period of 18 months, patients received mentalization-informed group and individual therapy. A broad array of measures was collected among which were number of suicide attempts and acts of self-harm, degree of symptom distress, and quality of interpersonal functioning. The investigators found that on all these measures, substantial improvement occurred at

---

[3]Whether we use the term *psychoanalytic* or *psychodynamic* in characterizing the research depends on what term was used in the research article.

6 months and continued to grow over the next year. In a first follow-up study (Bateman & Fonagy, 2001), participants in the earlier study were assessed posttreatment every 3 months over an 18-month period and maintained their gains. As Bateman and Fonagy (2001) noted, they also "showed a statistically significant continued improvement on most measures in contrast to the control group of patients who showed only limited change during the same period" (p. 45). In a subsequent follow-up study, Bateman and Fonagy (2008) assessed participants 5 years after the participants completed all treatment. They found that the mentalization group was superior to the TAU group on a range of variables including suicidality, diagnostic status, interpersonal functioning, and global functioning.

Bateman and Fonagy (2008) acknowledged that only a general conclusion could be drawn from this series of studies: The mentalization group fared better than the TAU group. No particular element of the package, including group psychotherapy, can be correctly identified as a causal agent in the positive change. However, group psychotherapy from the standpoint of the intensity of treatment was one of the major components of the package, and hence, their findings are promising for the usefulness of mentalization-based group psychotherapy with this patient population. Also encouraging is the fact that others have achieved similarly favorable findings. For example, in the Netherlands, Bales et al. (2012) tested a long-term mentalization program including a form of group psychotherapy (the authors labeled it *mentalizing cognitive group therapy*) with patients with severe borderline disorders, including those with comorbid substance abuse disorders, in the less restrictive day hospital setting. The PHP lasted for 18 months and was followed by 18 months of mentalizing group psychotherapy. On a host of outcome variables such as interpersonal functioning, symptom distress, suicide attempt, and care consumption, the investigators obtained ESs ranging from .7 to 1.7 when pretreatment and posttreatment measures were compared. The premature termination rate of 15.5% was relatively low, suggesting that the patients themselves saw the treatment as beneficial. This study's findings are important because they support the notion that a wide range of individuals with borderline disorders can be successfully treated with a mentalizing approach within a PHP setting.

In a pilot study, Laurenssen et al. (2014) explored the usefulness of a mentalization treatment with adolescents. In a Dutch IHP, participants—all female—received 4-week group sessions in addition to a variety of other treatment components for approximately a year. Over the course of program participation, participants showed less symptom distress (ES = 1.46), self-control (ES = 1.29), social concordance (ES = .70), identity integration (ES = 1.42), and responsibility (ES = .58). Notably, no patient in the study manifested deterioration. What establishes this investigation as a pilot study is the lack of a control group. Nonetheless, the severity of psychopathology of the participants makes unlikely the possibility that members improved primarily through spontaneous remission or some other nonspecific factor.

Brand, Hecke, Rietz, and Schultz-Venrath (2016) compared two of the models presented in this chapter—psychodynamic and mentalization based. A total of 174 participants in a PHP were randomly assigned to the two groups. The investigators found that the two groups were comparable in producing symptom relief and improved interpersonal functioning, but the mentalization group was superior in fostering mentalization of the self (as opposed to mentalization of others), including 12 months following the conclusion of therapy.

One emphasis in the mentalization research is on the level of personality organization rather than specific diagnostic categories. For example, as noted in this section, a number of studies can be found that look at borderline and psychotic levels of personality organization. Given that these levels correspond to those of individuals who enter IHPs, PHPs, and RTCs, this emphasis is convenient. However, those programs that focus on specific diagnostic conditions (e.g., an eating disorders unit) are likely to benefit from studies testing the effectiveness of the model with that category.

The Society of Clinical Psychology of the American Psychological Association rates mentalization-based treatment for borderline individuals as one with moderate support (Society of Clinical Psychology, 2016). For it to be deemed "strong," the effectiveness of mentalization-informed treatment would have to be established by independent investigators conducting well-designed studies. As Weber (2017) pointed out, mentalization treatments were developed in day hospitals in Great Britain in which the length of treatment spanned 18 months. He pointed to the need to determine the model's usefulness on a cross-cultural basis, recognizing that different cultures provide widely ranging spans of treatment. Mentalization treatment certainly merits the investment in well-designed studies that focus on the different components of mentalization programs within hospitals and RTCs. Only in this way will we know the criticalness of the group therapy modality to the successful delivery of this relatively new approach.

DEMANDS OF THE MODELS

Clinical Mission

None of the models featured in this chapter require that the unit or program at large embrace a psychoanalytic perspective on psychopathology. Nonetheless, it stands to reason that the potency of these approaches would be increased by the application within an environment that supports their goals and methods of intervention. Mentalization-based groups teach members new skills, and any skill profits from repetition in different settings. Therefore, members of a mentalization group who are exposed to mentalizing opportunities elsewhere in the program receive more substantial aid in moving toward treatment goals than clients who engage in this work primarily in their group time.

All the models described in this chapter could play a role in helping staff manage their reactions as they work with often highly challenging populations. The classic model continually reminds staff that patients engage in destructive behaviors for good reasons based on their early relationships with caregivers. The OR/S model helps staff recognize that aspects of the hospital environment add, often greatly, to the patients' stress loads. It also abets staff in setting more realistic goals for patients than they often embrace. Mentalizing approaches provide staff with skills to use when they find themselves affectively activated by patients. Knowledge of these potential benefits could help the therapist make a case for the broader use of a model.

Admittedly, procuring a staff's agreement to adopt a new model program wide is a tall order. At a minimum, the therapist has to ensure that the application of any of these models is not undermined by members' exposure in other parts of the program to ideas contrary to the assumptions of these models. For example, the OR/S model holds that the awareness and expression of negatively toned affect are useful to members. A program and its staff that conspire to assist patients in obtaining strict control over feelings through the institution of a highly structured regime would operate at cross-purposes in the group. Even an individual staff member could limit the group's effectiveness with a given member by expressing disapproval of particular exchanges:

> *Tom:* It was an exciting session today—we let Dr. Smith know how frustrated we've been with him.
>
> *Staff member:* But Dr. Smith is not responsible for your difficulties. Only you are. The only person with whom you should have frustration is yourself.

Within the framework of the OR/S approach, such a response on the part of the staff member would be antitherapeutic in that it would encourage any self-derogating tendency of Tom's. It would also undermine the effort of the group to help members link their feelings with precipitating events as a means of assisting in the restoration of the premorbid defense of splitting. Likewise, working at cross-purposes with a mentalization group would be staff encouragement for members to take immediate action on their feelings.

Context of the Group

The OR/S model requires that the psychotherapy group must be ensconced within an IHP, PHP, or RTC. The structure of the group assumes that the group has little autonomy from the larger program community. Any structural factor that increases the group's autonomy requires some adaptation of the model for its optimal application. This model can be applied most easily when the group takes place on the unit. A group that is held away from the unit and that combines members of different units is much more likely to achieve the status of a system rather than a subsystem. It might develop goals, values, and norms that differ from those of other systems in the hospital. Certainly, the dynamics of each residential unit, as well as those of the various departments and the broader institution itself, all affect the group. However, these influences are more indirect, interacting, and complicated. Linkages between in-the-group and on-the unit experiences to which all (or most) members can relate are less readily drawn.

Mentalization-based treatment presumes that the individual is receiving both individual and group psychotherapy, as well as, possibly, other treatments. Moreover, this approach requires therapists to share a theoretical system and to support one another in understanding the patient and meeting his or her needs. In other words, mentalization-based treatment requires a team approach (Karterud & Bateman, 2012). Not all IHPs, PHPs, and RTCs can accommodate such requirements. In such an instance, the group therapist would have to use mentalization-informed group psychotherapy. In this latter stand-alone approach, the members could be drawn from one or multiple units of the facility.

Temporal Variables

The psychodynamic family of models allows for a range of goals to be pursued. To the extent that a model entails intrapsychic change that has long-term ramifications for the individual's functioning, more time is needed. The Kibel group, which is based on a setting in which group members come and go, makes no temporal demands on the treatment. This model seeks only to restore members to their premorbid level of functioning. However, mentalization-informed group psychotherapy, which fosters a shift in how members respond internally to affective-interpersonal events requires considerably longer. In the research studies we cited, members remained in a PHP or RTC group for a year and then have an extended stint of outpatient group psychotherapy. However, it would be entirely possible for a brief IHP group to provide the psychoeducational component of mentalization-informed therapy while offering members resources to pursue this type of therapy in the community.

For most of these applications, the length of the session varies from 60 to 90 minutes. Fonagy et al. (2017) recommended 75 minutes, and a lesser period would accommodate with difficulty the structure of providing each member with a period of the group's time. The OR/S model does not make this same demand given that many of the interventions are at the level of the group.

Size of the Group

All these models could be used with a relatively small number of members (e.g., four members) or a much larger group (e.g., 10 members). For the OR/S group, because the most potent interventions are addressed to the group as a whole and deal with a common reality among members, the group can reach members who may not have had an opportunity to speak during the session. For the mentalization-informed group, the fact that each member is the focus of individual work necessitates careful consideration of expanding the group beyond nine. Fonagy et al. (2017) noted that six to nine members is an optimal size. Of course, as the length of the session increases so too does the number of members the group can accommodate. Also, for all types of groups, the therapist must attend to members' sense of safety—beyond a certain point, the intimidating character of the group might limit the good the group can accomplish. Also, as the level of ego functioning of members declines, so should the size of the group for members to experience safety in the sessions (Agazarian & Peters, 1981).

Composition of the Group

The OR/S and mentalization-informed models were developed with a particular population in mind: individuals organized at the borderline level. Both models have been adapted to persons at the psychotic levels as well (Weijers et al., 2016). Because mentalization difficulties have been demonstrated to figure into various other symptom patterns (see Allen, 2013; Rudden, Milrod, Target, Ackerman, & Graf, 2006), it seems that this model could accommodate a wide variety of types and levels of psychopathology. However, it is less clear whether the OR/S model as presented in this chapter could be useful to individuals who have milder forms of character pathology or who present with difficulties with anxiety, depression, or other symptom patterns. Although the restoration of splitting might not be an appropriate goal for some of these individuals, an alternate goal involving the restoration of their premorbid level of intrapsychic functioning might be developed. Such a change would have significant implications for the therapist's interventions, leading the therapist to shift from a supportive to a more exploratory style of intervening.

All applications of the psychoanalytic approach provide some technical resources to address a group in which cultural differences are present among the members. For example, to the extent that ethnic tensions that arise in the group are due to the members' need to export negative internal material on others, these dynamics can within all approaches be part of the group exploration. Mentalizing work can be particularly useful in its encouragement of members to be curious about one another's perspectives. However, for a psychoanalytic therapist to do the multicultural work that is sometimes demanded by the struggles that members present, certain modifications in psychodynamic technique might be needed. As Chen, Kakkad, and Balzano (2008) pointed out, often in process-oriented psychotherapy groups, members are encouraged to focus on the here and now and make a disclosure of a horizontal nature (i.e., what reactions are being currently stimulated by the other members). For individuals who have withstood experiences of stigmatization and discrimination, the opportunity to speak about these events and their effects on the person might be important both for therapeutic alliance and the individual's capacity to bond with other members. This model, like the cognitive behavior therapy model, was developed with Western values as its core. Restraint of feelings and reluctance to self-disclose are at the core of a more collectivist society. Disagreeing with authority would be even more difficult and might require some preparation on the part of the patient, many of whom would not want to disagree in the name of harmony. In contrast, this model offers a relational approach, which is a more natural fit for Latinos who value *personalismo* (personal relationships with individuals rather than institutions) and *confianza* (trust and closeness within a relationship).

Therapist Variables

Although none of the models presented in this chapter require a cotherapy team, all potentially benefit from it. For example, in the OR/S approach, therapists can assist one another in managing countertransference reactions. When one therapist is the object of members' emotional reactions, the other therapist can help members process it. Finally, the presence of two therapists lessens the strength of members' fears that they will be abandoned if they acknowledge aggression toward the leader. In the mentalization-informed group, a cotherapy team is invaluable in mentalizing the group before and after each session. Moreover, in a mentalization-informed group, attention must be given both to the individual whose event the group is considering and to other group members as they also process the event. These demands are better met when they are shared. Fonagy et al. (2017) recommended that cotherapy is particularly important when members with comorbid problems or propensities toward self-destructive behaviors populate the group. The mentalization-informed approach requires that cotherapists give attention to their functioning as a unit, and in fact, the mentalization-based Group Therapy Adherence and Quality Rating Scale includes an item specifically addressing cotherapists' functioning (Karterud, 2015).

Given the roots of the models presented in this chapter in psychodynamic theory, a good background in its principles abets therapists in using these models to best advantage. Still, both the OR/S and mentalization-informed models can be delivered, provided that one staff member who can serve in a supervisory role can provide oversight of the groups. Therapists-in-training can benefit from the high level of structure these models provide. Less structured applications of the psychodynamic approach are more demanding of the therapist's theoretical and technical knowledge.

All the models assume that the therapist has a capacity to recognize those inner events that the therapy situation stimulates in both the therapist and group members and use them to deepen the therapeutic work. The OR/S model requires therapists' ability to tolerate the expression of intense negative feelings that might be directed toward them. For new therapists, such tolerance might be difficult to achieve, and close supervision is likely necessary (Van Wagoner, 2000). Mentalization therapy demands that the therapist can mentalize. Karterud and Bateman (2012) noted, "The mental processes of the therapist are open to the group and become an important element in stimulating the mentalizing process" (p. 98). A positive development among the community of practitioners using mentalizing approaches is the effort to develop training modules in mentalization for trainees. For example, Ensink et al. (2013) compared trainees who were randomly assigned to a 2-hour session in either mentalization or didactic training on treatment plans for different types of psychopathology. Mentalization training involved "encouraging and training students to make effective use of their personal and affective reactions to the patient in order to gain a more nuanced and unique comprehension of the past and present experiences of the patient" (p. 530). The investigators found that although mentalization increased for those students obtaining training in mentalizing skills, it decreased in students receiving the lecture on the treatment of psychopathology. For our purposes, what is important is knowing that the cognitive and emotional skills are relevant to the delivery of these approaches and that efforts are underway to find training packages that foster them. Institutions that provide resources for training give the therapist leeway to choose a model that makes such a demand on the therapist's capabilities.

SUMMARY

Ever since psychotherapy groups have been conducted in inpatient settings, the psychodynamic approach has been one theoretical frame that has guided these groups. With the emergence of PHPs and RTCs, the psychodynamic approach has continued to exert a shaping role on the treatment terrain. In relation to other theoretical approaches, such as cognitive behavior therapy, the psychodynamic perspective has been slower to take into account some of the realities of these contemporary treatment environments. However, that is rapidly changing. Group psychotherapists who also happen to be psychodynamic are seeing the emergence of new models that are geared to the psychological problems of individuals in these settings and to the time frame of treatment and other contextual variables. Less structured versions of psychodynamic group psychotherapy would be most suitable in settings in which members' tenures are longer and in which members have the internal resources to take advantage of exploratory interventions.

The vast majority of IHP, PHP, and RTC patients are likely to be best served by a more structured psychodynamic model. This chapter featured two structured models. The OR/S model seeks to enhance members' functioning by reinstating those defenses that supported members' highest level of functioning in the community. A distinctive feature of the OR/S model is its capacity to be used in the briefest time frames—even one or two sessions of group participation. Unfortunately, this model has not been subjected to empirical scrutiny, even though certain elements of the model have received support. Approaches centered on mentalizing that have emerged on the group psychotherapy terrain share with the OR/S model the effort to take into account the customary intrapsychic pathologies of individuals who commonly present in IHP, PHP, and RTCs. This family of approaches targets that deficit or weakness that is associated with affective dysregulation and various dysfunctional behaviors—mentalization. The premise of the model is that by enhancing a group member's capacity to mentalize, the individual can achieve less distress, higher interpersonal functioning, diminished suicidality, greater vocational success, and a diminished need for ongoing care. Although these outcomes have been observed, what contribution group psychotherapy makes in a larger treatment program is yet to be determined.

REFERENCES

Agazarian, Y., & Peters, R. (1981). *The visible and invisible group: Two perspectives on group psychotherapy and group process.* London, England: Routledge & Kegan Paul.

Agazarian, Y. M. (2001). *Systems-centered approach to inpatient group psychotherapy.* London, England: Jessica Kingsley.

Ainsworth, M. D. S., Blehar, M. C., Waters, E., & Wall, S. N. (2015). *Patterns of attachment: A psychological study of the strange situation.* Hove, England: Psychology Press. (Original work published 1978)

Allen, J. G. (2013). *Restoring mentalizing in attachment relationships: Treating trauma with plain old therapy.* Arlington, VA: American Psychiatric Publishing.

American Psychiatric Association. (2013). *Diagnostic and statistical manual of mental disorders* (5th ed.). Arlington, VA: Author.

Astrachan, B. M., Harrow, M., & Flynn, H. R. (1968). Influence of the value-system of a psychiatric setting on behavior in group therapy meetings. *Social Psychiatry, 3*, 165–172. http://dx.doi.org/10.1007/BF00577947

Bakali, J. V., Wilberg, T., Klungsøyr, O., & Lorentzen, S. (2013). Development of group climate in short- and long-term psychodynamic group psychotherapy. *International Journal of Group Psychotherapy, 63*, 366–393. http://dx.doi.org/10.1521/ijgp.2013.63.3.366

Bales, D., van Beek, N., Smits, M., Willemsen, S., Busschbach, J. J., Verheul, R., & Andrea, H. (2012). Treatment outcome of 18-month, day hospital mentalization-based treatment (MBT) in patients with severe borderline personality disorder in the Netherlands. *Journal of Personality Disorders, 26*, 568–582. http://dx.doi.org/10.1521/pedi.2012.26.4.568

Bateman, A., & Fonagy, P. (2001). Treatment of borderline personality disorder with psychoanalytically oriented partial hospitalization: An 18-month follow-up. *The American Journal of Psychiatry, 158*, 36–42. http://dx.doi.org/10.1176/appi.ajp.158.1.36

Bateman, A., & Fonagy, P. (2004). *Psychotherapy for borderline personality disorder: Mentalization based treatment.* Oxford, England: Oxford University Press.

Bateman, A., & Fonagy, P. (2006). *Mentalization-based treatment for borderline personality disorder: A practical guide.* Oxford, England: Oxford University Press. http://dx.doi.org/10.1093/med/9780198570905.001.0001

Bateman, A., & Fonagy, P. (2008). 8-year follow-up of patients treated for borderline personality disorder: Mentalization-based treatment versus treatment as usual. *The American Journal of Psychiatry, 165*, 631–638. http://dx.doi.org/10.1176/appi.ajp.2007.07040636

Bateman, A., & Fonagy, P. (2010). Mentalization based treatment for borderline personality disorder. *World Psychiatry, 9*, 11–15. http://dx.doi.org/10.1002/j.2051-5545.2010.tb00255.x

Bion, W. R. (1959). *Experiences in groups.* New York, NY: Basic Books.

Bion, W. R. (1962). *Learning from experience.* New York, NY: Basic Books.

Blagys, M. D., & Hilsenroth, M. J. (2000). Distinctive features of short-term psychodynamic-interpersonal psychotherapy: A review of the comparative psychotherapy process literature. *Clinical Psychology: Science and Practice, 7*, 167–188. http://dx.doi.org/10.1093/clipsy.7.2.167

Brabender, V. (1988). A closed model of short-term inpatient group psychotherapy. *Psychiatric Services, 39*, 542–545. http://dx.doi.org/10.1176/ps.39.5.542

Brabender, V., & Fallon, A. (2009). *Group development in practice: Guidance for clinicians and researchers on stages and dynamics of change.* Washington, DC: American Psychological Association. http://dx.doi.org/10.1037/11858-000

Brabender, V. M., Fallon, A. E., & Smolar, A. I. (2004). *Essentials of group therapy.* Hoboken, NJ: Wiley.

Brand, T., Hecke, D., Rietz, C., & Schultz-Venrath, U. (2016). Therapy effects of mentalization-based and psychodynamic group psychotherapy in a randomized day clinic study. *Group Psychotherapy and Group Dynamics, 52,* 156–174.

Bretherton, I. (2006). The roots and growing points of attachment theory. In C. M. Parkes, J. Stevenson-Hinde, & P. Marris (Eds.), *Attachment across the life cycle* (pp. 9–32). New York, NY: Routledge.

Callahan, K. L., Price, J. L., & Hilsenroth, M. J. (2004). A review of interpersonal-psychodynamic group psychotherapy outcomes for adult survivors of childhood sexual abuse. *International Journal of Group Psychotherapy, 54,* 491–519. http://dx.doi.org/10.1521/ijgp.54.4.491.42770

Chen, E. C., Kakkad, D., & Balzano, J. (2008). Multicultural competence and evidence-based practice in group therapy. *Journal of Clinical Psychology, 64,* 1261–1278. http://dx.doi.org/10.1002/jclp.20533

Choi-Kain, L. W., & Gunderson, J. G. (2008). Mentalization: Ontogeny, assessment, and application in the treatment of borderline personality disorder. *The American Journal of Psychiatry, 165,* 1127–1135. http://dx.doi.org/10.1176/appi.ajp.2008.07081360

Coates, S. W. (2006). Foreword. In J. G. Allen & P. Fonagy (Eds.), *Handbook of mentalization-based treatment* (pp. xv–xvii). West Sussex, England: Wiley.

Dinger, U., & Schauenburg, H. (2010). Effects of individual cohesion and patient interpersonal style on outcome in psychodynamically oriented inpatient group psychotherapy. *Psychotherapy Research, 20,* 22–29. http://dx.doi.org/10.1080/10503300902855514

Durkin, H. (1972). Analytic group therapy and general systems theory. In C. Sager & H. Kaplan (Eds.), *Progress in group and family therapy* (pp. 9–17). New York, NY: Brunner/Mazel.

Ensink, K., Maheux, J., Normandin, L., Sabourin, S., Diguer, L., Berthelot, N., & Parent, K. (2013). The impact of mentalization training on the reflective function of novice therapists: A randomized controlled trial. *Psychotherapy Research, 23,* 526–538. http://dx.doi.org/10.1080/10503307.2013.800950

Fonagy, P., & Bateman, A. (2008). The development of borderline personality disorder: A mentalizing model. *Journal of Personality Disorders, 22,* 4–21. http://dx.doi.org/10.1521/pedi.2008.22.1.4

Fonagy, P., Campbell, C., & Bateman, A. (2017). Mentalizing, attachment, and epistemic trust in group therapy. *International Journal of Group Psychotherapy, 67,* 176–201. http://dx.doi.org/10.1080/00207284.2016.1263156

Fonagy, P., Gergely, G., Jurist, E. L., & Target, M. (2002). *Affect regulation, mentalization, and the development of self.* New York, NY: Other Press.

Fonagy, P., Luyten, P., & Bateman, A. (2015). Translation: Mentalizing as treatment target in borderline personality disorder. *Personality Disorders: Theory, Research, and Treatment, 6*, 380–392. http://dx.doi.org/10.1037/per0000113

Freud, S. (1958). The dynamics of transference. In J. Strachey (Ed. & Trans.), *The standard edition of the complete psychological works of Sigmund Freud* (Vol. 12, pp. 99–108). London, England: Hogarth. (Original work published 1912)

Freud, S. (1965). *The psychopathology of everyday life, standard edition.* New York, NY: Norton. (Original work published 1914)

Gergely, G. (2007). The social construction of the subjective self: The role of affect-mirroring, markedness, and ostensive communication in self-development. In L. Mayes, P. Fonagy, & M. Target (Eds.), *Developmental science and psychoanalysis: Integration and innovation* (pp. 45–82). London, England: Karnac.

Greene, L. R., & Cole, M. B. (1991). Level and form of psychopathology and the structure of group therapy. *International journal of group psychotherapy, 41*, 499–521. http://dx.doi.org/10.1080/00207284.1991.11490677

Greene, L. R., Rosenkrantz, J., & Muth, D. Y. (1985). Splitting dynamics, self-representations and boundary phenomena in the group psychotherapy of borderline personality disorders. *Psychiatry, 48*, 234–245. http://dx.doi.org/10.1080/00332747.1985.11024284

Harrow, M., Astrachan, B. M., Becker, R. E., Miller, J. C., & Schwartz, A. H. (1967). Influence of the psychotherapist on the emotional climate in group therapy. *Human Relations, 20*, 49–64. http://dx.doi.org/10.1177/001872676702000105

Haslam-Hopwood, G. T. G., Allen, J. G., Stein, A., & Bleiberg, E. (2006). Enhancing mentalizing through psycho-education. In J. Allen & P. Fonagy (Eds.), *Handbook of mentalization-based treatment* (pp. 249–267). West Sussex, England: Wiley. http://dx.doi.org/10.1002/9780470712986.ch13

Heinskou, T. (2010). Kibel groups and their dynamic perspective. In J. Radcliffe, K. Hajek, J. Carson, & O. Manor (Eds.), *Psychological groupwork with acute psychiatric patients* (pp. 254–260). London, England: Whiting & Birch.

Horowitz, H. (1996). Stress response syndromes: Character styles and dynamic psychotherapy. In J. E. Groves (Ed.), *Essential papers on short-term dynamic psychotherapy* (pp. 101–133). New York, NY: New York University Press. (Original work published 1974)

Karterud, S. (1989). A comparative study of six different inpatient groups with respect to their basic assumption functioning. *International Journal of Group Psychotherapy, 39*, 355–376. http://dx.doi.org/10.1080/00207284.1989.11491174

Karterud, S. (2015). *Mentalization-based group therapy (MBT-G).* Oxford, England: Oxford University Press. http://dx.doi.org/10.1093/med:psych/9780198753742.001.0001

Karterud, S., & Bateman, A. W. (2012). Group therapy techniques. In A. W. Bateman & P. Fonagy (Eds.), *Handbook of mentalizing in mental health practice* (pp. 81–105). Washington, DC: American Psychiatric Association.

Kauff, P. F. (2012). Psychoanalytic group psychotherapy: An overview. In J. L. Kleinberg (Ed.), *The Wiley-Blackwell handbook of group psychotherapy* (pp. 13–32). New York, NY: Wiley.

Kernberg, O. F. (1975a). *Borderline conditions and pathological narcissism*. New York, NY: Aronson.

Kernberg, O. (1975b). A systems approach to priority setting of interventions in groups. *International Journal of Group Psychotherapy, 25,* 251–275. http://dx.doi.org/10.1080/00207284.1975.11491899

Kibel, H. D. (1978). The rationale for the use of group psychotherapy for borderline patients on a short-term unit. *International Journal of Group Psychotherapy, 28,* 339–358. http://dx.doi.org/10.1080/00207284.1978.11491623

Kibel, H. D. (1981). A conceptual model for short-term inpatient group psychotherapy. *The American Journal of Psychiatry, 138,* 74–80. http://dx.doi.org/10.1176/ajp.138.1.74

Kibel, H. D. (1986). From acute to long-term inpatient group psychotherapy. *Psychiatric Journal of the University of Ottawa, 11,* 58–61.

Kibel, H. D. (1987a). Contributions of the group psychotherapist to education on the psychiatric unit: Teaching through group dynamics. *International Journal of Group Psychotherapy, 37,* 3–29. http://dx.doi.org/10.1080/00207284.1987.11491038

Kibel, H. D. (1987b). Inpatient group psychotherapy: Where treatment philosophies converge. In R. Langs (Ed.), *Yearbook of psychoanalysis and psychotherapy* (Vol. 2, pp. 94–116). New York, NY: Gardner Press.

Kibel, H. D. (1990). The inpatient psychotherapy group as a testing ground for theory. In B. E. Roth, W. N. Stone, & H. D. Kibel (Eds.), *The difficult patient in group: Group psychotherapy with borderline and narcissistic disorders* (pp. 245–264). Madison, CT: International Universities Press.

Kibel, H. D. (1992). Inpatient group psychotherapy. In A. Alonso & H. Swiller (Eds.), *Group therapy in clinical practice* (pp. 93–112). Washington, DC: American Psychiatric Press.

Kibel, H. D. (2003). Interpretive work in milieu groups. *International Journal of Group Psychotherapy, 53,* 303–329. http://dx.doi.org/10.1521/ijgp.53.3.303.42821

Kirchmann, H., Mestel, R., Schreiber-Willnow, K., Mattke, D., Seidler, K. P., Daudert, E., . . . Strauss, B. (2009). Associations among attachment characteristics, patients' assessment of therapeutic factors, and treatment outcome following inpatient psychodynamic group psychotherapy. *Psychotherapy Research, 19,* 234–248. http://dx.doi.org/10.1080/10503300902798367

Klein, M. (1952). *Contributions to psycho-analysis: 1921–1945*. New York, NY: Anglobooks.

Koch, H. C. H. (1983). Correlates of changes in personal construing of members of two psychotherapy groups: Changes in affective expression. *The British Journal of Medical Psychology, 56,* 323–327. http://dx.doi.org/10.1111/j.2044-8341.1983.tb01564.x

Kösters, M., Burlingame, G. M., Nachtigall, C., & Strauss, B. (2006). A meta-analytic review of the effectiveness of inpatient group psychotherapy. *Group Dynamics, 10,* 146–163. http://dx.doi.org/10.1037/1089-2699.10.2.146

Laurenssen, E. M., Hutsebaut, J., Feenstra, D. J., Bales, D. L., Noom, M. J., Busschbach, J. J., . . . & Luyten, P. (2014). Feasibility of mentalization-based treatment for adolescents with borderline symptoms: A pilot study. *Psychotherapy, 51,* 159–166. http://dx.doi.org/10.1037/a0033513

Leichsenring, F., & Leibing, E. (2003). The effectiveness of psychodynamic therapy and cognitive behavior therapy in the treatment of personality disorders: A meta-analysis. *The American Journal of Psychiatry, 160,* 1223–1232. http://dx.doi.org/10.1176/appi.ajp.160.7.1223

Leichsenring, F., & Rabung, S. (2008). Effectiveness of long-term psychodynamic psychotherapy: A meta-analysis. *JAMA, 300,* 1551–1565. http://dx.doi.org/10.1001/jama.300.13.1551

Lingiardi, V., & McWilliams, N. (Eds.). (2017). *Psychodynamic diagnostic manual: PDM-2.* New York, NY: Guilford Press.

Luyten, P., Fonagy, P., Lowyck, B., & Vermote, R. (2012). Assessment of mentalization. In A. W. Bateman & P. Fonagy (Eds.), *Handbook of mentalizing in mental health practice* (pp. 43–65). Arlington, VA: American Psychiatric Publishing.

MacKenzie, K. R., & Tschuschke, V. (1993). Relatedness, group work, and outcome in long-term inpatient psychotherapy groups. *The Journal of Psychotherapy Practice and Research, 2,* 147–156.

Marmarosh, C. L., & Markin, R. D. (2007). Group and personal attachments: Two is better than one when predicting college adjustment. *Group Dynamics, 11,* 153–164. http://dx.doi.org/10.1037/1089-2699.11.3.153

Ogden, T. (1979). On projective identification. *The International Journal of Psycho-Analysis, 60,* 357–373.

Radcliffe, J., & Diamond, D. (2007). Psychodynamically-informed discussion groups on acute inpatient wards. *Groupwork, 17*(1), 34–44. http://dx.doi.org/10.1921/0951824X.17.1.34

Rice, C. A., & Rutan, J. S. (1987). *Inpatient group psychotherapy: A psychodynamic perspective.* New York, NY: Macmillan.

Rudden, M., Milrod, B., Target, M., Ackerman, S., & Graf, E. (2006). Reflective functioning in panic disorder patients: A pilot study. *Journal of the American Psychoanalytic Association, 54,* 1339–1343. http://dx.doi.org/10.1177/00030651060540040109

Society of Clinical Psychology. (2016). *Mentalization-based treatment for borderline personality disorder.* Retrieved from http://www.div12.org/psychological-treatments/treatments/mentalization-based-treatment-for-borderline-personality-disorder/

Tschuschke, V., MacKenzie, K. R., Haaser, B., & Janke, G. (1996). Self-disclosure, feedback, and outcome in long-term inpatient psychotherapy groups. *The Journal of Psychotherapy Practice and Research, 5,* 35–44.

Van Wagoner, S. L. (2000). Anger in group therapy, countertransference and the novice group therapist. *Journal of Psychotherapy in Independent Practice, 1*, 63–75. http://dx.doi.org/10.1300/J288v01n02_08

von Bertalanffy, L. (1950). The theory of open systems in physics and biology. *Science, 111*, 23–29. http://dx.doi.org/10.1126/science.111.2872.23

von Bertalanffy, L. (1966). General system theory and psychiatry. In S. Arieti (Ed.), *American handbook of psychiatry* (Vol. 3, pp. 705–721). New York, NY: Basic Books.

Weber, R. (2017). Book review [Review of the book *Mentalization-based group therapy (MBT-G): A theoretical, clinical, and research manual*, by S. Karterud]. *International Journal of Group Psychotherapy, 67*, 288–290. http://dx.doi.org/10.1080/00207284.2016.1263503

Weijers, J., ten Kate, C., Eurelings-Bontekoe, E., Viechtbauer, W., Rampaart, R., Bateman, A., & Selten, J. P. (2016). Mentalization-based treatment for psychotic disorder: Protocol of a randomized controlled trial. *BMC Psychiatry, 16*(191). http://dx.doi.org/10.1186/s12888-016-0902-x

Wells, M. C., Glickauf-Hughes, C., & Buzzell, V. (1990). Treating obsessive-compulsive personalities in psychodynamic/interpersonal group therapy. *Psychotherapy: Theory, Research, & Practice, 27*(3), 366–379. http://dx.doi.org/10.1037/0033-3204.27.3.366

Yalom, I., & Leszcz, M. (2005). *The theory and practice of group therapy* (5th ed.). New York, NY: Basic Books.

5

COGNITIVE BEHAVIOR THERAPY

Many models or systems of psychotherapy take into account an individual's cognitions, including psychodynamic and interpersonal models. Even those who seek primarily to modify behavior accept that cognitive symbolic processes are often necessary mediators of behavior (Mahoney & Kazdin, 1979). Thus, although cognitions are now included in most therapeutic systems, the position accorded them varies substantially (Perris, 1988a). In this chapter, we review the cognitive and cognitive behavioral models in which cognitions are a central focus for change, particularly as they are relevant for inpatient hospital programs (IHPs), partial hospital programs (PHPs), and residential treatment centers (RTCs).

Cognitive behavior psychotherapy is a comprehensive and empirically based therapy that is historically grounded in two different theoretical schools—the behavioral and the psychoanalytic. The inception of cognitive psychotherapy as a separate school coincided with Beck and Ellis

http://dx.doi.org/10.1037/0000113-006
Group Psychotherapy in Inpatient, Partial Hospital, and Residential Care Settings, by V. Brabender and A. Fallon
Copyright © 2019 by the American Psychological Association. All rights reserved.

(traditionally trained psychoanalysts) departing from their psychoanalytic training (Perris, 1988a). From the behavioral school, cognitive behavior therapists have adopted the scientific method (i.e., clearly defined goals, emphasis on empirical outcome, low to moderate levels of inference from the behavior), a focus on behavioral change, and a variety of behavioral techniques and strategies, such as graded task assignments, scheduled behavior rehearsal, and role playing. Embraced from the psychoanalytic tradition, they maintained: the importance of understanding the individual's characteristic (subjective) perceptions of him- or herself and the world; the concomitant internal dialogue and process (often outside of awareness) that can influence one's perception of past, current, and future situations; and the importance of bringing these thoughts into awareness.

The influences of two very different traditions (psychoanalysis and behaviorism) have resulted in a number of different variations and combinations of cognitive and cognitive behavior therapy models. The term *cognitive behavior therapy* (CBT) could include Beck's cognitive therapy (Beck, 1967/1972, 1976; Beck, Rush, Shaw, & Emery, 1979) and Ellis's rational-emotive therapy (Ellis, 1962), as well as models developed in the 1970s and 1980s that were primarily designed as individual models but could be altered for a group format.[1] Newer developments such as dialectical behavior therapy (DBT; Linehan, 2014) and schema therapy (Young, Klosko, & Weishaar, 2003) have been specifically designed for more severe psychopathology.

All CBT models share three fundamentals: cognitions affect behavior; cognitions can be identified, monitored, and changed; and behavioral change can occur as the result of cognitive change (Dobson & Dozois, 2010). Hollon and Beck's (1986) model includes all those approaches that "attempt to modify existing or anticipate disorders by virtue of altering cognitions or cognitive processes" (p. 443). As this therapy has evolved, it has included experiential exercise (e.g., guided imagery) that aims to minimize dysfunctional affective states and maladaptive coping styles that interfere with rational cognitive processes. This definition excludes approaches that rely predominately on techniques that are considered more behavioral in focus (e.g., systematic desensitization).

---

[1] These included Goldfried's systematic rational restructuring (Goldfried, Decenteceo, & Weinberg, 1974), Meichenbaum's self-instructional training (Meichenbaum, 1977) and stress inoculation training (Meichenbaum, 1975), Maultsby's rational behavior therapy (Maultsby, 1975), Lazarus's multimodal therapy (Lazarus, 1981), cognitive appraisal therapy (Wessler & Hankin, 1988), interpersonal problem-solving therapy (Spivack, Platt, & Shure, 1976), Rehm's self-control therapy (Rehm, 1977), structural cognitive therapy (Liotti, 1987), covert conditioning (Mahoney & Arnoff, 1978), personal science (Mahoney, 1977), and Bandura's more cognitively mediated view of social learning (Bandura, 1977a, 1977b).

Originally developed for outpatient depressed individuals (Beck, 1967/1972; Dobson, 1989; Haaga & Davison, 1989), the use of a group format addressing a wider range of psychiatric problems, particularly the more severe disorders typically found in IHPs, PHPs, or longer term RTCs, has received increasing attention with regard to technique modification. It is less empirically validated than the individual format (Clarke & Wilson, 2008; Wright, Thase, Beck, & Ludgate, 1993).

The procedure and process of cognitive behavior group therapy vary depending on which model out of the diverse set available the therapist follows. The models differ on the goals, responsibilities, and styles of the leader; assessment and patient categorization; content and focus of the session; and importance of the therapeutic alliance; and attention to process. The models each can be broadly categorized into one of three classes of group approaches: a structured psychoeducational approach, a problem-solving approach, or an experiential–affective approach.

The psychoeducational group is a highly structured, time-limited approach in which the primary objective is imparting information and emphasizing self-help techniques, with the task of applying them left to the individual. By design, little or no attention is paid to the specific concerns of the individual. It can be an efficient way of teaching a large, highly motivated group a skill or issue known to plague the group of patients. Single-session groups can be designed to teach such topics as how to complete and use a thought record, how to recognize and manage stress, how to recognize a relapse, how to recognize an automatic thought, and the relationship between thought and emotion. Elements of cognitive strategies or behavioral interventions (see Appendixes 5.1 and 5.2) may be converted to a psychoeducational format. These single sessions are most effective when combined with other therapeutic techniques or used as an introduction to a more traditional CBT group.[2]

What has been reported more commonly in the recent literature is the use of 10 to 12 sessions of a closed-ended psychoeducational experience. These groups frequently enroll patients with specific symptoms, such as mania in bipolar disorders (R. Chen et al., 2018), or those with chronic mental illness (Duman, Yildirim, Ucok, Er, & Kanik, 2010; Long, Banyard, & Dolley, 2016). Cook, Arechiga, Dobson, and Boyd (2014) also presented an interesting variation in which the teaching of symptoms, triggers, and coping skills was combined with a "process component" emphasizing the promotion of self-disclosure, cohesion, universality, and socialization.

---

[2]See Sank and Shaffer (1984) for more specific information on how to conduct such groups.

The psychoeducational presentation can be modified to accommodate the background, values, and needs of a homogeneous minority group (Misurell & Springer, 2013). One interesting example was a psychoeducational group conducted for Korean Americans. With a Korean-speaking therapist, Korean perspectives on shamanism, disease, and illness were integrated with modules on relapse prevention, crisis management, stigma, and community resources (Shin & Lukens, 2002). The researchers reported that patients had a reduction in psychotic symptoms and perceived less stigma associated with mental illness.

Others have noted that content adaptation of a psychoeducational group for a specific minority group can have an increased therapeutic impact. Boyd-Franklin (1991) found that in groups with African American women there were recurring themes of racism, colorism, and sexism. Kohn, Oden, Muñoz, Robinson, and Leavitt (2002), working with a psychoeducational group of low-income African American women, emphasized topics such as creating healthy relationships, spirituality, family issues, and African American female identity. They reported that in the culturally adapted group, women reported significantly more symptom alleviation. Levy and O'Hara (2010), too, noted that the barriers to obtaining mental health care for low-income groups require an altered presentation to emphasize the relevance and benefits of overcoming the many obstacles (e.g., sporadic public transportation) required to engage in treatment.

Similarly, Stacciarini, O'Keeffe, and Mathews (2007), in their review of the literature on Latinos with depression, concluded that CBT with a psychoeducational component was the treatment of choice. Russell and Doucette (2012) indicated that acculturative stress is important to address in those patients who have immigrated. For Latinos, psychoeducational groups must incorporate the Latino values of *personalismo* (establishing and valuing the personal dimension of the relationship directly with the therapist, rather than the institution for which the therapist is a part), *respeto* (mutual respect and respect for authority), and *confianza* (trust that is built around a more informal social relationship rather than the impersonal structure of immediately starting with the problem). Indeed, many minority groups that value collectivism must have the engaged support of the extended social network for the patient to have a successful treatment (Misurell & Springer, 2013). Problem-solving groups, too, have educational aspects; however, the main objective is mastering an approach to solving the individual's practical and psychological problems. We discuss this type of group in more detail in Chapter 7.

The experiential–affective group relies on both direct teaching and more indirect methods (e.g., guided imagery, exercises, role playing). Its goals are to help patients identify and understand the connections between cognitive appraisals and resulting emotions and to promote changes in behavior, emotion, coping styles, and underlying schema. It is this latter class of models that is the focus of this chapter. The distinction between these classes of groups is, of course, an artificial one; various combinations of the techniques from each type can be flexibly combined depending on member characteristics and type of setting. Settings can also be differentiated based on whether the group operates independently of milieu support or the group operates in a context in which other staff members are capable of augmenting and implementing the techniques learned in group (Cowdrill & Dannahy, 2009; Sambrook, 2009).

THEORETICAL UNDERPINNINGS

Central to the cognitive behavioral model of therapy is the premise that there is an interaction in how individuals conceptualize and construe themselves, their worlds, and their futures. The focus is primarily on the correction of faulty cognitions and their infusion into behavioral patterns. The emphasis is on how cognition influences emotion and behavior rather than on the inverse, although reciprocal connections are also acknowledged in a cognition–emotion–motivation–behavior loop (Beck, 1991; Ellis, 1962).

Psychopathology involves the development of incorrect, unrealistic, or distorted thoughts and relational scripts during infancy or childhood. Referred to as *dysfunctional schemas*, they are often activated by particular external events that then warp newly acquired information and further distort the individual's self-perception and view of the world. A basic tenet of the theory is that individuals search for truth and strive for logical consistency. When individuals recognize that their views of themselves and contrary evidence clash, they evaluate the evidence and often change their self-perceptions. Changes in behavior and emotions result from such efforts to resolve inconsistencies and inaccuracies (Arkowitz & Hannah, 1989).

Although the theoretical contributions to the cognitive behavioral theory of emotion are many, we frame our theoretical discussion around the work of Beck and his colleagues (1979). The model proposes that an individual's perceptions or cognitions (usually negative) about themselves, the world, and the future (together referred to as the *cognitive triad*) are the result of cognitive distortions (i.e., thoughts, images of loss, negative interpretations of ambiguous events). These distortions arise when a stressor (either internal or external) activates an underlying cognitive structure or schema (i.e., an attitude or assumption, which can be an irrational or rational belief). These schemas become the substrate from which the cognitive distortions emerge. Central to the understanding of the formation and maintenance of psychological disorders are the three related concepts of the cognitive triad, cognitive distortions, and cognitive schemas (Beck et al., 1979).[3]

Core Concepts

Although these constructs are presented here abstractly, it is important for the therapist to be mindful that the way in which they unfold for the individual may be affected by social, cultural, ethnic, and religious beliefs of the particular population.

Cognitive Triad

The *cognitive triad* refers to the negative or distorted views that individuals may have about (a) themselves or themselves in relation to their group membership (e.g., "I'm a loser"), (b) the world (e.g., "Life's unfair"), and (c) the future (e.g., "It's hopeless"). The severity of the distortion and the extent to which the distortion is negative may vary for each element of the triad. The therapist can develop a refined conceptualization of the patient's problem by assessing the degree to which each of the three factors contributes to the patient's cognitions.

Cognitive Distortions

Because most environmental events have some ambiguity, people often have latitude in the meaning and value that they attribute to the events; thus, all people have a capacity to distort reality in significant ways. These distortions are the result of underlying schemas or belief systems. The ability to assess and monitor the veracity of the distortion becomes important. When a belief is held in spite of disconfirming evidence or when there is an inflexible application of a belief, the belief becomes dysfunctional (Ellis, 1962; Freeman, 1987).

Cognitive distortions are the dysfunctional thoughts and images generated by an event that activates a certain schema (Freeman, 1990). Thoughts or cognitions can be conscious or nonconscious. *Nonconscious cognitions*, or automatic thoughts, are ones that are outside one's awareness and are often not verbalized. However, the psychoanalytic notion of the unconscious is not applicable here (i.e., no emphasis is placed on hidden motives or "ego protecting" mechanisms). An example of a cognitive distortion is using a single example and evaluating oneself or situation in an all-or-nothing manner, such as having four to five tasks to complete and declaring that one cannot complete any of them correctly.

---

[3]For a more in-depth understanding of the theoretical underpinnings, see Dobson and Dozois (2010).

Schemas

Schemas are underlying assumptions and irrational beliefs that serve as the source of cognitive distortions. Schemas are inferential, deduced from automatic thoughts made conscious by exploration and from the observation of behavior.

Innate predispositions begin to influence cognitions and behavior from the earliest moments of life (Ellis, 1992). Traumas and deprivations contribute further to the development of core beliefs and schemas. For example, a young adult is admitted to the hospital after being picked up by police for screaming at his neighbors and waving a gun around, threatening to shoot anyone stealing his food. Born with an irritable and fussy temperament, he was neglected by his drug-addicted mother and placed in several foster care settings where older children stole his things and beat him up. As he grew up, he learned to trust no one, and if he was aggressive, others would shy away from him. He was recently fired for punching a coworker when the coworker moved the patient's lunch, presumably to find his own. The patient, however, thought the coworker was stealing it from him. The patient likely has schemas of abandonment, mistrust, and punishment. Assumptions continue to evolve and be modified throughout life; new assumptions can develop later in life in response to emotionally important events, even without childhood antecedents (Perris, 1988a). These beliefs are the accumulation of the individual's cultural, familial, social, gender, ethnic, generational, and religious values and experience. Schemas once adaptive become maladaptive when they no longer functionally protect the individual.

The totality of schemas an individual possesses constitutes a person's self-definition. Schemas can act individually or in combination with each other. For example, two contradictory schemas can coexist because one is dormant while the other governs day-to-day behavior. Some silent schemas may be activated only in certain situations by a specific external event. In the earlier example, the schema of mistrust was likely present, but the event of a coworker moving the food, perceived as stealing, reawakened the old traumas of deprivation and abandonment. The impact of a schema on an individual's thoughts, perceptions, emotions, and behavior depends on (a) how central to the individual's sense of self the schema is, (b) how important the individual perceives the schema to be for personal safety or well-being, (c) how actively the individual disputes or struggles with the schema when it is activated, (d) how young the individual was when the schema was internalized, (e) the relative importance and meaning of the individuals from whom the schema was acquired, and (f) how strongly the schema has been reinforced (Freeman, 1990).

As a schema develops, environmental information and experience are incorporated only to the extent that the individual can assimilate it into his or her subjective experiences. Schemas thus become self-selective because individuals may ignore data they are not able to render consistent with the schema. The greater the number of dysfunctional schemas a person has, the wider the range of situations that will activate one of them and thus the more vulnerable the individual will be to becoming disturbed. Once activated, schemas can produce biases in memory for past events, in the perception of current ambiguous situations, and in anticipation of future events.

Perceptions, beliefs, and other cognitive phenomena are considered important in the origin and maintenance of psychiatric disorders and in particular types of depression (Freeman, 1990). The cognitive behavioral model suggests that beliefs and schemas may render a person more vulnerable to a psychiatric disorder when faced with a stressor. For example, individuals with abandonment schemas (i.e., safety and love were not provided when young) and who as adults adapt by investing in warm, interpersonal relationships to satisfy those early abandonment needs may be more vulnerable to stressors such as interpersonal losses than may individuals who are high in autonomy and have more investment in the acquisition of personal power (Beck, 1991).

Controversy exists over whether cognitive distortions and underlying schemas cause psychiatric disorders or whether they are secondary to other causal agents. Regardless of the primary or secondary role of cognitions in causing symptoms, cognitive theory still has much to offer in the treatment of psychopathology. By whatever means psychiatric symptoms arise, negative thoughts, images, and interpretations do have subsequent effects on mood and behavior and can increase vulnerability to certain symptoms. Thus, even in cases in which such cognitive distortions are secondary to a biologically based psychiatric disorder, they can still play a role in maintaining disturbing emotions and behaviors (Williams & Moorey, 1989). For example, psychosis (as presented in the earlier example) and attention-deficit disorder in adolescents can be exacerbated, attenuated, or maintained by cognitions. Even though reality testing and rational thinking are particularly difficult for people with schizophrenia, identifying the dysfunctional thoughts and developing strategies to evaluate the omnipotence of the voices and hallucinations have helped people with schizophrenia become more functional (Chadwick, Sambrook, Rasch, & Davies, 2000).

GOALS OF TREATMENT

CBT is a coping model as opposed to a mastery model of psychotherapy (Freeman, 1987, 1990). The goal of the therapy is not to "cure" but to help the patient become more functional in the world and experience greater control and self-efficacy by developing better coping strategies to manage life's everyday problems. The task is to help patients replace distorted cognitions and dysfunctional behaviors with adaptive and healthier modes of functioning. Initially, patients learn the strength and impact their dysfunctional thoughts have on their lives. Therapists then help patients test the veracity or adaptiveness of their thinking and behavior and build more effective strategies or modes of functioning for responding both intrapersonally and interpersonally (Farrell, Reiss, & Shaw, 2014).[4] Later, more long-term goals include helping patients learn that their cognitive distortions are manifestations of their underlying schemas and that more long-lasting change will be the result of therapeutic work on the schemas.

Many of the CBT models have a significant educative function (the degree of emphasis depends on the model). The assumption is that misinformation and misconceptions are a source of psychopathology (e.g., depression results when one mistakenly sees a situation as hopeless) and can be attenuated by grasping new or corrective information. However, the introduction of new information alone often has little effect on changing the individual's behavior or cognitions because the organization of new information may be altered to fit preexisting schemas rather than new knowledge changing the cognition or schema. Hence, as illustrated in the methodological section, additional techniques (i.e., cognitive and behavioral strategies) are necessary to make cognitions and schemas more functional and accurate.

Target for Change and Process of Change

Cognitive behavioral therapies view factors within the individual rather than the individual's transactions with the environment as important causal agents. In CBT, the manifest cognitive distortions are the "thematic directional signs that point to the underlying cognitive schema" (Freeman, 1990, p. 66). The cognitive distortions (and underlying assumptions, coping styles, or schemas) are the causal mediators that are associated with different psychiatric symptoms. The automatic thoughts and schemas that underlie the problem have to be evaluated and modified because they are assumed to precipitate or at least maintain the symptoms.

---

[4]Versions of the cognitive behavior model vary in the breadth of change sought. At the most specific level, variants such as self-instructional training and stress inoculation offer particular techniques and have well-articulated steps, with the goal of acquiring specific behaviors. More broadly, variants such as Beck's cognitive therapy attempt to transform more dysfunctional cognitions and problematic schemas into more functional beliefs and schemas. Schema therapy attempts to reduce maladaptive modes of functioning with healthier ones (Farrell, Reiss, & Shaw, 2014). The variant that is most encompassing in its goals, rational-emotive therapy, seeks to present and modify a philosophy of life for patients to use on their own long after therapy has formally ended (Haaga & Davison, 1989).

Cognitions

At least two types of cognitive difficulties have been differentiated as targets for change (Kendall & Braswell, 1982): (a) distortions that are based on an existing but dysfunctional belief system and (b) deficits that result because the individual lacks appropriate mediating cognitions. With cognitive distortion, change occurs as a result of revising the current belief system. There are at least three ways of accomplishing this: *empirical disconfirmation* (presenting the patient with logic or evidence that contradicts current beliefs), *reconceptualization* (providing the patient with another construction to account for existing observations or experiences), and *process insight* (helping the patient understand and recognize the method or process followed to arrive at a belief; Hollon & Beck, 1986).

With cognitive deficits (e.g., impulsive children, explosive disorders), wherein the goal is to create or strengthen appropriate cognitive mediators when none currently exist, repetition-based approaches may be more effective. Approaches entailing the modifications of statements about the self such as self-instructional training and stress-inoculation training rely heavily on repetition and place less emphasis on influencing the validity of an individual's belief system. Repetition is thought to increase the likelihood that the individual will think a certain thought in a given situation (Hollon & Beck, 1986).

Although individuals' cognitions are a result of their past experiences, the focus of CBT is on what maintains or reinforces dysfunctional behavior (Freeman, 1987). CBT places little emphasis on insight or understanding the symbolic or historical meaning of one's maladaptive behavior. Difficulties are caused by the individual's evaluation of prior experience and the centrality of that evaluation (Ellis, 1962; Garfield, 1989).

With those patients presenting with personality disorders, schemas are strongly held ideas that have entrenched and maladaptive coping strategies closely connected to them. These schemas require a number of powerful cognitive, emotive, and behavioral techniques to change them (Beck et al., 1990). A purely cognitive strategy is not likely to change a schema because it would leave affect, motivation, and behavior untouched. Only limited exploration of schemas is possible in a short-term (acute inpatient or short-term day) setting. Models such as DBT and schema-focused therapy have attempted to use a multitude of techniques that engage cognitive, affective, and behavioral aspects of functioning and are presented later in the chapter as alternative models (Linehan, 2014; Martin & Young, 2010).

Cognition and Behavior

According to cognitive behavioral theorists, the modification of cognitions can occur in several ways. It can occur through the verbal analysis of experience, wherein patients are directed to report their automatic thoughts with a focus on what they say to themselves rather than to others (Beck, 1991). Rational-emotive therapists often use group exercises involving imagery or guided fantasy to invite the manifestations of "nonconscious algorithms" (Ellis, 1992). In both procedures, automatic thoughts are brought into the patient's awareness. This bringing into awareness may be similar to what Freud described as making conscious the preconscious material. However, unlike a psychodynamic therapist, the cognitive behavioral therapist does not attempt to uncover and deal with material that is defended against. Modification of cognitions can also occur with the use of behavioral techniques or experiments designed to allow the patient to have new experiences.[5] Various cognitive behavioral approaches differ in the manner in which and degree to which they incorporate behavioral procedures. Rational-emotive therapy and systematic restructuring combine a cognitive approach with behavioral interventions. The behavioral interventions, usually in the form of an assignment between sessions, serve as practice or behavioral rehearsal and strengthen the newly learned material. In contrast, other approaches integrate behavioral work with cognitive work by use of empirical hypothesis testing (e.g., Beck's cognitive therapy). The behavioral homework is an attempt to gather additional information concerning the validity of a particular belief.

Compared with a more psychodynamic or systems model, traditional CBT places little emphasis on affective disturbance as crucial to the evaluation of the dysfunction and as a target for change. However, there is recognition that an inability to tolerate distress is a significant factor in patients with personality disorders. These patients can use cognitive behavioral skills if they can develop interim strategies to manage the displeasure. DBT and schema-focused therapy both recognize the importance of managing the affective disturbance.

Cognitive Behavior Therapy in a Group Setting

The focus of the cognitive–behavioral group session is primarily the individual rather than group dynamics or relationships that develop among

---

[5]Even though cognitive behavioral and behavioral therapists may use behavioral interventions, the target for and mechanism of change differs. For example, both behavioral and cognitive behavioral therapists might choose the lack of social skills of the schizophrenic as their target symptoms. Behavioral therapists would develop therapeutic strategies to help patients learn and modify behaviors (see Chapter 8 for further discussion). Improvement of social skills for cognitive therapy is done in the context of attempting to correct the dysfunctional cognitions underlying these deficits. A role play, for example, in behavioral therapy is used to acquire and practice certain skills in a particular situation. The same role play in cognitive behavioral therapy is used primarily to elicit the patient's distorted thoughts and concomitant feelings, with the goal of bringing them into the conscious awareness rather than changing behavior itself (Perris, 1988a).

members of the group or with the therapist (Wessler & Hankin-Wessler, 1989). Despite the individual focus, the group is not regarded as inferior to an individual format (Burlingame, Fuhriman, & Mosier, 2003; Gaffan, Tsaousis, & Kemp-Wheeler, 1995; Huntley, Araya, & Salisbury, 2012; Moore, Carr, & Hartnett, 2017). Cognitive behavioral models are seen as suited to the group format for two reasons: (a) a number of patients can be taught efficiently by a single therapist, and (b) a group format allows patients to teach, supervise, and practice the model with others and thereby master it better themselves. In contrast to individual therapy, group therapy provides the added benefit of enabling members and the therapist to obtain information about a patient's beliefs and social behaviors by observing his or her interactions and by making comments about the beliefs and behaviors (Schachter, 2011; Wessler & Hankin-Wessler, 1989). The group can provide a supportive setting in which individuals can have corrective emotional experiences by being able to observe their own behaviors and receive feedback about them from both members and the therapist (Martin & Young, 2010). As was eloquently stated by Wessler and Hankin-Wessler (1989),

> A group provides a unique pool of experience that can prove to be very influential, a safe, shallow pool where, under the caring vigilance of experienced supporters, a person may learn to swim and develop style before plunging into the deep end of the real world. (p. 573)

Members can plan and practice novel responses within the group. This risk taking and behavioral rehearsal are likely to have a heightened generalization effect compared with that of a dyadic relationship (Covi, Roth, Pattison, & Lipman, 1988; McKain, 1984). Finally, as Bowers (2000) noted, in the CBT group, members have the opportunity to respond altruistically toward one another and can thereby be freed from unhealthy levels of self-absorption.

TECHNICAL CONSIDERATIONS

Cognitive behavior group therapy is active, directive, and collaborative (Freeman, 1990). It has an individualized focus on the contents of patients' problems, specifically "what is" and what maintains or reinforces dysfunctional thoughts and behaviors (Freeman, 1987). A here-and-now orientation is created by the use of tasks (both within and outside the session) designed specifically to create the everyday conditions wherein more information can be gathered to reality test attitudes, thoughts, and images (Williams & Moorey, 1989). Compared with other theoretical models, there is an abundance of treatment manuals available for various symptoms and diagnoses and different age populations. These manuals delineate a set of techniques; many of them spell out in observable and measurable terms the implementation of a wide range of techniques and their variants with the format and goals of each session and/or each treatment component (Aguilera, Bruehlman-Senecal, Liu, & Bravin, 2018; Aguilera, Garza, & Muñoz, 2010; Barley et al., 1993; Covi et al., 1988; Farrell et al., 2014; Heimberg & Becker, 2002; Linehan, 2014; Muñoz & Mendelson, 2005; Perris, 1988b; Van Noppen, Pato, Marsland, & Rasmussen, 1998). In the past 2 decades there has been significant progress in the recognition that diversity in race and cultural background (Brook, Gordon, & Meadow, 1998; Carter, 2004; E. C. Chen, Kakkad, & Balzano, 2008; De Las Nueces, Hacker, DiGirolamo, & Hicks, 2012; Kohn & Oden, 1997), economic status (Levy & O'Hara, 2010; Satterfield, 1998), and gender (Ghezelseflo & Esbati, 2013; Horne & Kiselica, 1999; Kohn et al., 2002; Long et al., 2016; Rose, 2002; Spencer & Vencill, 2017) may require alterations in language (Aguilera et al., 2010, 2018; Rosselló & Bernal, 1996; Shin & Lukens, 2002), format (Misurell & Springer, 2013; Russell & Doucette, 2012), and content (Balabanovic, Ayers, & Hunter, 2012; C. P. Chen, 1995; Cumba-Avilés, 2017; Ibrahim, Kamsani, & Champe, 2015; Rose, 2002; Rosselló & Jiménez-Chafey, 2006) of the group design.

A variety of cognitive behavioral techniques have been developed for different forms of psychopathology (Appendixes 5.1, 5.2, and 5.3 describe only a partial list of the strategies and exercises available for use in a group setting). The group therapist can plan to incorporate elements or processes from the various approaches, depending on the level of functioning, diagnostic composition, and length of stay. Even if a clinician chooses not to use one of these models in its entirety, mastery of these techniques can augment the clinician's clinical armamentarium. Most approaches incorporate elements of either Ellis's rational-emotive therapy or Beck's cognitive model.

Rational-emotive therapy (Ellis, 1962, 1992; Jacobsen, Tamkin, & Blount, 1987; Lyons & Woods, 1991) is both a cognitive theory of disorders and a set of procedures designed to alter a person's philosophy of life and reconstruct his or her personality. The procedures involve direct instruction, verbally forceful persuasion, and logical disputation. Patients are taught to recognize their irrational beliefs and dispute them. The therapist models rational thinking and provides feedback to the patient. Homework and behavioral assignments are used as practice rather than as a means of producing change. This therapy has been used with heterogeneous groups as well as homogeneous groups with sociopathy, schizophrenia, and substance abuse (Ellis, McInerney, DiGiuseppe, & Yeager, 1988; Garfield, 1989). It has been effectively used to reduce irrational beliefs and decrease psychiatric symptoms when at least nine sessions occur (Jacobsen et al., 1987; Nottingham & Neimeyer, 1992).

Cognitive therapy (Beck, 1976; Beck et al., 1979), like rational-emotive therapy, endorses a cognitive rationale and makes use of persuasion and logic. However, it differs from rational-emotive therapy in that it uses empirical hypothesis testing as a way of changing existing beliefs. Old beliefs are challenged, and new beliefs are proposed by having patients do prospective empirical testing of the validity of their beliefs through behavioral assignments and homework. Alternative conceptualizations often are developed before prospective hypothesis testing. There is also a focus on various systematic distortions in information processing; the content is differentiated from the way in which distortions are processed. Over the past 2 decades, there has been a burgeoning of application to specific populations with psychosis, personality disorders, substance abuse, and eating disorders.

Role of the Leader

The role and procedures a therapist uses vary in relation to the cognitive behavioral model chosen and the nature of the therapist–patient–group interaction. There are obvious procedural differences in the relative emphasis placed on the didactic presentation of material, problem-solving methods, the degree of encouragement of strong affect, insights, and level of activity. For example, rational-emotive group therapists are much more likely to use group exercises that involve guided imagery than are those who follow Beck's model. In addition, there are differences in the therapist's focus on content and the therapist's level of transparency. Nevertheless, there are some general principles about the role of the therapist. Comparatively, the cognitive behavior group therapist takes a verbally active approach, which may be even greater with certain patient populations such the elderly (Glantz, 1989; Yost, Beutler, Corbishley, & Allender, 1986), adolescents (Schrodt & Wright, 1987), and individuals with severe and chronic symptoms (Greenwood, 1987).

The therapist is highly directive in structuring the sessions, both in form and content. Therapists actively teach aspects of the model necessary for understanding dysfunction. They propose hypotheses and teach strategies for testing the veracity of members' newly discovered ways of viewing their "symptoms." They also give and direct feedback and propose homework (Freeman, 1987). Ellis is known to be forceful and sustained in his attack on patient irrationality (Becker & Rosenfeld, 1976). All actively highlight distortions and inaccuracies rather than restate feelings or cognitions (Freeman, 1987). The therapist monitors the intensity of the emotional expression and the level of distress. For example, members often endorse and escalate each other's gloomy perceptions. Rather than allowing members themselves to gradually establish realistic perceptions, the therapist Socratically guides patients to consider a more adaptive viewpoint (Covi et al., 1988). If the group cannot adequately maintain its focus on the task, the therapist intervenes rather than allowing members to struggle. The therapist orchestrates content and process so that antitherapeutic statements and actions by members are not permitted to affect other group members in a detrimental way (Wessler & Hankin-Wessler, 1989).

Some cognitive behavioral approaches encourage monitoring of relevant aspects of the patient–therapist relationship and attending to the dynamics and process of the group, despite the model's focus on individual change; at the very least, group dynamics are important insofar as they affect the individual's thinking, feelings, and actions (Covi et al., 1988). Group norms, communication patterns, and emerging leadership roles can be used to enhance the therapeutic process or can encourage continued maladaptive thinking, feelings, and actions (Schachter, 2011). For example, if group members begin to concentrate on only practical and not psychological and cognitive aspects of a problem, the group leader might comment on such a process and then propose an alternative (Ellis, 1992).

The cultural backgrounds of the patients may require alterations in the therapeutic stance. For instance, C. P. Chen (1995) suggested that many with Asian backgrounds view the therapist as an authoritative public figure with whom they may have difficulties disagreeing. This may be in contrast to Latinos, who value a therapist who has an informal and more personal connection and who prefer that the group atmosphere be more relational (Aguilera et al., 2018). Aguilera et al. (2018) described the importance of the therapist presenting an initial informal and more personal connection.

Role of the Patient–Therapist Relationship

Although the importance of a satisfactory patient–therapist relationship to the progression of therapy is recognized by most theoretical orientations presented in this book, the founders of the cognitive behavioral models did not strongly focus on the therapeutic alliance; however, most acknowledge its significance (Ellis, 1985; Garfield, 1989; Wessler & Hankin-Wessler, 1989). Rapport, empathy, genuine human caring, warmth, and active listening have been specified as being essential to the maintenance of a therapeutic alliance and successful treatment (Freeman, 1990).[6] In this model, the patient's specific reactions to the therapist are used in the context of examining distorted assumptions by having the patient look at the cognitions that are generating the response or behavior (Freeman, 1987). Similarly, the obstacle of noncompliance or resistance to treatment, which impedes collaboration, can be

---

[6]Rational-emotive therapy differentiates *acceptance* from *warmth* or *approval* and encourages the former. Warmth is given with extreme caution so that patients do not think that they are "good people" simply because the therapist approves of them (Ellis, 1980).

viewed as the result of irrational beliefs that the therapist can then actively confront and dispute (Ellis, 1985).[7]

One striking difference between cognitive behavioral models and the object relations and systems is the preponderance of validation, coaching, and even cheerleading that is felt to create a positive therapeutic climate and improve the patient's self-esteem (Swenson, 1989). Rather than setting the stage for an exploration of the patient's internal world, as the psychodynamic model might encourage, or focus on the interaction between members as the interpersonal model may do, the cognitive behavior therapist guides the patient to explore dysfunctional or deficit cognitions so that more functional cognitions and behaviors may replace them. From the cognitive behavioral perspective, technical neutrality would present an additional invalidating experience. Consonant with this lack of technical neutrality, cognitive behavioral models do not object to therapists' personal disclosures. The use of therapist self-disclosure, particularly when the therapist reveals the similarity of his or her problems to the patient's (e.g., communicating with others, feeling put down), is considered an appropriate intervention that can reduce a patient's denial, foster openness, and improve his or her self-esteem (Greenwood, 1987). Self-disclosure may be important for minority populations who experience marginalization within the larger community, especially if the therapist is of the same minority group.

Use of Cotherapists

The use of a cotherapy team is strongly advised, especially for groups with more than six members (Glantz, 1987; Hollon & Evans, 1983). The high level of therapist activity in the group session and the multiple tasks of the therapist are eased by a dyadic therapeutic team that can share the burden. In addition, some of the behavioral techniques, such as modeling and role playing, work best with the presence of at least two therapists. A division of therapeutic attention and labor helps therapists recognize and challenge distortions of the participant whose problem is being discussed while also monitoring other group members (Greenwood, 1987). The relative strengths of each therapist can be used in delineating roles. This model especially is accommodating to a training facility wherein a trainee may be paired with

---

[7]There is not adequate guidance for how to manage patients' reactions to the leader or the therapist's reactions to the patients. As an exception, Ellis (1992) viewed patients' reactions to the leader or other group members as samples of the distorted cognitions (e.g., overgeneralizations) that can be addressed. With regard to countertransference, Freeman advised the therapist to use the same techniques as the patient to explore and cope with what is evoked by the group experience (Freeman, Schrodt, Gilson, & Ludgate, 1993). In some circumstances, Ellis (1992) may even confront the patient (e.g., "I try not to hate you, but I really do dislike some of your behavior, and I hope for my sake, the group's sake, and especially your own sake, that you change it"; p. 68).

a senior therapist (Hill, Clarke, & Wilson, 2008).[8] The specificity of the role assignment enables the therapists to work together with ease. Covi et al. (1988) recommended that one member of the team assume the position of the primary therapist who begins and ends the session, initiates and directs the discussion of various agenda items, and summarizes the work of the session. The therapist reviews and organizes the homework, whereas the primary therapist asks members to describe their agendas (Hollon & Evans, 1983). The cotherapist also tracks the primary therapist's interactions with the group and monitors the group process (Covi et al., 1988). Despite the division of labor, the therapists should have a collaborative posture toward the group and equivalent access to each member of the group.

Role of Technique

The cognitive behavioral model presents an overall framework, not just a series of techniques. The followers of Ellis and Beck, in particular, rely heavily on the inductive method and a Socratic style of questioning to help members develop greater awareness of their distorted thinking and perceptions. The behavioral and cognitive techniques used are important devices for effecting cognitive change. Socratic dialogue, collaborative empiricism, and guided discovery most aptly describe the therapist's techniques (Schachter, 2011). The purpose is to bring into awareness nonconscious thoughts with specific structured exercises; monitor dysfunctional thoughts; recognize the link between thoughts, mood, and behavior; scrutinize the data supporting inaccurate or irrational assumptions; and substitute more accurate or realistic interpretations of their experiences. Behavioral techniques or assignments (e.g., role playing) are used primarily to elucidate the patient's thoughts and provide novel experiences. The emphasis is on discovering and changing cognitions, rather than changing the behavior (Arkowitz & Hannah, 1989). Available manuals help the therapist design each session.

The model was designed within the framework of a Westernized conceptualization of the world, which includes several assumptions that may not be embraced by those outside this cultural framework. First, there is an assumption that rationality will guide thinking, affect, and behavior. That is, once patients recognize that two thoughts are inconsistent with the "data," they change to maintain consistency. The "scientific method" is introduced

---

[8]Although therapist training is advised for the implementation of these models, trainees do not need tremendous psychological sophistication (Cowdrill & Dannahy, 2009; Sambrook, 2009). Research has indicated that a wide variety of support staff and therapists in training can be taught to deliver this type of treatment effectively in a group format (Rosebert & Hall, 2008). Objective measures of therapists' attitudes and competency (e.g., therapy preference scale, cognitive therapy scale) have been developed for this model (Shaw & Wilson-Smith, 1988).

at the grade-school level in American and European schools. Second, there is an assumption that when an individual develops more functional cognitions, they have the autonomy to change the circumstances that may empower the dysfunctional thought. However, this may not be true for immigrants, refugees, and others who have marginal status in their society (Carter, 2004; Salvendy, 1999). It also may not be true for those whose religious and cultural beliefs are strongly at odds with the notion that individuals have some control over their destiny (Ibrahim et al., 2015). Third, when the conception of the self includes a collective self, it may be more than resistance for an individual even to entertain the willingness to consider only their feelings and experiences. The terms *familism* and *respetos* in Spanish capture the importance of these issues in the Hispanic community (Rosselló & Bernal, 1996). Automatic and dysfunctional thoughts may be tightly tethered to the desire to accommodate important others rather than how the patient may view the world, and it may be threatening to the larger collective to have negative thoughts about important others (R. Chen et al., 2018).

Member Selection and Group Composition

The cognitive behavioral theory of emotion, symptoms, and psychopathology has much face validity for both patients and staff. It does not require the patient initially to have an understanding of beliefs outside his or her awareness. For patients, cooperation is clearly and concretely spelled out regarding the requirements for homework, participation, and attendance. The present problem-oriented focus of CBT reassures patients that their problems are being directly addressed. Patients readily experience themselves as actively involved from the start of treatment. Stylistically, patients appreciate and often request the active, reassuring, and encouraging stance of the therapist. The therapy allows the problems to be broken down into manageable steps. It facilitates the achievement of tangible results and provides the experience of success early in the course of therapy. It is an especially good set of models for those patients who like to feel that they are doing something for themselves.

In principle, a patient can benefit if his or her difficulties can be conceptualized in terms of irrational, unrealistic, or dysfunctional thoughts and beliefs. Those most likely to profit from this intervention are motivated to change (e.g., work hard in sessions and complete homework assignments), accept and understand the general cognitive behavior model, are able to use the theory to reframe their problems, can use the reconceptualizations to change dysfunctional thoughts, and are able and willing to complete tasks that require role playing and guided exercises in self-monitoring (Bowers, 1989; Glantz, 1987). Although the model is most effective when group attendance is voluntary, sanctions for nonattendance or privileges for attendance have not hindered its utility (Greenwood, 1987; Grossman & Freet, 1987).

Versatility in treating a wide range of human problems is one of the major strengths of this group of models as the myriad techniques give tremendous flexibility to the therapist's repertoire and style. There are reports of successful treatment for many diagnostic groups, such as severe depression (Chan, Sun, Tam, Tsoi, & Wong, 2017), general anxiety (Freeman & Simon, 1989), panic disorders (Barlow & Craske, 1991; Behenck, Wesner, Finkler, & Heldt, 2017), phobias (Heimberg, 1990; Hope, Herbert, & Bellack, 1991), eating disorders (Tchanturia, Doris, & Fleming, 2014), obsessional disorders (Salkovskis, 1989), alcohol dependency (Glantz, 1987), drug addiction (Ellis et al., 1988; Moorey, 1989), impulsive disorders (Meichenbaum & Asarnow, 1979), borderline personality and other personality disorders (Freeman, Pretzer, Fleming, & Simon, 1990; Linehan, 2014; Martin & Young, 2010; Tchanturia, Doris, & Fleming, 2014), and acute and chronic schizophrenia (Greenwood, 1987; Lecomte et al., 2008; Meichenbaum, 1977; Perris, 1988a).

Frequently, the structure of either an acute or longer term RTC necessitates the creation of a diagnostically heterogeneous group. The focus on the individual and the extent to which the treatment can be tailored to the specific dysfunction even in a group setting attenuates the central relevance of diagnostic composition more so than in approaches that emphasize group-level interventions. Both diagnostic homogeneous and heterogeneous groups have been successful (Freeman, 1987; Freeman, Schrodt, Gilson, & Ludgate, 1993). Groups with a heterogeneous composition more closely approximate real life and allow for a greater variety of perspectives. With respect to age, the successful use of cognitive behavior group therapy from adolescents to geriatric patients has been reported (Glantz, 1989; Grossman & Freet, 1987; Yost et al., 1986).

Initially, patients with extensive delusional systems or denied psychiatric impairment or whose interpersonal styles were verbally disruptive (e.g., overly verbose, hostile, demanding of attention) or whose cognitive deficits were significant (e.g., Alzheimer's disease, developmental delays, learning disabilities) were thought to be poor candidates for cognitive behavior group therapy. However, a number of modifications in techniques have permitted a wider range of patients to benefit from this form of therapy. For example, Williams and Moorey (1989) reported the successful use with individuals who had brain damage, if the procedures were simplified in such a way as to be comprehensible to these patients. The greater the severity of the cognitive deficit, the greater the ratio of behavioral to cognitive interventions needed, and most of the cognitive work has to be done during the session (Williams & Moorey, 1989). Some report success with patients who attribute their illnesses primarily to physical difficulties (Coleman & Gantman, 1991). A burgeoning of work over the past 2 decades with patients with psychosis has produced ways to reduce the perceived control of voices and other recalcitrant symptoms (see the research section). Similarly, significant model modifications by Young, Klosko, and Weishaar (2003) and Linehan (2014) have enabled successful outcomes for patients with borderline personality disorder.

Cognitive behavioral groups work best with four to 12 members, depending on the composition and availability of patients (Hollon & Evans, 1983). Sessions should range from 1 to 2 hours each, depending on the attention span of the members and the group size. The greater the number of members with individualized problems, the longer the time required to attend adequately to each member's agenda.

Assessment

Assessment before the member's first group meeting is highly recommended. Formal diagnosis is less important than the evaluation of the member's ability to understand the cognitive behavioral model and make use of feedback from the therapist and other members.

Motivation to complete homework assignments is crucial. If the patient is to join an ongoing group, assessment and preparation have to be done before the patient's first meeting. If a new group is forming, the assessment and preparation can be rendered more efficiently in the group rather than in an individual format. The use of questionnaires in the initial and ongoing assessments supplements the interview. The assessment begins with an exploration of each patient's presenting problems; formalized assessments such as the Beck Depression Inventory (BDI; Beck, 1978), the Beck Anxiety Inventory (BAI; Beck, Epstein, Brown, & Steer, 1988), and the Hopelessness Scale (Beck, Weissman, Lester, & Trexler, 1974) evaluate target symptoms. The Dysfunctional Attitude Scale (Oliver & Baumgart, 1985) and the Automatic Thoughts Questionnaire (ATQ; Hollon & Kendall, 1980) assess patients' main cognitions, appraisals, and irrational and unrealistic beliefs. The Young Schema Questionnaire (Version 3) assesses maladaptive schemas (Young, 2005). The Life History Questionnaire (Lazarus, 1981) collects background information (e.g., developmental, social, family history). In preparation, specificity of target symptoms and goal setting should be concretized collaboratively with the patient in the form of a detailed, prioritized problem list. The focus should be on problems that could be resolved in the length of time expected in the program.

For example, a 40-year-old man who has a 10-year history of alcohol abuse was hospitalized after a suicide gesture. Although he had made several attempts at outpatient treatment, he never stayed in treatment and found reasons not to attend Alcoholics Anonymous (AA) regularly. In interviewing the patient for group, the therapist found five possible areas for intervention: the drinking behavior itself; the concurrent depression (low mood, helplessness), although the direction of causation between the depression and drinking was unclear; the reliance on the use of alcohol as a primary coping mechanism; a highly critical self and overall hopelessness about his abilities to stay sober; and the social environment (his wife) that permitted and may even have supported his drinking (Glantz, 1987). Depending on the patient's length of stay, the patient's depression, and the concomitant automatic dysfunctional thoughts that were contributing to the depression or his reliance on alcohol as a primary coping mechanism to solve problems may be targeted as goals. This patient perceived his drinking as a means to "resolve" or "dissolve" dissatisfaction at work (lack of promotions, inability to assert himself) and conflicts with his wife. The alcohol also served to reduce his anxiety and anger by terminating fantasies and facilitating the forgetting of or distortion of a memory of past events (his drinking began 10 years ago after an affair). The therapist hypothesized that the maladaptive conceptualizations (both cognitive content and processes) had a central role in the etiology, maintenance, and exacerbation of the alcohol abuse. Both the maladaptive conceptualizations surrounding the development and maintenance of the alcoholism and depression were thus the primary targets of the group.

Further exploration with this patient revealed that his maladaptive processing included drawing arbitrary inferences, creating selective distortions, and making gross overgeneralizations; his thinking was either global, abstract, and undifferentiated or highly narrow, concretized, and specific, depending on the circumstance (Glantz, 1987). His self-evaluations were based on a single criterion (his affair 10 years ago), demonstrating a narrow focus of attention on a single aspect of the situation. He believed that alcohol was the only alternative to bad feelings and difficult problems. For this patient, the focus in the preparation and initial phases of therapy were his cognitive distortions in a specific area (e.g., his home life, wife, or job). As part of his assessment, he may complete the BDI, the BAI, the Hopelessness Scale, and perhaps the ATQ. He may then repeat all or some of these at regular intervals. He may also be given *Coping With Substance Abuse* (Beck & Emery, 1977) or *Coping With Depression* (Beck & Greenberg, 1974) to read as part of the initial preparation.

The initial goals for this patient in a longer term RTC in which he might attend six to 10 groups over a 2- to 4-week period are similar to those of other patients. Therapy works better if patients can be introduced to the following premises: (a) the way an individual thinks strongly affects the way he feels and behaves and therefore his ability to cope with and enjoy life, (b) there are alternative ways to view life that can lead to more desirable feelings and behaviors, and (c) by changing thinking, one can control feelings and behaviors (Glantz, 1987). The content chosen for therapy discussions should focus on one of a member's specific interpersonal problems, with the overall goal being to help the member identify his or her particular maladaptive conceptualization processes. The next step is to help the member understand the negative consequence of these maladaptive conceptualizations and to recognize alternatives and the concomitant improvement that will result from this reconceptualization. Members then have to be helped to develop more functional alternative coping and self-regulatory skills. In addition, patients are supported in replacing maladaptive conceptualizations and behavioral symptom patterns with more adaptive thoughts and behaviors rather than being encouraged simply to stop drinking (Glantz, 1987). This general intervention strategy applies to all patients with alcohol problems. However, the specific goals and techniques used for each individual are based on a patient's particular dysfunctional thinking, coping strategies, personality, symptoms, social resources, and drinking history. The primary goal is to generalize coping and reconceptualizing skills that extend beyond what is discussed in the group. If his stay is brief and he would be expected to attend outpatient treatment, then targeting cognitions that interfere with continued treatment would be the focus. Thus, the low self-esteem and highly critical self might be the most essential targets. This particular combination of symptoms is often resistant to traditional CBT, and patients could make better use of learning inner compassion and self-soothing. Hill et al. (2008) successfully developed a three-session group, "Making Friends With Yourself," that targets these attitudes specifically.

Preparation

The goal of preparation is to facilitate the patient's entry into group. If a new group is being formed, cognitive behavioral theory could be taught at the initial session. However, in short-term settings, the patient joins an ongoing group and must be given an education regarding the principles of CBT before beginning group. The emphasis of the preparation has to be adapted to the particular patient population and the resources that such a population brings to treatment. For example, with young disturbed chronic inpatients, the willingness to participate cannot be assured. The cognitive change desired during this initial phase would be from rejection (e.g., "I don't want to be here") to acceptance (e.g., "I can talk here"; Greenwood, 1987). However, with somewhat higher functioning, nonpsychotic patients, this issue may not be as relevant, and the initial focus may be on definitions and examples of automatic thoughts and schemas and the relation between thoughts and feelings (see Beck et al., 1979, for examples of how to present this material).

This introduction provides a common language and conceptual framework for group members. An essential part of the model is to conceptualize the relation of the members' target symptoms to their dysfunctional or irrational thought patterns. Once the member can identify the dysfunctional thought pattern, he or she is asked to develop an awareness of the frequency of this maladaptive thinking. To assist with this process, members can be given a relevant reading (see Appendix 5.2, Bibliotherapy), an activity schedule such as that included in *Mastery and Pleasure* (Blackburn, 1989) to rate their activities, or a thought record (Beck, 1976). The more completely the cognitive behavioral conceptual framework is understood at a practical level, the more able the patient will be to make use of the group experience. Adaptations of the language have to be made when patients are not fluent in English or their cultural lens does not allow for easy translation. For example, Aguilera et al. (2018) found that a direct translation for assertiveness, *asertivo*, was not well understood but was able to be captured in the concept of *firme* (being firm). Similarly explaining cognitive restructuring, the notion of cognitive distortion is more clearly understood when cast as "helpful" and "unhelpful" thoughts.

It is important to assess and review patients' expectations, particularly those related to concerns such as discomfort in groups, judgments about others' reactions to their problems, or fear of talking or getting help in the group. Although other models concentrate on exploring expectations, the emphasis in this model is on the cognitive distortions or irrationality of the cognitions that would preclude the patient's successful group participation. To instill hope, therapists sometimes talk about treatment effectiveness. Patients are also familiarized with the format of the session and the importance of the homework requirement.

If the therapist is not of the same ethnic background as the patient, knowledge of the social norms of his or her cultural group is essential. Having bicultural staff members who speak the language as sources for the therapist is especially important. For example, knowledge of the role of the family in South Asians and the stresses and traumas of a particular refugee group is essential in building trust for the group work to be successful.

Structured Agenda Format

Groups can be closed-ended or open-ended. If a group is closed-ended, both the course of therapy and each therapy session is structured. In an open-ended or ongoing group, it is possible to structure only the format of each session. Rather than permitting members' interactions or topics to emerge as the group progresses, sessions are framed with a consistent and structured format.

The session usually begins with members' completion of assessment instruments that evaluate their current status. As these forms are reviewed by one of the therapists for significant changes in clinical status, the other therapist may establish an agenda. The traditional CBT session begins by the therapist soliciting members' thoughts about the previous session and inviting members to review their activities since the previous session, to report on the success of the homework assignments, and to state briefly personal items on which they wish to work in the session.

Each of these segments can be divided into separate go-arounds or combined into one go-around. Agenda setting usually takes 5 to 15 minutes. A review of unfinished agenda items from previous sessions is also included. The therapists then attempt to highlight common experiences, illuminate complicated or difficult-to-grasp principles, or illustrate a topic that will be discussed during the session (Covi et al., 1988). This assumes that patients understand the frame and the model.

Most of the group session is devoted to discussing personal agenda items through the patient–therapist interchange.[9] An effort is made to cover all agenda items; a disproportionate amount of time spent with one or more members can be compensated for in subsequent sessions (Covi et al., 1988). The body of the session depends somewhat on group composition, the nature of the problems, how much each member has accomplished in previous sessions, and whether the group is closed ended or open ended. The therapists either work briefly with each member or concentrate in depth on a few members in a single session, recognizing that those members not receiving the group's attention will have their opportunity in the next session (Coleman & Gantman, 1991). Part of the group time may be spent introducing a new technique or concept. The particular cognitive behavioral strategies introduced and used by the therapist depend on the type and severity of the members' problems, their knowledge and understanding of their problems in cognitive behavioral terms, the number of sessions that the group has existed (if closed ended) or that an individual member has attended and the additional number he or she is expected to attend, and the therapist's preferences. The final few minutes of the session can be used as a wrap-up to evaluate the session, assign homework for the next session, get feedback from the members about the session, and have members summarize what they have learned

---

[9]While one member is actively working on his personal agenda, some therapists prefer to have other members involved initially by *active listening* (trying to understand the therapeutic principles used by the therapist and applying them to their own similar problems). At the end of the patient–therapist interchange, other members of the group can comment on what they discovered and offer feedback (Covi, Roth, Pattison, & Lipman, 1988). Other therapists request that members "jump in" whenever they feel that they can contribute (Coleman & Gantman, 1991).

during the session. The structured format permits patients to anticipate how the session will unfold and allows for a more gradual conclusion.

Homework[10]

A fundamental tenet of this approach is that much of the therapeutic change takes place outside the group therapy session (Covi et al., 1988). Individualized self-help exercises facilitate this process. Homework extends the therapy session and can reinforce newly learned skills. It is believed that the members who diligently complete self-help tasks make progress and are able to meet their stated therapy goals more quickly (Freeman, 1990).

In addition, the completion of written homework for each session makes this therapy available to many members who may be otherwise too uncontrolled and unskilled to participate actively in the group. For example, Grossman and Freet (1987) required adolescents to complete written homework as a prerequisite for attending group. The adolescents could get help on their homework from the hospital staff and teachers. Having written homework assignments completed ahead of time so that they were available to read during the session made social interaction possible for adolescents who were too reticent, psychotic, or socially inept to make spontaneous contributions. Structured homework made group sessions more productive, improved adolescents' relationships with staff, and increased their self-esteem.

The creation of the particular self-help exercise should be a collaborative effort relevant to the material discussed in the session and take into account a given member's behavioral repertoire and level of functioning. To increase compliance with assignment completion, other hospital staff should be aware of homework requirements and, ideally, be able to help with specific assignments. Patients might also be assisted either by the group or other staff members in scheduling time to complete their assignment during a day that may be full of other hospital activities (Clarke & Wilson, 2008). The assignment of homework is not always feasible. Certain groups, such as the elderly, do not readily do therapy work between sessions (Glantz, 1989). Time can be added to the beginning or end of group to complete the assignment, with attention to the techniques encouraged. For example, adolescent boys enjoy the role playing component (Rosselló & Bernal, 1996).

---

[10]This term can be modified for populations who experience the term as infantilizing or as too closely related to bad memories of school (Rosselló & Bernal, 1996). Aguilera, Bruehlman-Senecal, Liu, and Bravin (2018) used the term *proyecto personal*, which translates into *personal project*. Kohn, Oden, Muñoz, Robinson, and Leavitt (2002) used the term *therapeutic exercises*.

Course of Therapy and Content of the Session

Cognitive behavior group therapy is primarily problem rather than process oriented. This model usually does not focus on phenomena, such as cohesion, member-to-member interaction, group-as-a-whole dynamics, and affectivity, that are prominent in other models, unless they illustrate an individual's distortions or highlight the relevance of cognitive principles (Hollon & Evans, 1983).[11]

Cognitive and Behavioral Strategies

This model of therapy has a plethora of cognitive strategies and behavioral techniques available as part of its repertoire (see Appendixes 5.1 and 5.2). Although the format does not vary by setting for IHP, PHP, or outpatient therapy, the type of techniques used and how they are implemented depends on the group members' assets and demographics, skills, severities and symptom patterns, and treatment goals (Bowers, 1989). Suppose, for example, the therapist wishes to demonstrate to a group of young chronic schizophrenic patients the centrality of cognitions in determining one's reactions to an event. The therapist may use the strategy of performing skits that model an emotional episode wherein the activating event and emotional components are clearly labeled. The task of the group members would be to generate self-statements that would have led to the emotional sequence. Alternatively, after a short educational component that denotes auditory and visual hallucinations as part of a range of human experience and the continuum of shared and unshared experience, the therapist may have members examine their own shared and unshared experiences (Chadwick, Taylor, & Abba, 2005; Hill et al., 2008). From such exercises, members learn that they have particular cognitions that accompany their emotions.

Most types of CBT entail a characteristic plan of progression. In closed-ended groups, initial sessions are more behavioral in orientation, whereas later sessions involve more explicit cognitive techniques. For example, with adolescents in a state hospital, Grossman and Freet (1987) found that group sessions required specific and structured behavioral guidelines, which were referred to as *group therapy rules* and *constructive behavior tools*. The tools

---

[11]Although there are some exceptions, mostly in the outpatient setting (e.g., Bieling, McCabe, & Antony, 2013; Schachter, 2011), the focus is on the individual and not the group. Few writings address those aspects of treatment that are specific to a group setting, such as patients' interactions with and reactions to each other. This lack of articulation is in part because the model does not emphasize what is unique to a group format (e.g., patients' mutual support of, advice to, collaboration with, and reactions to other members). Thus, unless the cognitive behavioral group therapist has other additional training, there is little guidance for how to make use of patient-to-patient interaction and other group phenomena.

and rules became the foundation for teaching rudimentary social skills and provided guidelines for evaluating larger segments of behavior. After gaining behavioral control, the adolescents were encouraged to explore feelings and learn self-observational skills. In contrast, a group primarily composed of depressed adults might begin with exercises to improve self-observation.

In general, the particular behavioral techniques used change across sessions in a closed-ended group. Initially, specific behavioral tasks are assigned to increase activity, improve self-observational skills, and teach members that there is a connection between thoughts and resulting feelings. To accomplish these tasks, such techniques as activity scheduling, self-monitoring of mood events, mastery and pleasure ratings, and graded or partial task assignment are used. Iqbal and Bassett (2008) found that adding a single session that specifically focused on activity scheduling increased patient engagement in activities on the unit. As the sessions progress and the goals shift to focusing on discovery, evaluating, and empirically testing various automatic thoughts and underlying assumptions, the particular behavioral techniques change (e.g., shame-attacking exercises, role playing). Similarly, initial cognitive strategies (e.g., reattribution, advantages and disadvantages, alternative techniques, labeling distortions, identifying idiosyncratic meaning) are aimed at identifying specific automatic thoughts and gradually increasing attention toward discovering and changing underlying belief systems (e.g., through guided fantasy, as-if technique, downward-arrow technique; Hollon & Shaw, 1979).[12]

In an open-ended group, this cognitive and behavioral progression occurs at an individual level only. In the beginning or when the patient has more severe symptom patterns, a relatively greater proportion of behavioral techniques are used. As therapy progresses, more cognitive techniques are used. Within each of the cognitive and behavioral components, therapy proceeds from the relatively simple to the more complex. As therapy progresses, behavioral tasks proceed from graded or partial task assignments to whole task assignments. Similarly, cognitive strategies shift from processing current cognitive events or distortions (thoughts, images, particular interpretations) to accessing (if possible) nonconscious beliefs and schemas (Williams & Moorey, 1989). Similarly, there may be a higher number of patient–therapist interactions during the earlier part of the treatment than in the later phases when individual consolidation and self-initiation should be taking place (Covi et al., 1988).

---

[12]This latter cognitive shift seldom occurs during a short-term hospital stay. Patients are often discharged from the hospital having learned to recognize and correct specific faulty cognitions but not to change underlying beliefs or assumptions.

Course of Therapy

Many manuals detail the sequence and time frame of the sessions in closed-ended groups (Covi, Roth, & Lipman, 1982; Covi et al., 1988; Glantz, 1989; Moorey, 1989). In short-term IHPs, a closed-ended group with a specific time frame is less feasible. However, the phases are still somewhat applicable, and the progression can be followed at an individual level. The first phase of therapy is characterized by the process of understanding the basic tenets of cognitive behavioral theory and therapy and learning to think in cognitive and behavioral terms (Covi et al., 1982). The therapist facilitates members' understanding by illustrating the theory with examples from patients' experiences and by introducing techniques aimed at identifying distorted and irrational thoughts and modifying dysfunctional behavior (Covi et al., 1982). Members learn the relation between their target symptoms or problems and their dysfunctional thoughts. They are then trained to identify and test the accuracy of their cognitions and to dispute problematic cognitions through the use of structured exercises (Heimberg, 1990). This may be the limit of what can be accomplished in the three to six sessions available in short-term facilities.

During the next phase of group treatment, members use their newly acquired background of cognitive therapy to develop an understanding of their particular symptoms. This involves identifying the particular negative cognitions that accompany the symptoms, formulating the type of cognitive distortion they represent, and discovering the underlying assumptions that are at the core of such dysfunctional thinking (Covi et al., 1982). Therapy then proceeds on two levels: Techniques are taught and applied to the entire group (e.g., all members can be trained to identify, recall, and initiate mastery or pleasure activities), and treatment is individualized by matching techniques with personal goals (Covi et al., 1988).

For example, Grossman and Freet (1987) demonstrated how cognitive behavioral techniques could be adapted to the special needs of different diagnostic groups of IHP patients. They taught all adolescents in their group to differentiate among their thoughts, feelings, and actions and to then label their internal experiences and check feedback from other group members for accuracy so as to discover the systematic ways they distort what they hear. All group members were taught this skill even though the pace of learning for each member varied; members differed in the emphasis they required. Adolescents whose major problems were due to hyperactivity seemed to backslide easily even after they understood the whole process; practice at identifying and checking the accuracy of their thoughts was imperative to their success. With adolescents of below-average intelligence, the learning was slow; these members had to be helped to put their feelings into words and taught to use some alternative sentences that were chunked into small steps and then repeatedly practiced. However, once they understood their distortion processes, they were able to retain this understanding. For adolescents with psychosis, learning new sentences was only part of the task. They also had to learn to identify the exaggerations and the advantages gained by their distortions; because they had not learned basic coping skills, they had to be taught more effective ways to achieve their goals. Adolescents with personality disorders had distorted responses that were more consciously aimed at achieving some short-term objective than were those of the other adolescents. The task of these adolescents was to point out the exaggerations implicit in their distortions and to discuss the consequences of their behavior. Sentences that had enough emotional impact to be remembered were used to make the adolescents aware of how they gave themselves excuses to act out for immediate gratification but destroyed their long-term relationships with important people. Long-run consequences of their behaviors were thus emphasized (Grossman & Freet, 1987).

The last phase of the group treatment is consolidation and working on issues of termination. The cognitive behavioral model is mindful of relapse prevention as an essential part of the therapy. Preparation for termination begins in the first session. Members learn a model and a series of techniques they can use during stressful times. They are encouraged to understand the need for monitoring their moods and are taught how to be watchful for indications of the need for further cognitive therapy. Depending on the length of time in the session, at least one or two sessions should be devoted to an exploration of significant termination issues. Members are encouraged to express and discuss their concerns about leaving the setting and the group. The cognitive behavioral model is applied to termination issues in that the accuracy of members' posttreatment predictions (e.g., they will experience future symptoms, they are not yet well) has to be questioned. As part of this, a member's progress with respect to target symptoms is reviewed. Members identify procedures that were helpful in attenuating symptoms. They are also encouraged to design and implement their own self-help cognitive therapy programs for residual symptoms and possibly continue outpatient therapy to maximize the likelihood that therapeutic gains will be maintained (Covi et al., 1988).

In an open-ended, diagnostically heterogeneous group, pacing is one of the most arduous tasks the therapist faces. Experience and supervision are irreplaceable aids. Somehow, the healthier members' needs must be accommodated at the same time as those who are new or more severely disturbed are encouraged to learn the basics. Members' disparities can be somewhat attenuated if at each session basic principles are reviewed, the majority of the session is pitched to the "average patient," and remedial or advanced work is

TABLE 5.1
Cognitive Behavioral Approach

Elements of the model	Characteristics of the model
View of psychological problems	Problems due to cognitive distortions, which represent activated underlying early dysfunctional schema
Goals of model	Recognize the thought–emotion connection. Identify automatic thoughts that reveal underlying cognitive distortions. Develop more functional responses and reprogram dysfunctional modes of thought, affect, and behavior with more functional ones.
Methods of action	Cognitive techniques, behavioral strategies to effectively cope with symptoms
Therapeutic techniques	Use of the thought record, assignment of homework, structured agenda
Adaptation of the model to a brief time frame	Limit group to homogeneous symptoms. Teach and practice one cognitive strategy.
Use of group process	Group exercises to uncover aspects of distorted cognitions and dysfunctional coping modes. Patient's thoughts and responses to therapist are seen as representative of cognitive distortions.

done between sessions (Freeman et al., 1993). Table 5.1 presents the essential features of the cognitive behavioral approach.

ADAPTATIONS TO THE COGNITIVE BEHAVIOR THERAPY APPROACH

The CBT approach has remarkable flexibility. Over a 40-year period, a number of procedural adaptations have evolved to address setting limitations, particular symptoms, or problems of chronicity. Each is briefly covered in this section. Whether implemented in their entirety or incorporated into a more comprehensive group experience, they can augment the clinician's armamentarium of clinical skills.

Rotating Theme Group

This alternate form was developed to alleviate some problems inherent in settings in which there are a variety of diagnostic and educational backgrounds, variations in individual articulateness, different levels of comfort with social interaction and speaking in a group format, short patient stays, and the disruption in the group when members frequently come and go without notice (Freeman, 1987; Freeman et al., 1993). Homogeneity of age, severity of symptoms, and diagnosis is preferred but not essential to the utility of this approach. Its structured nature allows for patients with cognitive confusion to participate. Each group session is self-contained, with closure at the end of each session; sessions are not cumulative. The approach has maximum flexibility in design by estimating the average number of sessions attended by members (e.g., if the average length of stay is 5 days, and it is possible to have three sessions per week, the number of sessions in the cycle will be about three). Initially, staff members and, over time, members' input determines the most useful topics for the population served. Some examples of common topics include the stigma of mental illness, dealing with discrimination, impulse or anger control, family problems, relationships, reducing self-harm, stress management, emotional distress management, procrastination, how relationships affect mood, and healthy and unhealthy coping (see Freeman, 1987; Raune & Daddi, 2011, for other examples).

The topic for each session is posted on the unit before the meeting. Each group member is encouraged to prepare by writing two of his or her problems related to the topic of the day. Specific problems are written on the blackboard, and members read them at the beginning of the session. The therapist clusters issues to establish a group agenda. An educational component introduces relevant aspects of the CBT model. Grouped problems are then discussed using the principles and techniques previously described in this chapter (see Freeman, 1987; Freeman et al., 1993; Raune & Daddi, 2011, for more details of this model). Written notes can be brought to the session, especially for those less comfortable with talking in a group. Patients in short-term units overwhelmingly report that they find this group useful and look forward to future attendance.

Another variation of the rotating theme group is the *programmed group*, which is similar to a closed-ended structured psychoeducational group in that it is designed to teach specific information about cognitive therapy. Unlike the closed-ended group, it allows members to enter at any point. Freeman et al. (1993) provided a sample schedule for such a program. Skill in designing one of these programs requires presenting topics that do not require preexisting knowledge. This type of program is an efficient way of providing basic information about CBT but restricts the interactions among participants significantly.

Structural Variations

Systematic rational restructuring operationalizes rational-emotive therapy (Goldfried, Decenteceo, & Weinberg, 1974). There are four structured components to this procedure: a presentation of the rationale of treatment, an overview of basic (irrational) assumptions thought to underlie all symptoms and subjective distress, an analysis of specific instances of the patient's difficulties in rational-emotive terms to determine which irrational assumptions are operating, and teaching patients to modify their internal self-statements. As with rational-emotive therapy, logic, reason, and persuasion are the primary processes used to effect change. Although it offers promise for inpatient treatment, it has not developed much in the past 2 decades with the more severe disorders (Goldfried, Linehan, & Smith, 1978; Goldfried, Padawer, & Robins, 1984; Wise & Haynes, 1983).

Self-instructional training combines graduated practice with aspects of rational-emotive theory (Meichenbaum, 1977, 2017). Central to change is the repetition in which a sequence of overt verbalizations is transformed by the patient into covert self-verbalizations or thoughts. The procedure includes the therapist modeling the task by verbalizing the steps involved, the patient executing the task while the therapist articulates the steps, the patient performing the task while inaudibly moving his or her lips, and the patient completing the task while thinking the task through to him- or herself (Meichenbaum & Goodman, 1971). The repetition may facilitate the development of a mediating cognition. Similar to rational-emotive therapy, this therapy deals with distorted or irrational existing beliefs by relying largely on persuasion. Self-instructional training has been used most extensively with people with schizophrenia and impulsive, non–self-controlled children (Meichenbaum, 2017).

Stress-inoculation training combines a skills-training acquisition phase with subsequent practice (Meichenbaum, 1975). The procedure involves the following three main steps: educating the patient about the nature of stressful or fearful reactions and presenting a cognitive rationale for treatment; having the patient acquire and rehearse coping statements and behavioral self-control skills, such as progressive relaxation, that the patient can use when confronted by stress; and having the patient test and practice these skills in actual or stress-provoking role-play situations. The first two steps involve some combination of cognitive restructuring based on reason, persuasion, and the development of cognitive mediation or cognitive replacement achieved through repetition (Hollon & Beck, 1986). This approach has been used with elderly depressed patients in the consolidation phase of a more encompassing group treatment (Glantz, 1989).

Dialectical Behavior Therapy Skills Training

Since our 1993 book, *Models of Inpatient Group Psychotherapy*, DBT has evolved into a prominent treatment for individuals with suicidal behavior and borderline personality disorder (Reddy & Vijay, 2017; Verheul et al., 2003). DBT was developed as a yearlong comprehensive and intensive outpatient program that involved individual and group therapy for patients with suicidal and borderline personality disorders (Linehan, 2014). For RTC, PHP, and prison settings in which treatment can continue beyond a short-term interval, these treatment formats can be embraced in their entirety with proper staff training, collegial supervision, and administrative support. In settings that are typically short term (e.g., hospital inpatient programs) or in which a more multifaceted approach is embraced, some of the specific skills or philosophical elements of the treatment can be taught and practiced in a group format to improve patient functioning and therefore are worthy of a brief discussion here (Koerner, Dimeff, & Swenson, 2007).

At its theoretical core is *dialectics*. This element involves adopting a framework of reality that differentiates and accepts perspectives that are rigidly opposite, an approach that counters the black and white thinking that is dysfunctional for many patients. Therapeutically, it is a method of persuasion that challenges problematic beliefs. It "puts strong emphasis on dialogues that lead to synthesis" (Dimeff & Koerner, 2007, p. 12).

The comprehensive program involves psychoeducation, skills training, exposure procedures, contingency management, and cognitive restructuring (Dimeff & Koerner, 2007; Swenson, Sanderson, Dulit, & Linehan, 2001). Linehan's (2014) manual, an excellent and necessary resource, details elaborate instructions for teaching four modules (sets of skills) and provides a multitude of exercises and handouts for patients.

Mindfulness is the core and essential skill to be taught before all others. This skill helps patients focus their attention in the moment, teaching them to be aware of the present moment without judging or rejecting it (Linehan, 2014). Within this broad category, the main skills taught are *wise mind* (learning to balance reason and emotion), *what skills* (observing and describing self and self in relation to other and participating spontaneously in the present), and *how skills* (developing a nonjudgmental stance). An example of an exercise for developing wise mind involves having patients breathe in and out, noticing the pause after each breath in and out. At each pause, the patient is to "fall into the center space within the pause" (Linehan, 2014, Handout 3A). This exercise lends itself well to a group setting because it does not involve individual members' individual situations. An example of a *what skill* would be to have patients observing and describing their bodily sensations, including the contributions of each of the senses (e.g., ears, eyes). An example of developing the *how skill* is to have group members write out a nonjudgmental description of an event that was prompted by an emotion. This experience can be augmented by a group discussion of the event and its description. If time in a program is short, this skill would be among the more important to teach. A small study with chronic treatment-resistant hospitalized psychotic patients found that mindfulness exercises were well tolerated by these patients (Jacobsen, Morris, Johns, & Hodkinson, 2011).

Distress tolerance skills help patients tolerate their emotional distress when change is slow or not likely to occur. Patients learn impulse control and self-soothing strategies for surviving crises without engaging in dysfunctional or destructive behaviors. This work also involves accepting a reality that may be painful and having hope of moving forward in some way. An example of how to develop this skill is an exercise in which patients pick an experience in which they felt an overwhelming urge. They are then asked to write a list of pros and cons either individually or in discussion with the group. The individual is encouraged to imagine and talk about the positive consequences of resisting the urge and the negative consequences of giving into the urge or crisis (Linehan, 2014).

Interpersonal training focuses on teaching skills for maintaining relationships while preserving self-respect. This module includes 15 different handouts featuring skill evaluation, enhancement, and development. Exercises for this module highlight identifying priorities in relationships, building relationships and ending destructive ones, holding the dialectic (finding the middle ground), maintaining self-respect, and changing behaviors. These skills can easily be applied and practiced in an RTC as stressful encounters with family, staff, and other patients allow for in vivo practice.

The fourth set of skills aids in the development of *emotional regulation*. Patients are taught cognitive and behavioral strategies to learn to identify emotions, face negative emotions, develop more positive emotions, and improve strategies for decreasing unwanted affect and impulsive behaviors that accompany intense emotions. Twenty-five handouts and 16 worksheets comprehensively encourage skill development and practice.

There is good evidence for the efficacy of DBT when the program (2.5 hours per week of individual and group with telephone coaching, teaching, and practicing each of the skills twice over a 1-year period) is administered in an outpatient setting in its entirety (Dimeff & Koerner, 2007). Although the model shows promise, caution is also warranted. When the setting constrains full administration of the treatment package (such as the settings presented in this book), the results may be diminished, and decisions as to the most effective components are still somewhat speculative (Koerner et al., 2007). Complicating the effective use of DBT is that when hospitalization becomes the main strategy for managing distress, this option may interfere with strengthening more effective adaptive coping strategies (Swenson, Witterholt, & Bohus, 2007).

As the model has developed, many have attempted to adapt it to IHP (Kröger et al., 2006; Rendle & Wilson, 2009), PHP (Simpson et al., 1998; Yen, Johnson, Costello, & Simpson, 2009), RTC (Steil, Dyer, Priebe, Kleindienst, & Bohus, 2011), and forensic (McCann, Ball, & Ivanoff, 2000) settings, aware that a hierarchy may have to be developed for the priority of skills taught.

These applications include individual and group interventions. Settings vary in the range of time in the program and unitary commitment to a single treatment program. It has been used in IHPs with adolescents and adults in which stays range from 2 weeks to 3 months. Clinical studies and reports have shown positive findings, but results are best when the entire program uses a DBT model and all DBT skills are taught and reinforced by the nursing team throughout the day (Barley et al., 1993; Bohus et al., 2004; Katz, Cox, Gunasekara, & Miller, 2004; Kröger, Harbeck, Armbrust, & Kliem, 2013; Springer, Lohr, Buchtel, & Silk, 1995).

When the residence stay is shorter or the treatment program is a non–DBT-focused one, psychoeducation and skills training components of DBT can be most easily used in these settings. Some evidence exists that a DBT-focused group modality can enhance some of these skills (Nelson-Gray et al., 2006). For example, if the average length of stay is only 2 days, mindfulness, the core of DBT treatment, can be taught continuously, offering different exercises in each session (Swenson et al., 2007). If the stay is some-what longer (e.g., a 2-week PHP), a schedule of teaching a skill and assigning homework on Day 1 is followed by a detailed review of the homework on Day 2, followed by the teaching of a new skill and assignment of homework on Day 3, with review of homework on Day 4, ending with an overall review and practice at the end of the week. Teaching distress tolerance is usually considered the second priority, but it is particularly important for groups in which life circumstances are difficult. Both mindfulness and distress tolerance skills are perceived by patients to be most helpful (Miller, Wyman, Huppert, Glassman, & Rathus, 2000).

Originally designed for individuals with a borderline personality dis-order and those with suicidal behaviors, DBT can be further fine-tuned for other specific populations (Koons et al., 2006). For example, with eating disorder populations, DBT offers a more emotion regulation model of the symptoms than does traditional CBT treatment. DBT can be designed to focus on teaching more functional affect regulation and target binging and other impulsive dysfunctional behaviors that result from emotional dysregulation (Wisniewski, Safer, & Chen, 2007). For those suffering from addiction, out-patient studies have suggested that DBT is more effective than other treatments (McMain, Sayrs, Dimeff, & Linehan, 2007). For those with treatment-resistant depression, mindfulness with regard to relationships, distress tolerance, and self-soothing is emphasized (Harley, Sprich, Safren, Jacobo, & Fava, 2008). One unique aspect of the model is its conceptualization and focus on *dialectical abstinence*, which is the balance and the "synthesis of unrelenting insistence on total abstinence before any illicit drug abuse and radical acceptance, non-judgmental problems solving and effective relapse prevention after any drug use" (McMain et al., 2007, p. 151).

Some populations may require not only focus on specific target symptoms but also more lengthy, elaborate, and modified treatment. For example, in a forensic setting, focusing on symptoms of emotional insensitivity, apathy, and criminal identification would be important (McCann et al., 2000). Apathy, in particular, may be a critical target given its power to affect full engagement in the treatment. To ensure that patients learn the skill, videotapes and written materials with examples are presented first. Written quizzes are then used as motivators for further group participation (McCann, Ivanoff, Schmidt, & Beach, 2007).

Although DBT skills can help most psychiatric patients, this treatment is often considered and implemented when patients exhibit recalcitrant symptoms. Several important considerations emerge from the literature. The first is that staff and therapists need support and supervision. Without it, a demoralized staff can quickly emerge. Attending to opportunities for patients to practice on the unit requires a motivated staff. McCann et al. (2007) suggested "contests" among staff to improve motivation. Second, the teaching of skills does not have to be left entirely to therapists and staff. Videotapes, written examples, and worksheets can augment the intense psychoeducation staff must provide. Third, groups work best with two staff trainers, one to teach a skill and the second to track the process and provide support for patients.

Schema Therapy

Developed by Young et al. (2003) as an individual therapy, schema therapy evolved from Beck's model to treat patients whose chronic and persistent psychopathology is severe and often resistant to traditional cognitive behavioral techniques described earlier in this chapter. Although Beck's theory acknowledged the importance of schemas as the origin of dysfunctional thoughts, the focus in practice has been on the identification of automatic dysfunctional thoughts and the rejection of them through empirical testing.

In schema therapy, the main constructs are schemas, modes, and coping styles. In this therapy *schemas*, usually outside of awareness, are more broadly conceptualized as consisting of memories, bodily sensations, emotions, and cognitions about the self, the world, and other people. Originating in childhood, they are elaborated, reinforced, or extinguished throughout a person's life. They are heavily determined by the interaction of temperament and whether the environment met core childhood needs. The theoretical foundation and basis of therapy is that unmet core childhood needs (e.g., through early rejection, abandonment, neglect, and abuse) result in the development of maladaptive schemas. These early childhood schemas may have been adaptive at the time but have become inaccurate, dysfunctional, and limiting by adulthood (Farrell et al., 2014). For example, a child who experiences significant trauma may develop schemas of distrust, subjugation, or defectiveness that may have been protective in an unsafe environment. Over time, however, these schemas become codified as everyone is perceived as untrustworthy. Or they may have become relatively dormant until a new traumatic event, perceived to be similar (e.g., a partner's affair), triggers the activation of the schema. Eighteen early maladaptive schemas have been identified (Martin & Young, 2010).

The strategies used to cope with schemas, referred to as *coping styles*, may vary by temperament, situation, and life stage. Three common maladaptive coping styles are surrender, avoidance, and overcompensation. Consider a child who, due to early physical abuse, develops a schema of mistrust. If the child regards him- or herself as deserving this toxic environment, as an adult, that person will select abusive partners and allow the abuse. The adult could also avoid vulnerability by not trusting anyone and keeping secrets, both from important others as well as in therapy. In contrast, overcompensating adults use and abuse others in a preemptive attempt to protect their vulnerabilities. A patient could also cycle through all three of these coping styles, allowing abuse, then avoiding further involvement with others, and eventually becoming the abuser.

Modes are states, activated when specific schemas or coping responses arouse overwhelming emotions. Four types of modes shape experience: child mode, maladaptive coping mode, dysfunctional parent mode, and healthy adult mode (Martin & Young, 2010). *Child modes* include the vulnerable child (e.g., sad, misunderstood, defective, fragile), the angry child, the impulsive child, and the contented child. *Maladaptive coping modes* correspond to the three coping styles: compliant surrender, detached protector, and overcompensator. *Maladaptive parent modes* include the punitive parent (feeling that self or others deserve punishment) and the demanding, critical parent (internalized high standards for self and others). When in *healthy adult mode*, the person engages in taking responsibility, manages and limits maladaptive coping, and seeks pleasurable, healthy, and age-appropriate activities. Modes can shift rapidly, whereas schemas and coping styles are more enduring. For example, patients with borderline personality disorder can be functioning in healthy adult mode when a perceived neglect or inattention suddenly shifts the person to the abandoned and angry child modes and then the punitive parent mode who punishes for expression of neediness.

The goals of therapy involve the following: identifying and labeling maladaptive modes as they arise in and outside of therapy; linking these modes to problems and symptoms; exploring the origin and function of each mode; attenuating the intensity of intrusive memories, negative emotions and bodily sensations, and maladaptive cognitions and behaviors; exposing the dysfunctional and interfering nature of these schemas, coping styles, and modes; and replacing dysfunctional modes with healthy ones.

Schema therapy is effective when patients have any of the following: vague, entrenched, chronic symptoms; maladaptive thoughts, feelings, and behaviors; dysfunctional relationships; and/or ambivalent and avoidant motivations for treatment. Schema therapy expands the therapist's CBT repertoire with the integration of psychodynamic (object relations and attachment) and gestalt theory and techniques. Cognitive, behavioral, and psychoeducation techniques are augmented in several ways. First, schema therapy recognizes the significance of the therapeutic relationships as an internal source of support and as it enables and facilitates the unfolding of the maladaptive schemas, coping styles, and modes. In a group setting this includes the importance of group cohesiveness and the containing functions of the group. Second, schema therapy values the affective, emotive, and defensive elements of the patient's modes of functioning.

An essential ingredient in the treatment is *limited reparenting*. Within the bounds of an appropriate therapeutic relationship, the therapist provides validation and comfort for the vulnerable child mode, the space to vent for the angry child mode, and empathic confrontation and limit setting for the impulsive child mode (Farrell et al., 2014). *Empathic confrontation*, a technique that empathizes with patients' deep-seated pain while challenging the behavior, has been further articulated by Farrell and Shaw (2013) and may be useful across a variety of theoretical orientations in the group setting for disruptive patients. The steps include the following:

1. Strengthen the therapeutic alliance and name the maladaptive mode. Farrell and Shaw (2013) suggested, "I am not saying this to be critical. I am saying it because I am concerned that your old protective behavior will not get your needs met today" (p. 2).
2. Acknowledge the origins of the behavior but that the behavior will not get their needs met now. For example, "We know that you were bullied as a youngster, and this bully-attack mode takes charge when you feel vulnerable and hurt. However, I am worried that this way of handling your feelings will frighten others. They even might avoid you. Your needs for having relationships and receiving love and caring won't be met."
3. Offer an alternative and assistance in practicing a more adaptive behavior. For example,

   You could decide in the group to let safe people know when they hurt your feelings and see if they mean to or if it was a misunderstanding before letting the old coping behavior take over and protect you by hurting them. That way your need for companionship has a chance of being met. The old way you will stay alone. . . . We can work on how to let someone know when you are hurt and even role play that in the group. (Farrell & Shaw, 2013, p. 2)

Although manuals have been published describing structured treatment that adapt to a group-only or individual-only format, a comprehensive treatment includes both group and individual therapy and requires training and/or supervision to achieve proficiency (Dickhaut & Arntz, 2014; Farrell et al., 2014). We focus here only on the group treatment. Young et al.'s (2003) model was modified for a group outpatient setting by Farrell, Reiss, and Shaw (2014). One 8-month outpatient treatment program was designed with thirty 90-minute group sessions. It included emotional awareness training, psychoeducation, distress management and schema change, traditional CBT techniques, experiential work, and focus on relations inside and outside therapy that helped identify and modify schemas, coping styles, and modes. In a pre–post design, Farrell, Shaw, and Webber (2009) found significant changes in impulsive and self-harm behaviors and in self-hatred and emptiness.

The full program of 42 group sessions can be adapted to a short-term IHP with a minimum of 10 hours per week for 6 weeks. When stays are longer (as often occurs in European countries) or in a PHP or RTC, 5 hours per week for 12 weeks is suggested (Farrell et al., 2014). Both include five sessions of psychoeducation teaching the lexicon of schema therapy, 12 sessions of helping patients develop awareness of each of their modes of functioning, 12 sessions of learning to manage their maladaptive modes, and 12 sessions of practicing more adaptive functioning to stressful life situations. All sessions are structured and include worksheets, experiential exercises, imagery work, and homework. This model focuses more on identifying and modifying modes rather than the underlying schemas. Another variation specifically developed for eating disorders (van Vreeswijk, Broersen, Bloo, & Haeyen, 2012; van Vreeswijk, Spinhoven, Eurelings-Bontekoe, & Broersen, 2014) emphasizes underlying schemas rather than modes and is more structured than the Farrell et al. (2014) model.

The use of this treatment in RTCs shows promise, as suggested by recent research on patients with intermediate or long-term stays (e.g., Borge et al., 2008; Shorey, Stuart, Anderson, & Strong, 2013) and those staying for brief or short-term intervals (Roper, Dickson, Tinwell, Booth, & McGuire, 2010). In IHPs, three studies using a pre–post design examined the utility of schema group therapy (Nenadić, Lamberth, & Reiss, 2017; Reiss, Lieb, Arntz, Shaw, & Farrell, 2014; Schaap, Chakhssi, & Westerhof, 2016). All patients had chronic dysfunctional and unremitting symptoms and carried diagnoses of personality disorders. In addition to group, all settings offered one to two sessions per week with individual therapists and/or other adjunctive therapies.[13] All

---

[13]Nenadić, Lamberth, and Reiss (2017) offered 12 to 15 sessions (45–50 minutes) for 6 to 7 weeks. Reiss, Lieb, Arntz, Shaw, and Farrell (2014) conducted groups for 8 hours per week over 10 to 12 weeks. Schaap, Chakhssi, and Westerhof (2016) delivered a twice-weekly group (1.25 hours per session) over 12 months.

studies demonstrated a general improvement in distress or symptomatology. However, maladaptive schemas when measured were not reduced (Nenadić et al., 2017). Within a PHP, schema therapy was used with eight women with chronic eating disorders over a 6-month period. Although symptom reduction did not occur, women showed an increase in motivation over the course of treatment and a low dropout rate, unusual for this patient population (George, Thornton, Touyz, Waller, & Beumont, 2004; Simpson, Morrow, van Vreeswijk, & Reid, 2010).

CLINICAL ILLUSTRATION OF A COGNITIVE BEHAVIOR THERAPY APPROACH

This example takes place in a PHP where patients average a 2-week stay. The group meets five times per week for 90 minutes each session. New members enter at the beginning of the week and are interviewed in a group format before beginning group. Patients who cannot complete at least a week or are disruptive are not included. Patients are given information about the group, taught cognitive behavioral theory, given handouts and reading material, and make a commitment to attend and do homework. They also complete the Beck Depression Inventory–2 (BDI-II; Beck, Steer, & Brown, 1996) and the BAI (Steer & Beck, 1997) before beginning and before every session. The cotherapist collects the responses and reviews them as the therapist begins each session.

The first half of the first day of the week is dedicated to again reviewing the basic Beck model: identifying automatic thoughts, the relationship between thought and feeling, and how to complete the automatic thought record. The second half of the session is helping each patient apply the model to his or her symptoms or problems and assigning homework. The illustration is the second session for each of these patients.

Group Members

Al is a 45-year-old Caucasian construction worker, with a 25-year history of alcohol abuse but who had stopped drinking 6 months prior. He had been experiencing increasing anxiety since he had stopped drinking, feeling overwhelmed at work and yelling at his children and wife. He was hospitalized after he had gotten into a physical fight with one of his coworkers, had gone on a drinking binge, and then, had made a suicide gesture because he felt hopeless about his ability to keep from drinking. He was hospitalized overnight. He agreed to attend a 2-week PHP and Alcoholics Anonymous before returning to work. The therapist assessed him as having inadequate skills to cope with the difficulties of daily life and exhibiting some distorted cognitions (e.g., all-or-nothing thinking). His case illustrates how drug and alcohol problems may be tackled within a cognitive behavioral framework.

Nicole is a 60-year-old widow who had been in long-term treatment for anxiety and depression. She complained that she was lonely and that her siblings and children did not visit her. A number of antidepressants had been unsuccessful in ameliorating her chronic dysphoria (she regularly called her psychiatrist and had numerous physical complaints). She had been hospitalized many times over the years. She was referred to the PHP because the number of complaints to her psychiatrist and relatives had increased dramatically, with no significant physical findings. This member illustrates how one can work with a patient who has little acceptance of her difficulties (e.g., Coleman & Gantman, 1991).

Patricia is a 39-year-old African American mother of 8-month-old twin boys. After recovering from postpartum psychosis, she returned to her job full-time as an administrative assistant when the boys were 6 months old. Two months later she was hospitalized after an overdose of the psychotropic medications given her by her general practitioner (she had complained of weight loss, insomnia, and loss of concentration on her job). This suicide attempt resulted in a 48-hour comatose state. After being cleared medically, she was referred to the PHP. She had no other psychiatric history or experience with therapy. The therapist assessed her to be passive, hopeless, and overwhelmed. This member is included to show how the cognitive behavioral model can be used with a depressed patient.

The Session

Therapist: This is a cognitive behavior therapy group. Last time we learned about automatic thoughts and how they affect the way you feel. We learned how some thoughts are distorted and how they can lead us to feel bad. When you get upset, it is often related to what you are thinking. If you think differently, you will often feel better and be able to do things differently. This group is structured. We have an agenda [*Cotherapist writes this on the blackboard.*]. First, we check with everyone and find out what has been happening since last we met. Make a brief comment about how your homework went. Then after touching base with everyone, we'll go over homework in more detail and continue working on our goals by developing specific strategies to help you think, feel, and behave differently. Then, we will collaboratively decide on each of your assignments for tomorrow. Does anyone have any questions about what I said right now or thoughts or questions from yesterday? [*Therapist structures the session format.*]

Nicole: I have a question about something I noticed in our last meeting. It sounds like this is more between doctor and patient than other therapies that I've had. [*Patient articulates one of the differences between this group and the psychodynamic group she had been involved with in her last hospitalization.*]

Therapist: You mean the therapist is more active here? In other types of groups, the therapist may be quieter, and group members are free to talk about whatever seems important at the time. Yes, that's perceptive. We have a structured format. Let's go around and find out how everyone is doing and how their efforts on the homework went. It's important for us to iden-tify a manageable chunk of your goal that you can accom-plish today. Please feel free to give feedback when other people present what they are working on. After all, we have so much collective wisdom here. Let's start with Patricia. Did you do your homework? [*Homework was to pick two times when she felt upset and write what the automatic thoughts were. She was to complete a form that she had been given the previous group meeting requiring the specification of the situation, her feelings, and her automatic thoughts.*]

Patricia: Yes, it went okay. I feel fine.

Therapist: Good. How about you Nicole?

Nicole: Oh, no, I forgot. What was I supposed to do? I left it at home. I've been having a bad day. I was just so upset after talking to my doctor on the phone.

Therapist: Did you write it down?

Nicole: Well, I guess. Some of it. I started to anyway. I have such a bad memory. I just can't seem to remember anything anymore.

Therapist: I'm glad that you wrote it down [*reinforcing the importance of written homework*].

Cotherapist: [*takes a piece of paper from a nearby pile*] Here is some paper. Today you can write your assignment down so that you do not forget. Homework is important because it's like continuing the therapy after you leave. The more a person is participating in the therapy process, the more likely and sooner that they can achieve their goals. [*Cotherapist uses this as an opportunity to reinforce the essential aspect of homework, reinforcing Nicole for her attempts without exposing her.*]

Therapist: Al, how about you?

Al: I'm jangled. I'm constantly being bombarded with these events, thoughts. I wrote it down as part of my homework.

Therapist: Great. I'm glad you wrote them down so we can review them. We'll talk about your jangledness when we go over your homework in detail.

[*Therapist continues with four other patients. When this finishes, therapist works with those receiving the least attention the previous day.*]

Therapist: Good job, everyone! You remembered a lot from yesterday. You were able to apply it to yourself. Al, we didn't have much chance to work with you last time. You told us last time that you drank your whole life and that you had stopped drinking 6 months ago and that work was overwhelming.

Al: Yeah. I don't know who I am anymore.

Therapist: What's being abstinent feel like?

Al: I used to just drink and let life go by. I didn't know what it was like not to drink. I guess these problems used to be around, but I didn't know about them. I was too drunk all the time. Without the booze, I feel lost. Don't know how to do anything.

Therapist: So you were using alcohol so you wouldn't see and feel life's difficult issues.

Al: Sounds good.

Therapist: So now he's a baby. [*Group members giggle.*] Al has a million upsets each day because he doesn't have booze. [*To Al*] All those things that you shielded yourself from you're going to have to deal with in new ways other than drinking the booze. For homework, you were going to write down two events, and we were going to scrutinize them in our cognitive behavior therapy way.

[*Cotherapist goes to board and draws four columns labeled situation, feelings, automatic thoughts, and rational responses and enters members' responses in the appropriate columns.*]

Al: Yesterday, here, after group, I was supposed to go to psychological testing at the same time as I was supposed to go to the AA meeting, and shoot, they [*staff*] don't know where I'm supposed to be. I was getting nervous, but I know I have to leave this building and go to another.

Therapist: So we have upset with the staff for not knowing where to send you [*entered under* situation]. How were you were feeling?

Al: Sad, nervous. I could use a drink.

Therapist: Automatic thoughts are brief, fleeting thoughts of which you may be barely aware.

Al: I thought, I gotta be somewhere for two activities at the same time.

Therapist: Anything else?

Al: I started saying the Serenity Prayer.

Therapist: Okay. You made a rational response to this situation. Or another way to look at it is to say that you developed a behavioral strategy to manage the situation. The behavioral strategy was saying the Serenity Prayer. The automatic thought is one step earlier. Do you remember, however fleeting, what the thought might have been?

Al: I can't control this situation. How can I be at two places at the same time?

Patient X: What would happen if you weren't able to?

Al: I don't know. I feel like maybe I could get into trouble.

Therapist: Al says, "I got to be in two places at once. I can't control it. What am I supposed to do? What are they going to think of me?" He thought he could get into trouble. [*To Al*] Evaluate whether the thought is a faulty one. Sometimes just putting out the thought—recognizing and labeling it is helpful. Let's develop a treatment plan for Al. Let's say that without booze, you're a worrier. You have to learn how to handle a lot of these situations without worrying. Does that seem like a reasonable and realistic plan to you?

Al: Sounds good to me.

Therapist: First you frame the situation. Label your feelings. Then focus on that automatic thought that you may never have concentrated on before. Then evaluate whether that thought is a reasonable or an accurate one. You are on your way to understanding how to use cognitive behavior therapy. Let's go on to your other homework situation.

Al: The situation was that yesterday since I had to go to psych testing, I could not attend the AA day meeting, so I went to the early evening one which is just next door. I was with Joe [*another patient*], and we left our stuff here at the center. When the meeting was over, the doors to enter the center were locked. I felt anxious. I thought I'm going to have to go through all this garbage to get in. I'll draw attention to myself. They'll ask me a lot of questions.

Therapist: This is a good one. What's the issue around being the center of attention?

Al: I don't like being the center of attention. I don't know why. They'll ask me a lot of questions. Everyone will be wondering about me. I won't be able to explain myself. I don't like to draw attention to myself. What will they think of me?

Therapist: What would happen if you did? What's wrong with a lot of questions?

Al: I just wouldn't like to do it. It's like I couldn't explain myself. Like they would think, "What was I doing?" Fooling around? Was I trying to steal something? Would they think I'm a loser?

Therapist: Al predicts everyone will think badly of him. You feel guilty. Al is afraid he will be accused of something. Al predicts trouble for himself. How did you get back in?

Al: Well, that's the crazy thing. Joe, the guy I was with, he had the right idea. I wish that I could have reacted like he did. He was mad. He said, "Why the heck did they lock the doors? They know we went to a meeting and left our stuff in the center." He just rang the doorbell, which was right there, and the guard let us in, and he didn't even ask any questions.

Cotherapist: Your tests indicated yesterday and today that you get anxious about a lot of things and that you are anxious much of the time.

Therapist: Now that you've stopped drinking, you're raw in the world. You're anxious, and you don't know how to manage it. Al had thought of saying the Serenity Prayer. What other rational response can he say to himself?

Nicole: Well, you can ask, "What is the worst that could happen?"

Al: Well, I know. I could kick myself for getting so bent out of shape.

Therapist: It's a good thought, but it doesn't work for Al. He just feels worse. Could you stand being anxious for 3 to 6 months and not give yourself such a tough time?

Al: Well, I have to.

Therapist: If you are able to put up with being anxious for a few months as you get more experience in the world without drinking, that anxious feeling will lessen to some degree. It's going to be many months of work, and you're going to have to do it yourself. Some people don't want to work on it, but with a lot of effort and cognitive behavior therapy, it will get better. So your rational response would be to say, "Let me step back and see if I can handle this. I don't need booze to handle this" [*writes on board*]. You anticipate many bad things happening. You're like a weatherman predicting rain 95% of the time. Remind yourself of your ability to predict.

Al: Not great.

Therapist: You are working very hard. Continue to collect examples and automatic thoughts for next time [*assigns homework*]. Over the next few days, we will work on more strategies to help you cope with the anxiety. Let's talk to Nicole. Yesterday, she told us that she has no problems that we could help with [*Nicole giggles*]. [*To Nicole*] You're depressed. You think that you have pain from the medication. Your doctor thinks you have something else.

Nicole: Well, she knows I have pain, but she says it's not due to the medication. But every time I take my medication, I get sick, physically sick. I have a lot of pain. She wanted me to come into the hospital, but I felt that we could have done this on an outpatient basis.

Therapist: So you compromised and came to our program. Now you've met us!

Nicole: Yes, well. She says that I am psychosomatic. I don't see it that way. I think that my case is much more complicated than she says. But she intimidates me. I think we should be partners. She should take me seriously and think that these symptoms are real or at least evaluate them.

Patricia: It scares me because she is my doctor also. How long have you been seeing her? Did you trust her in the past?

Nicole: I've seen her for years, off and on. I trusted her. Maybe you won't have the same problem with her. [*They appear to wander. The therapist returns them to the agenda.*]

Therapist: Let's talk about your homework that you forgot. You felt your psychiatrist doesn't listen to you. That makes you feel frustrated and helpless. Your automatic thought was, "She doesn't respect me." Last time, other members helped to evaluate that response. Is it a reasonable response to feel frustrated if you feel that you have not been listened to?

[*Patient X and Al nod yes.*] So then we were going to have you check out the accuracy of your perception that your psychiatrist wouldn't listen to you. So the group suggested seeing if she would talk with you about your symptoms, and you agreed that it was a reasonable test of whether she listens. Part of your homework was to see if your psychiatrist would talk with you about your symptoms.

Nicole: Well, that's why I'm so upset and forgot my homework, because of my meeting with her before group. I can't be right with her. She thinks she's the doctor—she knows best, and she doesn't listen. [*Laughing*] I'm laughing because she says that I don't listen to her. I wrote her this letter, which she told me to bring here and share with the group. It says I think that we should be partners. I know my body better than she does. I know when things are real, and she should listen and take what I say seriously. I think that sounds reasonable.

Therapist: Does it to you?

Al: Nah. The doctor is always right.

Nicole: She says that I don't admit to my problems. She says that I'm angry. I don't feel angry. I'm willing to work on it, but how can I work on something I don't feel?

Therapist: [*Breaks in to stay on track*] Part of your homework was to test whether she would listen to you. She listened to you by reading the letter. You may not like her opinion, but your idea of collaboration was that she was to listen to you, which she did by allowing you to present your case through the letter. You feel that your symptoms are real side effects, and it sounds like she thinks that they are due to your depression. [*Having a specific criterion for evaluating whether someone is listening helps eliminate the "yes–but" response from the patient.*]

Al: Isn't it a matter of perspective? My wife is a pharmacy assistant, and if I get a drug from a doc, I just take it. I say the doctor is an authority—she went to medical school, and she should know. My wife says, "What are you crazy? Taking a drug without knowing anything about it?"

Therapist: [*To Al*] So you would take the drug, and if you had these pains, you would say to yourself that you were not going to worry about it. The drug is supposed to work, and these pains must be something else, or you would just ignore them. [*Al nods.*]

Nicole:	I told her that I had pains in my body, but she said these pains are not the usual side effects for medicines I am taking.
Therapist:	So she listened to your complaint and told you that these pains you have aren't side effects. You checked out what the usual side effects are?

[*The cognitive distortion in question, "My psychiatrist doesn't listen to me," has been disproved through this empirical demonstration. The patient then attempts to go on to another complaint about her doctor, which implicitly takes a yes–but form. Some therapists may attempt to handle this new complaint in the same manner as the previous one. Nicole, however, had a two-part assignment. This deliberate shift, although appearing to take the focus away from the patient's complaint about her psychiatrist, removes the therapist from the yes–but struggle that is beginning to emerge in the interaction with this patient. The question about the side effects begins the transition into the second part of Nicole's assignment, which was to write down the circumstances surrounding the pains. That is, when Nicole developed these pains, she was to write down the situation around the development and termination of these symptoms and what she was thinking and feeling.*]

Nicole:	Well, yes, she told me.
Therapist:	Which symptoms did you write down that make you sick?
Nicole:	Well, I feel sick in my stomach, and I have lots of pain here in my shoulder, and my neck hurts, and I sometimes have tingling in my feet, and I feel like sometimes that there is this tight collar around my neck and . . .
Therapist:	These were all from yesterday, and you wrote them down? [*Nicole shakes her head no.*] Which ones were from yesterday? [*Therapist attempts to narrow the field of discussion and keep it specific.*]
Nicole:	Throat burning, weakness in the legs, but the symptoms seemed to have lessened. I know these are side effects.
Therapist:	Which ones?
Nicole:	I had them before, the weakness in the legs.
Therapist:	What was the feeling like?
Nicole:	I don't know if I can describe it. It's like a drawing feeling, the energy just drawing away.
Therapist:	What do you mean by a "drawing feeling"? [*Again, the therapist tries to get the patient to be as behaviorally specific as possible*

and focus on the specific qualities of the feeling rather than on the pervasive feeling of not being listened to.]

Nicole: I don't know. Like a draining feeling.

Therapist: [*Cotherapist writing on the chalkboard in the appropriate columns* situation, feelings, *and* thoughts.] So what did you do? [*The therapist also could have addressed what else was doing on at that moment.*]

Nicole: I just tried to ignore it.

Therapist: Good. What were you doing at that moment?

Nicole: Well, I was listening to the radio, and then I decided to take a nap and went to bed.

Therapist: Good. You had these symptoms. Your rational response was to ignore it and to think that it would go away. This went better than I thought. [*To the group*] Her bodily symptoms are diminishing, and the ones that she still has she copes with by ignoring them. We asked her to talk with her psychiatrist. Nicole wrote her a letter and was able to get her psychiatrist to listen to her. If this progress continues, we will need to revise your goals. Let's move on to Patricia. Do you have your homework?

Patricia: Yes. I wanted to ask you a question. Do I have a goal? We were talking about goals last time and today.

Therapist: Good point. The goal for Al is to be able to cope with worrying. The goal for Nicole is to learn how to evaluate whether her symptoms are side effects or masking her anxiety and depression. Her other goal is to learn to communicate better with her psychiatrist. For you, Patricia, yesterday we were talking about your perfectionism and doing two things at once. What would you say your goals are? [*This summary is a useful way to keep a simple focus.*]

Patricia: Maybe the inadequacies I feel and realizing they are normal?

Therapist: Is the inadequacy you feel the result of your pessimism or are you really inadequate? In other words, you feel you haven't done a good job with any task. But an outsider would say that the job is fine, or would they agree that you haven't done a good job? We have to figure out whether your thoughts are erroneous. Or if they are accurate, we need to problem solve so that you feel more adequate. We'll have to gather more data and look at situations to see whether you are inadequate or are not. Let's look at your first situation and set of feelings.

Patricia:	I feel down and depressed. I can't be what I am supposed to be.
Therapist:	What do you mean more specifically?
Patricia:	I am not a good mother. Jason and Jacob seem totally dependent on me. I can't do anything right. I can't seem to do everything that I used to do. If I had been a better mother, then they would have developed a little more independence. I haven't done a good job.
Therapist:	[*Cotherapist writes on the board.*] So you think, "My little boys are dependent upon me." What is the feeling?
Patricia:	I feel anxious, scared, and overwhelmed. I thought everything would be instinctive. I thought I should be a loving mother.
Therapist:	Did you think that you were not?
Patricia:	I guess I was at first, but not now.
Therapist:	You thought you were supposed to be loving all the time? [*Patricia nods.*] You're supposed to be loving all the time, and if you are not, you're terrible? [*Patricia nods.*] You are a terrible person for not being a loving mother 100% of the time?
Nicole:	You're trying to be a supermom. Trying to be perfect. If you're not perfect, you are horrible. No room to be human.
Al:	You're feeling guilty. You're like me: If it rains, I feel guilty and worry even though I know it's not my fault really. You got it in your head that you're supposed to be super all the time. Well, that just ain't possible. My kid is now 18. When he was young, he was a royal pain. I remember when he was 5 on a Saturday watching these boring cartoons. I would rather have been doing something else. If you think that you're not supposed to be bored some of the time, well, it is boring. You gotta admit it.
Therapist:	[*Turning back to Patricia*] Maybe you're a perfectionist. You want to do it 100% of the time. Be a loving mother, be perfect at your job.
Patricia:	I have a problem with doing two things at once. If I'm not with my sons, I can't concentrate on what I'm doing. I feel like I should be with them. I feel like they need me even if they are doing okay without me. When I'm in the office, I feel like I should be home.
Nicole:	You're very hard on yourself.

Therapist: You have trouble dividing your time, doing two things 100% of the time perfectly. [*Patricia nods.*] What was the second situation?

Patricia: Working.

Therapist: What is your feeling about your work situation?

Patricia: Anxiety.

Therapist: What was the automatic thought?

Patricia: I can't do it. I'm not smart enough to do this anymore.

Therapist: Anymore?

Patricia: That's it. Can I bring up something stupid? The major problem with me is that I can't do it.

Therapist: You said, "I can't do it." What can't you do?

Patricia: Before I had children, I could stay after work to finish.

Therapist: Before you had children, you would spend extra time, and that would help you feel that you did a good job. Now when you went back to work were you depressed? [*Patricia says yes.*] So you were already handicapped. Do you know what I am talking about? Part of the depressive symptoms are that you don't feel motivated, you can't concentrate. [*Therapist educates.*] What part of the job was overwhelming?

Patricia: I don't have time to finish now. Our company is trying to cut back, and I have more to do.

Therapist: Before your children, you worked until you finished. Now there is more to do, and you need to stay even longer to finish. Is that okay with you?

Patricia: No, it's not okay with me. It can't take longer. I have babies to get home to. Maybe I'm not being honest. I don't want the responsibility that I used to have anymore.

Therapist: Sounds okay to me. Does it sound reasonable for a woman who just had twins to not want the responsibility at work that she had before? What stopped you from talking to your boss?

Patricia: Well, I feel my boss pulling on me. She had to go to bat for me being out so long on a pregnancy leave. She told her boss that I was a very hard worker and that I would come back and more than pull my weight in the company. She said she's doing everything she can to keep me, and then I'm going to tell her that I don't want to work like I used to. I'm afraid she will be disappointed in me.

Therapist:	You don't like to disappoint people, or maybe you don't like them to get angry? [*Patricia nods.*] You'd be like Nicole, who can't talk to her psychiatrist. You wouldn't be able to talk to the psychiatrist either.
Patricia:	No, I wouldn't. That's why I was asking her about her experience with her doctor.
Therapist:	I'd like you to write rational responses to automatic thoughts and collect more data.
Patricia:	You mean you'd like me to call my boss?
Therapist:	Well, you can think about doing it, but for next time, for each of the two situations you presented today, the one about feeling inadequate at work and feeling inadequate as a mother, I want you to list a rational response to them. Then collect two more situations. Was that helpful? [*Patricia nods.*] Are you saying that so you won't disappoint me? [*Patricia laughs and says no.*] Okay. Let's move on.

[Group continues with other patients. At the end, homework for each is again reviewed, and brief feedback about how the session was for each group member was solicited.]

Comment on the Session

This example features work with mixed diagnoses in a single group. This is likely to be the situation in a PHP and acute IHP. Because this model has many specific interventions that are often used with particular disorders, an effort was made to endow the clinical example with a diversity of patients to illustrate how interventions vary regarding the special problems of each member. For example, Nicole illustrated the difficult somaticizing patient and how she might be successfully managed in a diagnostically mixed group (Coleman & Gantman, 1991). Al represents a method of conceptualizing and working with patients who have problems with addiction (Glantz, 1987). Finally, Patricia illustrates how a bright, seriously depressed, and passive individual begins to identify some of her dysfunctional perfectionistic cognitions that may have been contributing to her helplessness. As a demonstration of technique, what was not addressed in this session, but might be considered in a future session, was the social reality of economic vulnerability. As a single working-class mother without spousal support, Patricia has limited options if she does not want to enter the welfare system. It is not clear the extent to which she perceives herself as a minority, having to work harder than her Caucasian peers.

Given the short-term stay, goals involved learning to identify problematic situations, identification of distorted thinking, developing rational responses to the distorted and automatic thoughts using the framework of thought record. The therapist was active in keeping a focus when patients' conversation wandered, at the same time allowing for some flexibility, which revealed patients' curiosities about each other and the application of their problems to their situations, allowing them to learn from each other.

STATUS OF THE RESEARCH

In our 1993 book and in the additional work published since then, it has been established that inpatients with a wide range of psychiatric disorders have benefited from individual CBT (Stuart & Bowers, 1995). Similarly, the group format is successful in an outpatient setting (Brabender & Fallon, 1993; Moore et al., 2017). Although there was much enthusiasm about the utility of an IHP CBT group, at the time, only two research studies could support its efficacy. One study compared a 12-session (8-week) CBT regimen to a treatment-as-usual intervention with adolescents and found the CBT group to be superior in increasing both verbal and behavioral self-control (Feindler, Ecton, Kingsley, & Dubey, 1986). A second study with moderate severely depressed geriatric patients in a nursing home found a 20-session (10-week) CBT group superior in decreasing depression compared with a music group or standard care (Zerhusen, Boyle, & Wilson, 1991).

In the past 2 decades, efforts to demonstrate the utility of group using a cognitive behavioral model in both RTC and IHP settings have come to fruition as a number of outcome studies have yielded positive findings. Still, only a few studies have compared two active treatments (Bechdolf, Köhn, Knost, Pukrop, & Klosterkötter, 2005; Drury, Birchwood, & Cochrane, 2000; Wiseman, Sunday, Klapper, Klein, & Halmi, 2002). Even these had a number of flaws, such as nonrandom assignment and unequal numbers of sessions per treatment. A few studies used a treatment as usual comparison (Owen, Sellwood, Kan, Murray, & Sarsam, 2015; Rosner, Lumbeck, & Geissner, 2011; Veltro et al., 2008; Wykes, Parr, & Landau, 1999). The rest compared before and after measurements to show positive results (Bellus et al., 2003; Chadwick et al., 2000; Hodel & West, 2003; Long et al., 2016; Lynch, Berry, & Sirey, 2011; Manning, Hooke, Tannenbaum, Blythe, & Clarke, 1994; McInnis, Sellwood, & Jones, 2006; Newton et al., 2005; Pinkham, Gloege, Flanagan, & Penn, 2004; Wykes et al., 1999). Most were admittedly pilot programs. All published studies we found had some measurable positive findings. Here, we report the trends, acknowledging that significant criticism could be marshaled against any one of the studies.

Outcome Findings

Two studies that compared two active treatments are worth noting. In one acute IHP, patients with schizophrenia received either 16 sessions of group CBT or eight sessions of psychoeducation (Bechdolf et al., 2005). Sessions were 60 to 90 minutes. Both groups improved in symptoms, but the CBT group improved more. At 6-month follow-up, both groups had high compliance for medication, but the CBT group had fewer rehospitalizations. At 2-year follow-up, the CBT group trended toward fewer hospitalizations, decreased days in the hospital, and greater compliance with medications.

The second study compared CBT with recreational and support therapy (Drury et al., 2000; Drury, Birchwood, Cochrane, & Macmillan, 1996). Each group of patients received 3 hours a week of group treatment, with a maximum of 6 months of treatment—the term of their hospital stay. Those in the CBT group had fewer positive symptoms (hallucinations, delusions) and greater perceived control over them at discharge and 9-month follow-up. At 5-year follow-up, for those patients with fewer than two relapses, those receiving CBT still perceived greater control over illness and had fewer delusions and hallucinations than those receiving the other therapies.

It is most exciting that even a modest intervention can improve functionality for those with psychotic symptoms. These studies provide an interesting contrast in that the first was a closed-ended group in an acute setting, whereas the second was an open-ended group in a longer term setting, where a greater number of patients were more likely to have chronic psychotic symptomatology. Both initially measured symptoms, but on follow-up, the first only compared compliance and rehospitalization, whereas the second measured symptoms as well. The comparison of these two studies illustrates how differences in symptom acuity, chronicity of illness, setting, length of stay, and goals of treatment muddy the clarity of relevant mechanisms of change. Healthier patients recover quicker and are likely to be discharged sooner, thus having exposure to fewer cognitive behavioral group sessions (Frederiksen, 2010). In addition to these IHP studies, CBT group has been effective in PHP (Manning et al., 1994; Wykes et al., 1999), mixed IHP and PHP (Hagen, Nordahl, & Gråwe, 2005; McInnis, Sellwood, & Jones, 2006), and forensic unit settings (Hodel & West, 2003).

Symptoms and Goals of Treatment

The scope of symptom acuity that responded positively to CBT group ranges from first break adolescents (Newton et al., 2005) to chronic psychotic patients hospitalized for more than 2 years (Bellus et al., 2003). The studies suggested that a broad array of realistic goals is accomplished in CBT group.

With both acute and chronic patients, increases in attendance, self-care, and participation have been found (Bellus et al., 2003; Raune & Daddi, 2011). Several studies have demonstrated that CBT group improves knowledge and awareness of the illness (Long et al., 2016; McInnis et al., 2006). Acknowledgment and awareness open the door for evaluating the reality and omnipotence of the voices (Chadwick et al., 2000; Manning et al., 1994; Pinkham et al., 2004) and finding strategies to help focus and organize thoughts and process information (Hodel & West, 2003). These skills, in turn, enable patients to perceive themselves to have more control over their hallucinations and delusions and be more optimistic about the future (Chadwick et al., 2000; Drury et al., 2000, 1996; McInnis et al., 2006; Newton et al., 2005; Owen et al., 2015). Overall, the distress of the voices and stress of the illness are lessened and compassion toward the self and self-esteem increases (Hagen et al., 2005; Long et al., 2016; Manning et al., 1994; Owen et al., 2015).

Number of Sessions

In acute short-term settings it is difficult to have closed-ended groups. In longer term programs in which, presumably, the patients' problems were more chronic and severe, it is possible to have closed-ended groups with a greater number of sessions. Studies range in the number of sessions offered and the number that patients attended. Raune and Daddi (2011) described a stand-alone session model in which they tracked whether patients reported group to be helpful and desired to attend in the future (43% did reattend). Because some psychoeducation is necessary for the implementation of the model, it is difficult to teach these concepts and then have patients identify these in themselves in a brief stay. However, when patients have a good experience, albeit brief, it is more likely that they will be amenable to the outpatient treatment needed for continued mental health (Rosen, Katzoff, Carrillo, & Klein, 1976). One way to augment the time needed for this education is to increase the length of the group and offer it daily. When CBT group is extended to 105 minutes per group and patients attend at least 3 days, rates of symptom improvement were higher than treatment as usual (Veltro et al., 2008). Although it is not clear how many sessions each patient attended, the symptom improvement lasted up to 18 months. Unfortunately, at 18 months, the symptom readmission rate did not differentiate the groups. Similarly, another study offered weekly 90-minute sessions over 4 weeks and found that compared with treatment as usual, confidence in managing symptoms improved along with reduced stress around the illness (Owen et al., 2015).

For patients with chronic schizophrenia in longer term care, CBT group has been shown to have some positive effect for sessions that range from seven (Chadwick et al., 2000; Pinkham et al., 2004) to as many as 50 (Bellus et al., 2003). One study found that there was no additional benefit to increasing the number of sessions from seven to 20 (Pinkham et al., 2004). Other studies have suggested that a minimum of 10 sessions was required for positive results (Long et al., 2016). Most studies have used weekly groups, but some have used twice-weekly groups (Hodel & West, 2003).

Outcome Studies With Other Disorders

A number of studies using pre–post research designs have conducted groups with heterogeneous diagnoses in PHP (Neuhaus, Christopher, Jacob, Guillaumot, & Burns, 2007), mixed PHP and IHP (Hagen, Nordahl, Kristiansen, & Morken, 2005), and IHP settings (Strong, Gilbert, Cassidy, & Bennett, 1995). Groups were open ended, with patients attending from 12 to 20 groups lasting up to 8 weeks. All studies reported positive effects ranging from decreases in psychiatric symptomatology to relationship improvement.

Mood-Related Disorders

Four studies examined the effects of a cognitive behavioral group treatment on mood disorders, both using pre–post design. As previously reviewed in alternative models, inpatients diagnosed with mood disorders (bipolar and mixed) attended a diagnostically mixed CBT group that used Freeman's programmed model in a 5-day rotation. Patients averaged five to six sessions during their inpatient stay. If they attended three or more, functioning at discharge improved significantly (Raune & Daddi, 2011).

Nielsen (2015) conducted closed-ended groups in which patients began as inpatients and completed as outpatients if discharged before completing the 12 sessions. Booster sessions at 3 and 6 months aimed at maintaining gains. She reported a significant decrease in depressive symptomatology throughout the treatment despite significant cognitive and motivational impairments.

A large study of mixed diagnostic categories (mostly anxiety and depression) had PHP patients attend 60 hours of group over 2 weeks, with follow-up at 6 weeks and 3 months. There was a significant improvement in depression, self-esteem, and anxiety at discharge and these gains were maintained at 1 year (Manning et al., 1994).

A cognitive behavioral group (nine 90-minute sessions) designed specifically for complicated grief was compared with treatment as usual in an inpatient setting (Rosner et al., 2011). The treatment group had significant improvement in grief symptoms, although overall mental distress or other depressive symptoms were not significantly different for the two groups.

Anxiety Disorders

Page and Hooke (2003), using a pre–post measure design, conducted a manualized CBT group for IHP and PHP patients diagnosed with anxiety and/or mood disorder. Anxiety was the focus and measurement of treatment even though diagnoses were mixed.[14] Patients attended 40 sessions (90 minutes each) over 10 days of their stay. The focus was on psychoeducation, behavioral interventions to reduce anxiety and stress, self-esteem, assertiveness and communication, and relapse prevention. Both PHP and IHP patients' anxiety improved equally. However, at 3-month follow-up, PHP patients had better outcomes on anxiety than did inpatients, which makes sense given that the former were overall likely to be more functional at the beginning of treatment.

Eating Disorders

Two studies examined the effectiveness of cognitive behavioral group therapy with IHP eating-disordered patients in modifying different aspects of the disorder. Wiseman et al. (2002) compared CBT with psychoeducation. In eight sessions over 2 weeks, the CBT group monitored participants' food records, identified problematic beliefs, and used cognitive restructuring. The psychoeducation group provided information on medical and social consequences of disordered eating and nutritional education. Although there was no symptom difference between the groups at the end of 2 weeks, patients preferred the CBT group and found the psychoeducation group repetitive and less valuable (Wiseman, 2002). Lloyd, Fleming, Schmidt, and Tchanturia (2014), using a pre–post design, administered a six-session weekly CBT group to reduce perfectionism and doubts about actions. There was a significant change in overall perfectionism and concern about mistakes; however, this was independent of body mass index change.

It is likely that for this disorder, more sessions are necessary for change. In support of this, Bowers, Evans, and Andersen (1997) examined a hospitalized anorectic population (average 2-month stay). Patients received a psychoeducation group geared toward distorted cognitions about body image and eating 5 days per week and a cognitive behavioral group (which also included process and relational elements) 90 minutes twice a week (Bowers et al., 1997). Thus, group members on average received over 60 hours of group. At discharge, attitudes toward eating, body image, and perfectionism had changed and body mass index increased. At 1-year follow-up, many of these gains were maintained (Bowers & Ansher, 2008). Similarly, in a mixed IHP and PHP sample with a mixed group of eating disorder patients, patients

---

[14]Depression and anxiety frequently co-occur, and successful treatment of one often attenuates the other.

attended groups 8 hours per day 7 days a week for an average of 13 weeks (Gerlinghoff, Gross, & Backmund, 2003). At discharge and follow-up (17 months average), body mass index improved and was maintained, symptoms improved, and disordered eating attitudes and behaviors changed (Gerlinghoff, Backmund, & Franzen, 1998).

Alcohol Abuse

In a pre–post design, Ness and Oei (2005) examined the effectiveness of a cognitive restructuring and social skills group in reducing alcohol abuse, anxiety, and overall psychopathology. Forty-two group sessions based on a model specifically for alcohol dependence (Monti, Abrams, Kadden, & Cooney, 1989) were conducted over a 3-week RTC stay after detoxification. There was a reduction of alcohol consumption, anxiety, and overall psychiatric symptoms at treatment's end 1 and 3 months later. The rate of attendance was related to improvement in anxiety and psychopathology but not alcohol consumption at 1- and 3-month follow-up. This finding is similar to another study that added 12 sessions of cognitive behavioral group for those with comorbid panic disorder. There was a significant improvement by the end of treatment, but the small number of sessions did not provide additional benefit in reducing drinking (Bowen, D'Arcy, Keegan, & Senthilselvan, 2000).

DEMANDS OF THE MODEL

Clinical Mission

The utility of the cognitive behavioral model is marginally limited by the clinical mission of the setting. It is not highly compatible with an environment that exclusively endorses the biological etiology of all symptoms given that the CBT model requires that patients view dysfunctional or irrational cognitions as important causes in the etiology and maintenance of their symptoms. The success of this model requires, at the very least, a supportive environment and, preferably, an explicit collaborative interface with the rest of the treatment. That is, without a supportive milieu, its efficacy is compromised. The development of a supportive milieu may require additional staff training, supervision, and discussions to increase the acceptance of the model within the treatment setting (Hanna, 2008; Kinderman, 2008; Schrodt & Wright, 1987). The model is best suited for a setting in which the group therapy is just one component within the framework of an entire cognitive behavioral program in which formulation and teaching of the model are provided by individual therapists and supported and reinforced by staff (Cowdrill & Dannahy, 2009; Kennedy, 2008; Rosebert & Hall, 2008).

Context of the Group

The cognitive behavioral group functions autonomously from other setting activities, and thus it does not require group members to live together. It does not presuppose that the therapist knows the day-to-day happenings of the RTC; these events do not have to be a part of the content of the session. This independence from setting life permits the group therapist to be an outside consultant rather than a member of the core treatment team. It remains valuable for the therapist to liaise with the treatment staff to inform them about the current efforts and problems being discussed in group and get feedback from them about patients' behaviors. Knowledge of group goals and aims also enables staff to more readily encourage patients to complete homework or to aid them in carrying out the assignments (savvy staff may know to help patients without the group therapist's specific instructions). Conversely, it is not necessary that the patient's goals in group exactly parallel those of the rest of his or her treatment. However, it is an asset if formulations are aligned and supported by other treatment aspects (Kennedy, 2008; Sambrook, 2009).

Temporal Variables

The most limiting factor is the required time frame. The implementation of cognitive behavioral group therapies as currently reported in the literature requires a time frame that most acute inpatient facilities cannot accommodate. There have been some advances in the development of groups that operate as single sessions (Freeman et al., 1993; Raune & Daddi, 2011) and specific skills that can be taught in a few sessions (Hill et al., 2008; Rendle & Wilson, 2009). However, most studies have suggested four to 10 sessions or more to be effective; hence, the PHP and RTC settings are most appropriate for this model. Schema-focused therapy and DBT suggest either a weekly yearlong commitment or the equivalent number of sessions.

The amount of group time required by this model depends on the patient composition, whether other concurrent treatments use the cognitive behavioral model, the number of group members, the stability of the group, whether assessment and formulation has been accomplished and introduced before beginning group, how extensive the preparation is, and individual goals to be accomplished. If treatment is individualized (as opposed to preestablished topics or skills), the completion of an assessment and then preparation for group are strongly advised, particularly with populations who find some of the assumptions and constructs foreign. It is possible to minimize preparation before beginning a closed-ended group.

Descriptions of cognitive behavioral group therapy have included both closed-ended and open-ended groups. Membership stability is important and can be accomplished more readily if the group is closed-ended. Most of the shorter term groups described in the literature were closed-ended. Although there are some exceptions, the open-ended groups work much better if there is at least a three-session commitment (often more for patients with psychotic disorders). Even if the group is open ended, turnover at every session can be chaotic, unless the leader structures into the session an introduction of new members and teaches the relevant techniques and theory. However, if goals can be limited, there may be clinical benefit even if only a few sessions can be attended (Hill et al., 2008).

Size of the Group

Group size constraints are between four and 12 members. The greater the turnover, the more difficult it is to accommodate the upper range of members. This is because time is not available to adequately work on all the problems and handle the initial sessions for new members who may require much teaching. Group size is also constrained by the availability of a cotherapist. A single therapist cannot manage more than six patients.

Composition of the Group

CBT was designed for higher functioning patients. However, in the last 25 years, the model has been modified and successfully applied to individuals with chronic and acute schizophrenia, psychotic and nonpsychotic mood disorders, borderline personality, anxiety, eating disorders, and alcohol abuse. Although most examples of cognitive behavioral groups in the literature have been homogeneous, it is not clear the extent to which this bias reflects a demand of the model. The model seems best suited for homogeneous groups given that the focus of the teaching may be vastly different depending on members' intelligence, levels of ego strength, and presenting symptoms. It takes considerable skill for a therapist to have a group with mixed ego strength and mixed diagnostic categories, although there is sufficient evidence for the value of these groups. The model does not require that members be psychologically sophisticated. It does require time to prepare and teach theory and have patients apply it to their lives. There is little research to suggest that gender is a factor in efficacy. Although voluntariness is desired, tethering attendance to privileges and discharge does not hinder the model's utility. With some modification, this model can be suited to a wide age range (from adolescents to elderly patients). One major strength of this model is that it has been adapted to diverse cultural groups; manuals have been translated into a number of languages (see Muñoz & Mendelson, 2005).

Therapist Variables

The use of a cotherapist is highly recommended. The role of the therapist is articulated more than in most models so that it is possible to have different cotherapists if the therapist remains the same (e.g., nurses on rotating shifts or trainees).

The successful use of the cognitive behavioral model requires that both patients and staff understand principles of CBT. This means that staff must be trained in CBT techniques (which may require the organization to provide formal training and supervision). Data from a National Institute of Mental Health collaborative study by Shaw and Wilson-Smith (1988) suggested that this model requires therapists to see patients in therapy for 72 to 100 hours and have 34 to 54 hours of supervision to learn this model. However, individuals with less than advanced degrees (e.g., nurse trainees and other mental health students) can be successfully trained. Competency of the therapist and members' improvement is significantly correlated, which suggests therapists' competency is an important variable in CBT (Chaisson, Beutler, Yost, & Allender, 1984; Clarke & Wilson, 2008).

SUMMARY

The cognitive behavioral model is aimed at enabling the patient to cope better with his or her symptoms and problems in life. The target of change is the individual's dysfunctional cognitions and behaviors. The focus of the group is on the individual patient. The therapist uses a wide variety of cognitive and behavioral strategies to aid each member in identifying dysfunctional cognitions, testing their accuracy, and practicing new ways of thinking and acting that will enable the patient to function better.

Different versions of the models are well documented and well articulated in Procedure manuals. There is a growing body of empirical support for the efficacy of the cognitive behavioral model with various diagnostic populations and both diagnostically heterogeneous and homogeneous populated groups in both acute and longer term settings. The most severe constraint on the use of this model is tenure in the group. It can be useful in short-term settings if goals are more modest. The approach requires assessment and preparation before beginning group. Clinicians report that some stability of membership is best and more than a few sessions are required for members to benefit from the group experience. If these demands of the model can be fulfilled, this model is likely to show much promise regarding its contribution to the care of psychiatric patients in both shorter- and longer-term settings.

APPENDIX 5.1: COGNITIVE STRATEGIES[15]

- *Rational coping statements.* These statements are also referred to as *constructive adaptive self-statements.* Patients are taught to use self-statements or instructions (first verbally out loud and then silently) to help them through a stressful situation. These statements should be meaningful to the patient and ideally should be chosen by them. This technique can be the entire therapy, or it can be used in combination with other techniques (Meichenbaum, 1977).
- *Cognitive distraction.* This technique enables the individual to temporarily stop ruminating by having him or her focus on complex counting, addition, or subtraction. Engaging in mental imagery, physical activity, or humor are also used as distractions that provide temporary relief and allow patients to detach from their anxiety and establish control over their thoughts (Freeman, 1990). Ellis (1980) cautioned that cognitive distraction should always be used as an adjunct to other methods given that patients may not want to continue to work on their problems if this alleviates the majority of their distress.
- *Thought stopping.* This technique teaches patients to stop dysfunctional thoughts at their inception rather than letting them accrue. Patients are usually taught to use a sensory cue (e.g., visualizing a stop sign) as a way to stop the thoughts (Wolpe, 1973).
- *Semantic analysis.* This technique challenges patients who overgeneralize and misuse language (Ellis, 1990).
- *Guided imagery or guided fantasy.* This technique is specifically designed to raise certain issues such as anxiety, guilt, shame, and joy. Initially, the technique is used to illustrate the relationship between cognitions and resulting emotions. Later in the therapy process, each member works separately on his or her problem area during the guided group fantasy and then participates in a group discussion. Group members who had similar emotional experiences find that they had similar cognitions, whereas others are surprised that they responded in unpredictable ways (Wessler & Hankin-Wessler, 1989).
- *The discomfort anxiety concept.* A technique used especially by rational-emotive therapists to dispute the irrational belief that

[15]Adapted from *Models of Inpatient Group Psychotherapy* (pp. 415–418), by V. Brabender and A. Fallon, 1993, Washington, DC: American Psychological Association. Copyright 1993 by the American Psychological Association.

one should not experience discomfort or unease. For some patients, this is manifested in their low frustration tolerance of their symptoms (e.g., depression and anxiety) and a desire for immediate relief. Rational-emotive therapists philosophically endorse long-term rather than short-term hedonism. Patients are encouraged to remain in an uncomfortable situation for discrete periods of time to encourage the development of frustration tolerance (Ellis, 1977a, 1977b, 1990). Discomfort anxiety can take an interpersonal form as well, manifesting itself as a manipulation to obtain immediate gratification. Grossman and Freet (1987) attempted to help adolescents deal with this by listing as one of the goals "Building up your emotional bank accounts [with people]" (p. 142). The goal was to have enough in one's "emotional bank accounts" to get what one wants from them "off the interest." When adolescents manifested discomfort anxiety and manipulated the situation, therapists asked, "What must you have been thinking to allow yourself to get away with that?" (Grossman & Freet, 1987, p. 147).

- *Realistic appraisal.* Patients use index cards or a smartphone to record thoughts and realistic responses to them, and practice responses to thoughts (Friedberg, Fidaleo, & Mikules, 1992).
- *Active disputing.* This popular technique of rational-emotive therapy involves vigorous disputing or debating by challenging, questioning, and expressing skepticism about the patient's irrational and absolutist thinking and then teaching patients how to do their own disputing. This technique is less applicable for intellectually disabled and severely psychotic individuals (Ellis, 1980).[16] This technique may need significant modification in those cultural groups in which this is an unacceptable way to communicate or where harmony is important (Chen, 1995).
- *Idiosyncratic meaning.* This technique involves the clarification of terms and statements to ensure that the group, the patient, and the therapist have the same understanding (Freeman, 1987). By doing this, the therapist models the importance of "active listening" and provides a method for questioning and confirming assumptions. This is particularly essential in ethnically diverse groups in which the meaning of certain terms may differ. Alternative language may be used to improve

---

[16]Freeman (1990) advocated using this technique only when suicidality is prominent. In his opinion, this technique has the potential to lead to a power struggle with the patient; patients with chronic symptoms are often reluctant to give up a problem that will leave them with no way to cope.

understanding, as when automatic thoughts are viewed as "helpful or unhelpful" thoughts (Aguilera, Bruehlman-Senecal, Liu, & Bravin, 2018).

- *Questioning the evidence.* This technique teaches patients to question the "data" they are using to continue a belief or strengthen an idea. It is a less confrontational technique than is active disputing (Freeman, Schrodt, Gilson, & Ludgate, 1993). This may be more acceptable in groups that value *respeto* and *simpatia* (Rosselló & Bernal, 1996).

- *Reattribution.* This technique is used when patients inaccurately attribute negative events to a personal deficiency (e.g., "It's all my fault that my son did not get into Harvard"). The therapist guides the patient to recognize all responsible individuals (Freeman, 1987). This technique may need some fine tuning in cultural groups in which the individual is encouraged to take responsibility for the collective (Chen, 1995).

- *Examining alternatives.* This technique helps patients learn to solve problems by using additional options. Other group members' participation can be particularly helpful in this regard.

- *De-catastrophizing* (also called the *what-if technique*). This helps patients recognize that they are overestimating the catastrophic nature of a situation. The therapist asks the patient questions such as "What if it did occur?" and "What is the worst that would happen?" (Freeman, 1987). Imagined events or interactions that might happen often illustrate the dysfunctional thinking that distorts patients' perceptions.

- *The "as-if" attitude.* This technique can be used when the patient appears to be following some nonconscious belief or holding a particular cognition that is irrational or dysfunctional. The therapist states that the patient is acting "as if" he or she holds a belief and then presents evidence to support the "as-if" statement. Other group members can add further support for the therapists' interpretation and offer speculations about each other's nonconscious cognitions (Wessler & Hankin-Wessler, 1989). This is a difficult construct to use when patients have not achieved formal operations.

- *Advantages and disadvantages* (also called *referenting*). Patients list the pros and cons of a belief or behavior to help gain a balanced perspective. This is often effective with adolescents (Schrodt & Wright, 1987).

- *Reframing.* This technique helps patients reframe a negative experience. Patients learn to see the positive side of unfortunate events. For example, losing one's job may be seen as an opportunity for growth (Ellis, 1990).

- *Labeling of distortions.* Identifying and labeling cognitions aids in monitoring dysfunctional thinking. Often, patients are given a list and description of types of distortions that can be referred to during the session (Heimberg, 1990).
- *Downward arrow.* In this guided association approach, patients articulate their thoughts and fears of the significance of events so they can understand the underlying assumptions. The technique follows each patient's statement with questions such as "Then what?" or "What would happen then if that were true?" (Freeman, 1987). This technique requires the cognitive achievement of formal operations.
- *Replacement imagery.* This technique helps patients develop more effective positive imagery and dreams to replace the ones that generate anxiety or depression (Freeman, 1987). Here, familiarity with the culture's stories, myths, folktales, parables, and *dichos* is essential (Carter, 2004).
- *Cognitive rehearsal.* Patients imagine each step in a sequence to an event or task as a way to rehearse cognitively before a task is behaviorally performed (Freeman, 1987).
- *Direct questioning.* This technique can be used when a patient does not acknowledge a feeling that is apparent from his or her demeanor. The patient is asked what just went through his or her mind (Williams & Moorey, 1989).

APPENDIX 5.2: EXAMPLES OF BEHAVIORAL TECHNIQUES[17]

The goal of using behavior techniques is threefold: (a) to change behavior through the introduction and practice of a broad range of behavioral techniques (Beck, Rush, Shaw, & Emery, 1979; Beck & Weishaar, 1989), (b) to use the behavioral techniques as short-term interventions with the goal of long-term cognitive change, and (c) to collect data and then empirically test the veracity the underlying assumptions and beliefs. (Followers of rational-emotive therapy do not use empirical testing because they tend to believe that irrationality is ultimately not testable.)

- *Activity scheduling.* This technique assesses the patient's current use of time. It can be used in the preparatory phase of group

---

[17]Adapted from *Models of Inpatient Group Psychotherapy* (pp. 413–414), by V. Brabender and A. Fallon, 1993, Washington, DC: American Psychological Association. Copyright 1993 by the American Psychological Association.

as an assignment to get the patient accustomed to the idea of doing homework outside the group session. It can also be used prospectively to plan the more productive use of time later in the course of therapy (Freeman, 1987). It is particularly helpful with depressed patients (Iqbal & Bassett, 2008). This form and assignment may need modification because of living circumstances (Organista & Muñoz, 1996).

- *Mastery and pleasure ratings.* The patient can begin to examine his or her mastery (the sense of accomplishment in doing the activities) and pleasure (how much he or she enjoys the activities) using the activity schedule. These ratings are made using a 5- or 10-point scale and can be used to plan more mastery and pleasure activities as well. This schedule provides data with which to identify cognitive distortions by exploring the discrepancies between what was accomplished and the feeling of mastery and whether the reasons for this difference are realistic or distorted (Beck et al., 1979). *Pleasure* can be broadened to include satisfaction for the family or larger social group for those who believe that individual pleasure is a decadent western construct.

- *Behavioral rehearsal.* This technique allows the patient to practice interactions with other group members. The therapist and group can coach and model new behaviors. Both group members and the therapist can give feedback on the patient's performance (see Chapter 9).

- *Externalization of voices.* This technique has the therapist role play the patient's dysfunctional voice and then an adaptive response. Patient and therapist role play together so that the therapist can, in a stepwise manner, become an increasingly more dysfunctional voice of the patient, and the patient, through successive approximation, can get practice in adaptively responding.

- *Bibliotherapy.* For some patients, reading can aid in the induction phase to educate the patient about principles of cognitive behavior therapy. Books such as *Feeling Good* (Burns, 1980), *Coping With Substance Abuse* (Beck & Emery, 1977), *Own Your Own Life* (Emery, 1984), and *How to Stubbornly Refuse to Make Yourself Miserable About Anything—Yes, Anything* (Ellis, 1988). Bibliotherapy is only a small part of the therapy unless the group is mostly an educational one. The reading material chosen should be carefully selected with the characteristics and limitations of the patient population in mind (see Irish College of General Practitioners, 2013, for examples). Worksheets and reading should be presented in the language in which the patient feels conversant (Aguilera, Garza, & Muñoz, 2010).

- *Graded task assignments.* The therapist assigns tasks in a stepwise fashion from simpler to more complex. Each assignment is accompanied by an exploration of the patient's doubts and encouragement of realistic evaluation of his or her accomplishment (Freeman, 1987).

- *In vivo work.* This technique consists of having the patient practice his or her newly learned skills outside the group setting. It is often used with those who have social and interactional difficulties. It also can be used within the session to simulate real-life circumstances (e.g., having the patient hyperventilate to learn that many symptoms he or she has are the result of the hyperventilation; Williams & Moorey, 1989). Without staff support, this is not often accomplished because patients' anxieties overwhelm their desire to complete the task.

- *Progressive relaxation.* The use of progressive relaxation, focused breathing, and meditation helps anxious patients begin to gain a sense of control over their anxiety. *The Relation and Stress Reduction Workbook* (Davis, Eshelman, & McKay, 1988) is an excellent resource for both patients and therapists.

- *Shame-attacking exercises.* This technique consists of having patients test their distorted beliefs regarding how others view them by performing shameful or foolish activities. The goal is for the patient to realize that others tend not to scrutinize and evaluate his or her behavior with the same critical eye that he or she does (Ellis, 1985). For those patients for whom their social behavior is a reflection of their larger social group, the larger social group must be on board with these activities.

- *Journal writing.* This involves daily detailing of experiences in the program. Patients record thoughts, feelings, and self-revelations. Patients have the option of sharing entries with the group (Witt-Browder, 2000).

APPENDIX 5.3: GROUP EXERCISES

Exercises are listed in relative developmental phase of the group life. Each exercise includes the therapeutic purpose and a description of administration.

Experiential Focusing Exercise

When: First session
Purpose: Increase patients' awareness of any sensation, thought, or feeling
Part of the Experiential Mode Work Sessions. Maladaptive coping modes are identified. Individual members stand approximately 12 feet from one another and one member slowly walks toward the other. Members are directed to record their physical sensations, thoughts, and feelings that occur at each step. This is done silently, and members record their observations at the completion of the exercise. This unstructured exercise sometimes triggers their maladaptive coping mode. They are not initially told of this possibility because therapists do not want to bias what they experience (Farrell, Reiss, & Shaw, 2014).

Safe Place Imagery

When: First sessions
Purpose: Develop a safe place image
The group develops individual safe-place images in the group setting. Therapists begin by describing their own safe place images in addition to providing images used by previous patients as examples. As a group, therapists lead members through an exercise in which they develop in great detail the different parts of their safe place image by using smells, physical sensations, sounds, and as much visual information as possible.

Group Safety Bubble

When: Beginning of group or when group needs reminding of the group as a safe place
Purpose: Establish safety and protection of the group through their initial role as protectors
The group safety bubble is a simpler, more general form of the safe-place imagery that is developed in later sessions in group schema therapy. The therapists lead the group through a guided imagery session that describes the safety of the group setting (Farrell et al., 2014).

Web Connecting Exercise

When: Early sessions or whenever support of the group is needed or when empathically confronting
Purpose: For group to provide emotional and physical support

In the first session, a ball of yarn is exchanged between group members until a web of connections is formed between members. Members provide their names and where they are from. The ball is passed by making eye contact (Farrell et al., 2014). In later sessions, experiment with tugs, loosening and tightening, and how physical connections feel (Farrell & Shaw, 2013). The issue of eye contact may be problematic for some cultural groups where direct eye contact is discouraged.

Wise Mind Exercise—Expanding Awareness

When: Early sessions
Purpose: Develop WISE MIND
Patients are asked to observe the sensations they have about one of their senses (vision, hearing, smell, taste, touch). They then are asked to breathe and open their eyes, and patients discuss their sensations (Harley, Sprich, Safren, Jacobo, & Fava, 2008; Linehan, 2014).

Distress Reduction Techniques

When: Early to middle phase of group
Purpose: Develop a personalized distress reduction plan
Members are encouraged to develop better kinesthetic awareness. Examples include feeling the hard edges of their chairs or handling smooth objects, and so forth. This is in opposition to focusing on cognition or imagery. Individuals then complete worksheets measuring distress ratings before and after techniques were tried and the kind of technique they tried. Different techniques are tried and assessed (Farrell & Shaw, 2013).

Wise Mind Puzzle Making Exercise

When: Middle sessions
Purpose: Helping patients develop "wise mind"—grasping the whole picture when before only parts were understood
Each group member was given puzzle pieces and told to help assemble the puzzle; the members were told to raise their hand when they "got" what the puzzle was. Wise mind was equated with understanding what the puzzle was. This is an exercise that was adapted for use with adolescents (Nelson-Gray et al., 2006).

Balloon Work

When: Any time after the initial sessions
Purpose: To release anger during stuck times
Patients inflate a balloon while imagining they are filling it with angry feelings and thoughts. Together, everyone releases their balloons (Farrell et al., 2014).

Tug of War Exercise

When: Patient is in angry child mode or cannot easily be reached with words
Purpose: To communicate that group is with them
Toss a towel or fleece strip to a patient in angry child mode who cannot be easily reached by words. When he or she grabs it, initiate a tug of war (Farrell & Shaw, 2013).

Group Identity Bracelet

When: Throughout the group
Purpose: To reinforce cohesion
Members are given a bracelet to signify their membership in the group. These can be given out at different times throughout the group to signify different achievements or at the beginning of the group (Farrell et al., 2014).

REFERENCES

Aguilera, A., Bruehlman-Senecal, E., Liu, N., & Bravin, J. (2018). Implementing group CBT for depression among Latinos in a primary care clinic. *Cognitive and Behavioral Practice, 25,* 135–144. http://dx.doi.org/10.1016/j.cbpra.2017.03.002

Aguilera, A., Garza, M. J., & Muñoz, R. F. (2010). Group cognitive-behavioral therapy for depression in Spanish: Culture-sensitive manualized treatment in practice. *Journal of Clinical Psychology, 66,* 857–867. http://dx.doi.org/10.1002/jclp.20706

Arkowitz, H., & Hannah, M. T. (1989). Cognitive, behavioral, and psychodynamic therapies: Converging or diverging pathways to change? In A. Freeman, K. M. Simon, L. E. Beutler, & H. Arkowitz (Eds.), *Comprehensive handbook of cognitive therapy* (pp. 143–167). New York, NY: Plenum Press. http://dx.doi.org/10.1007/978-1-4757-9779-4_8

Balabanovic, J., Ayers, B., & Hunter, M. S. (2012). Women's experiences of group cognitive behaviour therapy for hot flushes and night sweats following breast cancer treatment: An interpretative phenomenological analysis. *Maturitas, 72,* 236–242. http://dx.doi.org/10.1016/j.maturitas.2012.03.013

Bandura, A. (1977a). Self-efficacy: Toward a unifying theory of behavioral change. *Psychological Review, 84,* 191–215. http://dx.doi.org/10.1037/0033-295X.84.2.191

Bandura, A. (1977b). *Social learning theory.* Englewood Cliffs, NJ: Prentice-Hall.

Barley, W. D., Buie, S. E., Peterson, E. W., Hollingsworth, A. S., Griva, M., Hickerson, S. C., . . . Bailey, B. J. (1993). Development of an inpatient cognitive-behavioral treatment program for borderline personality disorder. *Journal of Personality Disorders, 7,* 232–240. http://dx.doi.org/10.1521/pedi.1993.7.3.232

Barlow, D. H., & Craske, M. G. (1991). *Mastery of your anxiety and panic.* Albany, NY: Graywind.

Bechdolf, A., Köhn, D., Knost, B., Pukrop, R., & Klosterkötter, J. (2005). A randomized comparison of group cognitive-behavioural therapy and group psycho-education in acute patients with schizophrenia: Outcome at 24 months. *Acta Psychiatrica Scandinavica, 112,* 173–179. http://dx.doi.org/10.1111/j.1600-0447.2005.00581.x

Beck, A. T. (1972). *Depression: Causes and treatment.* Philadelphia: University of Pennsylvania Press. (Original work published 1967)

Beck, A. T. (1976). *Cognitive theory and the emotional disorders.* Madison, CT: International Universities Press.

Beck, A. T. (1978). *Depression inventory.* Philadelphia, PA: Center for Cognitive Therapy.

Beck, A. T. (1991). Cognitive therapy: A 30-year retrospective. *American Psychologist, 46,* 368–375.

Beck, A. T., & Emery, G. (1977). *Cognitive therapy of substance abuse.* Philadelphia, PA: Center for Cognitive Therapy.

Beck, A. T., Epstein, N., Brown, G., & Steer, R. A. (1988). An inventory for measuring clinical anxiety: Psychometric properties. *Journal of Consulting and Clinical Psychology, 56,* 893–897. http://dx.doi.org/10.1037/0022-006X.56.6.893

Beck, A. T., Freeman, A., Pretzer, J., Davis, D. D., Fleming, B., Ottoviani, R., . . . Trexler, L. (1990). *Cognitive therapy of personality disorders.* New York, NY: Guilford Press.

Beck, A. T., & Greenberg, R. L. (1974). *Coping with depression.* New York, NY: Institute for Rational Living.

Beck, A. T., Rush, A. J., Shaw, B. F., & Emery, G. (1979). *Cognitive therapy of depression.* New York, NY: Guilford Press.

Beck, A. T., Steer, R. A., & Brown, G. K. (1996). *Beck Depression Inventory* (2nd ed.). San Antonio, TX: Psychological Corporation.

Beck, A. T., & Weishaar, M. (1989). Cognitive therapy. In A. Freeman, K. M. Simon, L. E. Beutler, & H. Arkowitz (Eds.), *Comprehensive handbook of cognitive therapy* (pp. 21–36). New York, NY: Plenum Press. http://dx.doi.org/10.1007/978-1-4757-9779-4_2

Beck, A. T., Weissman, A., Lester, D., & Trexler, L. (1974). The measurement of pessimism: The hopelessness scale. *Journal of Consulting and Clinical Psychology, 42,* 861–865. http://dx.doi.org/10.1037/h0037562

Becker, I. M., & Rosenfeld, J. G. (1976). Rational emotive therapy: A study of initial therapy sessions of Albert Ellis. *Journal of Clinical Psychology, 32,* 872–876. http://dx.doi.org/10.1002/1097-4679(197610)32:4<872::AID-JCLP2270320431>3.0.CO;2-9

Behenck, A., Wesner, A. C., Finkler, D., & Heldt, E. (2017). Contribution of group therapeutic factors to the outcome of cognitive–behavioral therapy for patients with panic disorder. *Archives of Psychiatric Nursing, 31,* 142–146. http://dx.doi.org/10.1016/j.apnu.2016.09.001

Bellus, S. B., Donovan, S. M., Kost, P. P., Vergo, J. G., Gramse, R. A., Bross, A., & Tervit, S. L. (2003). Behavior change ad achieving hospital discharge in persons with severe, chronic psychiatric disabilities. *Psychiatric Quarterly, 74,* 31–42. http://dx.doi.org/10.1023/A:1021189505212

Bieling, P. J., McCabe, R. E., & Antony, M. M. (2013). *Cognitive-behavioral therapy in groups.* New York, NY: Guilford Press.

Blackburn, I. M. (1989). Severely depressed in-patients. In J. Scott, J. M. G. Williams, & A. T. Beck (Eds.), *Cognitive therapy in clinical practice* (pp. 1–24). New York, NY: Routledge. http://dx.doi.org/10.4324/9780203359365_chapter_one

Bohus, M., Haaf, B., Simms, T., Limberger, M. F., Schmahl, C., Unckel, C., . . . Linehan, M. M. (2004). Effectiveness of inpatient dialectical behavioral therapy for borderline personality disorder: A controlled trial. *Behaviour Research and Therapy, 42,* 487–499. http://dx.doi.org/10.1016/S0005-7967(03)00174-8

Borge, F. M., Hoffart, A., Sexton, H., Clark, D. M., Markowitz, J. C., & McManus, F. (2008). Residential cognitive therapy versus residential interpersonal therapy for social phobia: A randomized clinical trial. *Journal of Anxiety Disorders, 22,* 991–1010. http://dx.doi.org/10.1016/j.janxdis.2007.10.002

Bowen, R. C., D'Arcy, C., Keegan, D., & Senthilselvan, A. (2000). A controlled trial of cognitive behavioral treatment of panic in alcoholic inpatients with comorbid panic disorder. *Addictive Behaviors, 25,* 593–597. http://dx.doi.org/10.1016/S0306-4603(99)00017-9

Bowers, W. A. (1989). Cognitive therapy with inpatients. In A. Freeman, K. M. Simon, L. E. Beutler, & H. Arkowitz (Eds.), *Comprehensive handbook of cognitive therapy* (pp. 583–596). New York, NY: Plenum Press. http://dx.doi.org/10.1007/978-1-4757-9779-4_29

Bowers, W. A. (2000). Eating disorders. In J. R. White & A. S. Freeman (Eds.), *Cognitive–behavioral group therapy for specific problems and populations* (pp. 127–148). Washington, DC: American Psychological Association.

Bowers, W. A., & Ansher, L. S. (2008). The effectiveness of cognitive behavioral therapy on changing eating disorder symptoms and psychopathology of

32 anorexia nervosa patients at hospital discharge and one year follow-up. *Annals of Clinical Psychiatry, 20*, 79–86. http://dx.doi.org/10.1080/10401230802017068

Bowers, W. A., Evans, K., & Andersen, A. E. (1997). Inpatient treatment of eating disorders: A cognitive therapy milieu. *Cognitive and Behavioral Practice, 4*, 291–323. http://dx.doi.org/10.1016/S1077-7229(97)80005-3

Boyd-Franklin, N. (1991). Recurrent themes in the treatment of African-American women in group psychotherapy. *Women & Therapy, 11*, 25–40. http://dx.doi.org/10.1300/J015V11N02_04

Brabender, V., & Fallon, A. (1993). *Models of inpatient group psychotherapy.* Washington, DC: American Psychological Association.

Brook, D., Gordon, C., & Meadow, H. (1998). Ethnicity, culture, and group psychotherapy. *Group, 22*, 53–80. http://dx.doi.org/10.1023/A:1022123428746

Burlingame, G. M., Fuhriman, A., & Mosier, J. (2003). The differential effectiveness of group psychotherapy: A meta-analytic perspective. *Group Dynamics: Theory, Research, and Practice, 7*, 3–12. http://dx.doi.org/10.1037/1089-2699.7.1.3

Burns, D. (1980). *Feeling good.* New York, NY: Morrow.

Carter, R. T. (2004). *Handbook of racial–cultural psychology and counseling, training and practice: Training and practice.* Hoboken, NJ: Wiley.

Chadwick, P., Sambrook, S., Rasch, S., & Davies, E. (2000). Challenging the omnipotence of voices: Group cognitive behavior therapy for voices. *Behaviour Research and Therapy, 38*, 993–1003. http://dx.doi.org/10.1016/S0005-7967(99)00126-6

Chadwick, P., Taylor, K. N., & Abba, N. (2005). Mindfulness groups for people with psychosis. *Behavioural and Cognitive Psychotherapy, 33*, 351–359. http://dx.doi.org/10.1017/S1352465805002158

Chaisson, M., Beutler, L., Yost, E., & Allender, J. (1984). Treating the depressed elderly. *Journal of Psychosocial Nursing and Mental Health Services, 22*, 25–30.

Chan, A. T. Y., Sun, G. Y. Y., Tam, W. W. S., Tsoi, K. K. F., & Wong, S. Y. S. (2017). The effectiveness of group-based behavioral activation in the treatment of depression: An updated meta-analysis of randomized controlled trial. *Journal of Affective Disorders, 208*, 345–354. http://dx.doi.org/10.1016/j.jad.2016.08.026

Chen, C. P. (1995). Group counseling in a different cultural context: Several primary issues in dealing with Chinese clients. *Group, 19*, 45–55. http://dx.doi.org/10.1007/BF01458190

Chen, E. C., Kakkad, D., & Balzano, J. (2008). Multicultural competence and evidence-based practice in group therapy. *Journal of Clinical Psychology, 64*, 1261–1278. http://dx.doi.org/10.1002/jclp.20533

Chen, R., Xi, Y., Wang, X., Li, Y., He, Y., & Luo, J. (2018). Perception of inpatients following remission of a manic episode in bipolar I disorder on a group-based psychoeducation program: A qualitative study. *BMC Psychiatry, 18*, 26. http://dx.doi.org/10.1186/s12888-018-1614-1

Clarke, I., & Wilson, H. (Eds.). (2008). *Cognitive behaviour therapy for acute inpatient mental health units: Working with clients, staff and the milieu.* New York, NY: Routledge.

Coleman, R., & Gantman, C. (1991, February). *Inpatient cognitive-behavioral groups*. Paper presented at the meeting of the American Group Psychotherapy Association, San Antonio, TX.

Cook, W. G., Arechiga, A., Dobson, L. A. V., & Boyd, K. (2014). Brief heterogeneous inpatient psychotherapy groups: A process-oriented psychoeducational (POP) model. *International Journal of Group Psychotherapy, 64*, 180–206. http://dx.doi.org/10.1521/ijgp.2014.64.2.180

Covi, L., Roth, D., & Lipman, R. S. (1982). Cognitive group psychotherapy of depression: The close-ended group. *American Journal of Psychotherapy, 36*, 459–469.

Covi, L., Roth, D. M., Pattison, J. H., & Lipman, R. S. (1988). Group cognitive-behavioral therapy of depression: Two parallel treatment manuals for a controlled study. In C. Perris, I. M. Blackburn, & H. Perris (Eds.), *Cognitive psychotherapy: Theory and practice* (pp. 198–222). New York, NY: Springer. http://dx.doi.org/10.1007/978-3-642-73393-2_10

Cowdrill, V., & Dannahy, L. (2009). Running reflective practice groups on an inpatient unit. In I. Clarke & H. Wilson (Eds.), *Cognitive behaviour therapy for acute inpatient mental health units: Working with clients, staff and the milieu* (pp. 115–128). New York, NY: Routledge.

Cumba-Avilés, E. (2017). Cognitive-behavioral group therapy for Latino youth with type 1 diabetes and depression: A case study. *Clinical Case Studies, 16*, 58–75. http://dx.doi.org/10.1177/1534650116668270

Davis, M., Eshelman, E. R., & McKay, M. (1988). *The relaxation and stress reduction workbook* (3rd ed.). Oakland, CA: New Harbinger.

De Las Nueces, D., Hacker, K., DiGirolamo, A., & Hicks, L. S. (2012). A systematic review of community-based participatory research to enhance clinical trials in racial and ethnic minority groups. *Health Services Research, 47*, 1363–1386. http://dx.doi.org/10.1111/j.1475-6773.2012.01386.x

Dickhaut, V., & Arntz, A. (2014). Combined group and individual schema therapy for borderline personality disorder: A pilot study. *Journal of Behavior Therapy and Experimental Psychiatry, 45*, 242–251. http://dx.doi.org/10.1016/j.jbtep.2013.11.004

Dimeff, L. A., & Koerner, K. (Eds.). (2007). *Dialectical behavior therapy in clinical practice: Applications across disorders and settings*. New York, NY: Guilford Press.

Dobson, K. S. (1989). A meta-analysis of the efficacy of cognitive therapy for depression. *Journal of Consulting and Clinical Psychology, 57*, 414–419. http://dx.doi.org/10.1037/0022-006X.57.3.414

Dobson, K. S., & Dozois, D. J. (2010). Historical and philosophical bases of the cognitive-behavorial therapies. In K. S. Dobson (Ed.), *Handbook of cognitive-behavioral therapies* (pp. 3–38). New York, NY: Guilford Press.

Drury, V., Birchwood, M., & Cochrane, R. (2000). Cognitive therapy and recovery from acute psychosis: A controlled trial: 3. Five-year follow-up. *The British Journal of Psychiatry, 177*, 8–14. http://dx.doi.org/10.1192/bjp.177.1.8

Drury, V., Birchwood, M., Cochrane, R., & Macmillan, F. (1996). Cognitive therapy and recovery from acute psychosis: A controlled trial: I. Impact on psychotic symptoms. *The British Journal of Psychiatry, 169*, 593–601. http://dx.doi.org/10.1192/bjp.169.5.593

Duman, Z. C., Yildirim, N. K., Ucok, A., Er, F., & Kanik, T. (2010). The effectiveness of a psychoeducational group program with inpatients being treated for chronic mental illness. *Social Behavior and Personality, 38*, 657–666. http://dx.doi.org/10.2224/sbp.2010.38.5.657

Ellis, A. (1962). *Reason and emotion in psychotherapy*. Secaucus, NJ: Lyle Stuart and Citadel Press.

Ellis, A. (1977a). Discomfort anxiety: A new cognitive-behavioral construct. In A. Ellis & R. Grieger (Eds.), *Handbook of rational-emotive therapy* (Vol. 2, pp. 105–120). New York, NY: Springer.

Ellis, A. (1977b). Rational-emotive therapy and cognitive behavior therapy: Similarities and differences. In A. Ellis & R. Grieger (Eds.), *Handbook of rational-emotive therapy* (Vol. 2, pp. 31–45). New York, NY: Springer.

Ellis, A. (1980). Rational-emotive therapy and cognitive-behavior therapy: Similarities and differences. *Cognitive Therapy and Research, 4*, 325–340. http://dx.doi.org/10.1007/BF01178210

Ellis, A. (1985). *Overcoming resistance: Rational-emotive therapy with difficult clients*. New York, NY: Springer.

Ellis, A. (1988). *How to stubbornly refuse to make yourself miserable about anything— Yes, anything*. New York, NY: Carol.

Ellis, A. (1990). Rational-emotive therapy. In I. L. Kutash & A. Wolf (Eds.), *The group psychotherapist's handbook* (pp. 289–315). New York, NY: Columbia University Press.

Ellis, A. (1992). Group rational-emotive and cognitive-behavioral therapy. *International Journal of Group Psychotherapy, 42*, 63–80. http://dx.doi.org/10.1080/00207284.1992.11732580

Ellis, A., McInerney, J. F., DiGiuseppe, R., & Yeager, R. J. (1988). *Rational-emotive therapy with alcoholics and substance abusers*. New York, NY: Pergamon Press.

Emery, G. (1984). *On your own life: How the new cognitive therapy can make you feel wonderful*. New York, NY: NAL/Dutton.

Farrell, J. M., Reiss, N., & Shaw, I. A. (2014). *The schema therapy clinician's guide: A complete resource for building and delivering individual, group and integrated schema mode treatment programs*. Chichester, England: Wiley. http://dx.doi.org/10.1002/9781118510018

Farrell, J. M., & Shaw, I. A. (2013). Empathic confrontation in group schema therapy. In N. Reiss & F. Vogel (Eds.), *Empathic confrontation*. Retrieved from https://www.researchgate.net/publication/281108601_Empathic_Confrontation_in_Group_Schema_Therapy

Farrell, J. M., Shaw, I. A., & Webber, M. A. (2009). A schema-focused approach to group psychotherapy for outpatients with borderline personality disorder: A randomized controlled trial. *Journal of Behavior Therapy and Experimental Psychiatry, 40*, 317–328. http://dx.doi.org/10.1016/j.jbtep.2009.01.002

Feindler, E. L., Ecton, R. B., Kingsley, D., & Dubey, D. R. (1986). Group anger-control training for institutionalized psychiatric male adolescents. *Behavior Therapy, 17*, 109–123. http://dx.doi.org/10.1016/S0005-7894(86)80079-X

Frederiksen, B. (2010). *Cognitive-behavioral group therapy in an acute inpatient setting* (Unpublished doctoral dissertation). Palo Alto University, Palo Alto, CA.

Freeman, A. (1987). Cognitive therapy: An overview. In A. Freeman & V. Greenwood (Eds.), *Cognitive therapy: Applications in psychiatric and medical settings* (pp. 19–35). New York, NY: Human Sciences Press.

Freeman, A. (1990). Cognitive therapy. In A. Bellack & M. Hersen (Eds.), *Handbook of comparative treatments for adult disorders* (pp. 64–87). New York, NY: Wiley.

Freeman, A., Pretzer, J., Fleming, B., & Simon, K. M. (1990). *Clinical applications of cognitive therapy*. New York, NY: Plenum Press. http://dx.doi.org/10.1007/978-1-4684-0007-6

Freeman, A., Schrodt, G., Gilson, M., & Ludgate, J. (1993). Group cognitive therapy with inpatients. In J. Wright, A. Beck, M. These, & J. Ludgate (Eds.), *Cognitive therapy with inpatient populations* (pp. 121–153). New York, NY: Guilford Press.

Freeman, A., & Simon, K. M. (1989). Cognitive therapy of anxiety. In A. Freeman, K. M. Simon, L. E. Beutler, & H. Arkowitz (Eds.), *Comprehensive handbook of cognitive therapy* (pp. 347–366). New York, NY: Plenum Press. http://dx.doi.org/10.1007/978-1-4757-9779-4_18

Friedberg, R. D., Fidaleo, R. A., & Mikules, M. M. (1992). Inpatient cognitive therapy: Detours, potholes, and roadblocks along the routes of progress. *Journal of Rational-Emotive and Cognitive-Behavior Therapy, 10*, 83–93. http://dx.doi.org/10.1007/BF01061384

Gaffan, E. A., Tsaousis, I., & Kemp-Wheeler, S. M. (1995). Researcher allegiance and meta-analysis: The case of cognitive therapy for depression. *Journal of Consulting and Clinical Psychology, 63*, 966–980. http://dx.doi.org/10.1037/0022-006X.63.6.966

Garfield, S. L. (1989). The client–therapist relationship in rational-emotive therapy. In M. E. Bernard & R. DiGiuseppe (Eds.), *Inside rational-emotive therapy* (pp. 113–125). San Diego, CA: Academic Press.

George, L., Thornton, C., Touyz, S. W., Waller, G., & Beumont, P. J. V. (2004). Motivational enhancement and schema-focused cognitive behaviour therapy in the treatment of chronic eating disorders. *Clinical Psychologist, 8*, 81–85. http://dx.doi.org/10.1080/13284200412331304054

Gerlinghoff, M., Backmund, H., & Franzen, U. (1998). Evaluation of a day treatment programme for eating disorders. *European Eating Disorders Review*, 6, 96–106. http://dx.doi.org/10.1002/(SICI)1099-0968(199806)6:2<96::AID-ERV236> 3.0.CO;2-P

Gerlinghoff, M., Gross, G., & Backmund, H. (2003). Eating disorder therapy concepts with a preventive goal. *European Child & Adolescent Psychiatry*, 12, 72–77. http://dx.doi.org/10.1007/s00787-003-1110-z

Ghezelseflo, M., & Esbati, M. (2013). Effectiveness of hope-oriented group therapy on improving quality of life in HIV+ male patients. *Procedia—Social and Behavioral Sciences*, 84, 534–537. http://dx.doi.org/10.1016/j.sbspro.2013.06.599

Glantz, M. (1987). Day hospital treatment of alcoholics. In A. Freeman & V. Greenwood (Eds.), *Cognitive therapy: Applications in psychiatric and medical settings* (pp. 51–68). New York, NY: Human Sciences Press.

Glantz, M. (1989). Cognitive therapy with the elderly. In A. Freeman, K. M. Simon, L. E. Beutler, & H. Arkowitz (Eds.), *Comprehensive handbook of cognitive therapy* (pp. 467–489). New York, NY: Plenum Press. http://dx.doi.org/10.1007/ 978-1-4757-9779-4_24

Goldfried, M. R., Decenteceo, T., & Weinberg, L. (1974). Systematic rational restructuring as a self-control technique. *Behavior Therapy*, 5, 247–254. http:// dx.doi.org/10.1016/S0005-7894(74)80140-1

Goldfried, M. R., Linehan, M. M., & Smith, J. L. (1978). Reduction of test anxiety through cognitive restructuring. *Journal of Consulting and Clinical Psychology*, 46, 32–39. http://dx.doi.org/10.1037/0022-006X.46.1.32

Goldfried, M. R., Padawer, W., & Robins, C. (1984). Social anxiety and the semantic structure of heterosocial interactions. *Journal of Abnormal Psychology*, 93, 87–97. http://dx.doi.org/10.1037/0021-843X.93.1.87

Greenwood, V. B. (1987). Cognitive therapy with the young adult chronic patient. In A. Freeman & V. Greenwood (Eds.), *Cognitive therapy: Applications in psychiatric and medical settings* (pp. 103–116). New York, NY: Human Sciences Press.

Grossman, R., & Freet, B. (1987). Cognitive approach to group with hospitalized adolescents. In A. Freedman & V. Greenwood (Eds.), *Cognitive therapy: Applications in psychiatric and medical settings* (pp. 132–151). New York, NY: Human Sciences Press.

Haaga, D. A. F., & Davison, G. C. (1989). Outcome studies of rational-emotive therapy. In M. E. Bernard & R. DiGiuseppe (Eds.), *Inside rational-emotive therapy* (pp. 155–198). San Diego, CA: Academic Press.

Hagen, R., Nordahl, H. M., & Gråwe, R. W. (2005). Cognitive-behavioural group treatment of depression in patients with psychotic disorders. *Clinical Psychology & Psychotherapy*, 12, 465–474. http://dx.doi.org/10.1002/cpp.474

Hagen, R., Nordahl, H. M., Kristiansen, L., & Morken, G. (2005). A randomized trial of cognitive group therapy vs. waiting list for patients with co-morbid psychiatric disorders: Effect of cognitive group therapy after treatment and six and twelve months follow-up. *Behavioural and Cognitive Psychotherapy, 33*, 33–44. http://dx.doi.org/10.1017/S1352465804001754

Hanna, J. (2008). CBT on the wards: Standards and aspirations. In I. Clarke & H. Wilson (Eds.), *Cognitive behaviour therapy for acute inpatient mental health units: Working with clients, staff and the milieu* (pp. 11–21). New York, NY: Routledge.

Harley, R., Sprich, S., Safren, S., Jacobo, M., & Fava, M. (2008). Adaptation of dialectical behavior therapy skills training group for treatment-resistant depression. *The Journal of Nervous and Mental Disease, 196*, 136–143. http://dx.doi.org/10.1097/NMD.0b013e318162aa3f

Heimberg, R. G. (1990). Cognitive behavior therapy. In A. Bellack & M. Hersen (Eds.), *Handbook of comparative treatments* (pp. 203–218). New York, NY: Wiley.

Heimberg, R. G., & Becker, R. E. (2002). *Cognitive-behavioral group therapy for social phobia: Basic mechanisms and clinical strategies.* New York, NY: Guilford Press.

Hill, G., Clarke, I., & Wilson, H. (2008). The "Making friends with yourself" and the "What is real and what is not" groups. In I. Clarke & H. Wilson (Eds.), *Cognitive behaviour therapy for acute inpatient mental health units: Working with clients, staff and the milieu* (pp. 161–172). New York, NY: Routledge.

Hodel, B., & West, A. (2003). A cognitive training for mentally ill offenders with treatment-resistant schizophrenia. *Journal of Forensic Psychiatry & Psychology, 14*, 554–568. http://dx.doi.org/10.1080/14789940310001527745

Hollon, S. D., & Beck, A. T. (1986). Cognitive and cognitive-behavioral therapies. In S. L. Garfield & A. E. Bergin (Eds.), *Handbook of psychotherapy and behavior change* (3rd ed., pp. 443–482). New York, NY: Wiley.

Hollon, S. D., & Evans, M. D. (1983). Cognitive therapy for depression in a group format. In A. Freeman (Ed.), *Cognitive therapy with couples and groups* (pp. 11–41). New York, NY: Plenum Press. http://dx.doi.org/10.1007/978-1-4757-9736-7_2

Hollon, S. D., & Kendall, P. C. (1980). Cognitive self-statements in depression: Development of an automatic thoughts questionnaire. *Cognitive Therapy and Research, 4*, 383–395. http://dx.doi.org/10.1007/BF01178214

Hollon, S. D., & Shaw, B. F. (1979). Group cognitive therapy for depressed patients. In A. T. Beck, A. J. Rush, B. F. Shaw, & G. Emery (Eds.), *Cognitive therapy of depression* (pp. 328–353). New York, NY: Guilford Press.

Hope, D. A., Herbert, J. A., & Bellack, A. S. (1991, November). *Social phobia subtype, avoidant personality disorder and psychotherapy outcome.* Poster presented at the meeting of the Association for the Advancement of Behavior Therapy, New York, NY.

Horne, A. M., & Kiselica, M. S. (1999). *Handbook of counseling boys and adolescent males: A practitioner's guide.* Thousand Oaks, CA: Sage.

Huntley, A. L., Araya, R., & Salisbury, C. (2012). Group psychological therapies for depression in the community: Systematic review and meta-analysis. *The British Journal of Psychiatry, 200*, 184–190. http://dx.doi.org/10.1192/bjp.bp.111.092049

Ibrahim, N., Kamsani, S. R., & Champe, J. (2015). Understanding the Islamic concept of usrah and its application to group work. *Journal for Specialists in Group Work*, 40, 163–186. http://dx.doi.org/10.1080/01933922.2015.1017067

Iqbal, S., & Bassett, M. (2008). Evaluation of perceived usefulness of activity scheduling in an inpatient depression group. *Journal of Psychiatric and Mental Health Nursing*, 15, 393–398.

Irish College of General Practitioners. (2013). *Bibliotherapy booklet: The power of words (2013)*. Retrieved from https://www.icgp.ie/go/courses/mental_health/articles_publications/1BE52354-19B9-E185-8339BDC253FAD21C.html

Jacobsen, P., Morris, E., Johns, L., & Hodkinson, K. (2011). Mindfulness groups for psychosis; key issues for implementation on an inpatient unit. *Behavioural and Cognitive Psychotherapy*, 39, 349–353. http://dx.doi.org/10.1017/S1352465810000639

Jacobsen, R. H., Tamkin, A. S., & Blount, J. B. (1987). The efficacy of rational-emotive group therapy in psychiatric inpatients. *Journal of Rational Emotive Therapy*, 5, 22–31. http://dx.doi.org/10.1007/BF01080517

Katz, L. Y., Cox, B. J., Gunasekara, S., & Miller, A. L. (2004). Feasibility of dialectical behavior therapy for suicidal adolescent inpatients. *Journal of the American Academy of Child & Adolescent Psychiatry*, 43, 276–282. http://dx.doi.org/10.1097/00004583-200403000-00008

Kendall, P. C., & Braswell, L. (1982). Cognitive-behavioral self-control therapy for children: A components analysis. *Journal of Consulting and Clinical Psychology*, 50, 672–689. http://dx.doi.org/10.1037/0022-006X.50.5.672

Kennedy, F. (2008). The use of formulation in inpatient settings. In I. Clarke & H. Wilson (Eds.), *Cognitive behaviour therapy for acute inpatient mental health units: Working with clients, staff and the milieu* (pp. 39–62). New York, NY: Routledge.

Kinderman, P. (2008). New ways of working and the provision of CBT in the inpatient setting. In I. Clarke & H. Wilson (Eds.), *Cognitive behaviour therapy for acute inpatient mental health units: Working with clients, staff and the milieu* (pp. 22–29). New York, NY: Routledge.

Koerner, K., Dimeff, L., & Swenson, C. (2007). Adopt or adapt? Fidelity matters. In L. A. Dimeff & K. Koerner (Eds.), *Dialectical behavior therapy in clinical practice: Applications across disorders and settings* (pp. 19–36). New York, NY: Guilford Press.

Kohn, L., & Oden, T. (1997). *Group therapy manual for African American women's group*. San Francisco, CA: San Francisco General Hospital, Division of Psychosocial Medicine.

Kohn, L. P., Oden, T., Muñoz, R. F., Robinson, A., & Leavitt, D. (2002). Brief report: Adapted cognitive behavioral group therapy for depressed low-income African American women. *Community Mental Health Journal*, 38, 497–504. http://dx.doi.org/10.1023/A:1020884202677

Koons, C. R., Chapman, A. L., Betts, B. B., Morse, N., & Robins, C. J. (2006). Dialectical behavior therapy adapted for the vocational rehabilitation of significantly disabled mentally ill adults. *Cognitive and Behavioral Practice, 13,* 146–156. http://dx.doi.org/10.1016/j.cbpra.2005.04.003

Kröger, C., Harbeck, S., Armbrust, M., & Kliem, S. (2013). Effectiveness, response, and dropout of dialectical behavior therapy for borderline personality disorder in an inpatient setting. *Behaviour Research and Therapy, 51,* 411–416. http://dx.doi.org/10.1016/j.brat.2013.04.008

Kröger, C., Schweiger, U., Sipos, V., Arnold, R., Kahl, K. G., Schunert, T., . . . Reinecker, H. (2006). Effectiveness of dialectical behaviour therapy for border-line personality disorder in an inpatient setting. *Behaviour Research and Therapy, 44,* 1211–1217. http://dx.doi.org/10.1016/j.brat.2005.08.012

Lazarus, A. A. (1981). *The practice of multimodal therapy.* New York, NY: McGraw-Hill.

Lecomte, T., Leclerc, C., Corbière, M., Wykes, T., Wallace, C. J., & Spidel, A. (2008). Group cognitive behavior therapy or social skills training for individuals with a recent onset of psychosis? Results of a randomized controlled trial. *Journal of Nervous and Mental Disease, 196,* 866–875. http://dx.doi.org/10.1097/NMD.0b013e31818ee231

Levy, L. B., & O'Hara, M. W. (2010). Psychotherapeutic interventions for depressed, low-income women: A review of the literature. *Clinical Psychology Review, 30,* 934–950. http://dx.doi.org/10.1016/j.cpr.2010.06.006

Linehan, M. M. (2014). *DBT skills training manual* (2nd ed.). New York, NY: Guilford Press.

Liotti, G. (1987). Structural cognitive therapy. In W. Dryden & W. L. Golden (Eds.), *Cognitive-behavioral approaches to psychotherapy* (pp. 92–128). New York, NY: Hemisphere.

Lloyd, S., Fleming, C., Schmidt, U., & Tchanturia, K. (2014). Targeting perfection-ism in anorexia nervosa using a group-based cognitive behavioural approach: A pilot study. *European Eating Disorders Review, 22,* 366–372. http://dx.doi.org/10.1002/erv.2313

Long, C. G., Banyard, E., & Dolley, O. (2016). Living with mental illness: A cog-nitive behavioural group psycho-education programme with women in secure settings. *Clinical Psychology & Psychotherapy, 23,* 368–376. http://dx.doi.org/10.1002/cpp.1967

Lynch, K., Berry, C., & Sirey, J. (2011). A group-oriented inpatient CBT programme: A pilot study. *The Cognitive Behaviour Therapist, 4,* 38–51. http://dx.doi.org/10.1017/S1754470X10000152

Lyons, L. C., & Woods, P. J. (1991). The efficacy of rational-emotive therapy: A quantitative review of the outcome research. *Clinical Psychology Review, 11,* 357–369. http://dx.doi.org/10.1016/0272-7358(91)90113-9

Mahoney, M. J. (1977). Personal science: A cognitive learning therapy. In A. Ellis & R. Grieger (Eds.), *Handbook of rational psychotherapy* (pp. 352–366). New York, NY: Springer.

Mahoney, M. J., & Arnoff, D. B. (1978). Cognitive and self-control therapies. In S. L. Garfield & A. E. Bergin (Eds.), *Handbook of psychotherapy and behavioral change: An empirical analysis* (2nd ed., pp. 689–722). New York, NY: Wiley.

Mahoney, M. J., & Kazdin, A. E. (1979). Cognitive behavior modification: Misconceptions and premature evaluation. *Psychological Bulletin, 86,* 1044–1049. http://dx.doi.org/10.1037/0033-2909.86.5.1044

Manning, J. J., Hooke, G. R., Tannenbaum, D. A., Blythe, T. H., & Clarke, T. M. (1994). Intensive cognitive-behaviour group therapy for diagnostically heterogeneous groups of patients with psychiatric disorder. *The Australian and New Zealand Journal of Psychiatry, 28,* 667–674. http://dx.doi.org/10.1080/00048679409080790

Martin, R., & Young, J. (2010). Schema therapy. In K. S. Dobson (Ed.), *Handbook of cognitive-behavioral therapies* (3rd ed., pp. 317–346). New York, NY: Guilford Press.

Maultsby, M. C., Jr. (1975). *Help yourself to happiness.* New York, NY: Institute for Rational-Emotive Therapy.

McCann, R. A., Ball, E. M., & Ivanoff, A. (2000). DBT with an inpatient forensic population: The CMHIP forensic model. *Cognitive and Behavioral Practice, 7,* 447–456. http://dx.doi.org/10.1016/S1077-7229(00)80056-5

McCann, R. A., Ivanoff, A., Schmidt, H., & Beach, B. (2007). Implementing dialectical behavior therapy in residential forensic settings with adults and juveniles. In L. A. Dimeff & K. Koerner (Eds.), *Dialectical behavior therapy in clinical practice: Applications across disorders and settings* (pp. 112–144). New York, NY: Guilford Press.

McInnis, E., Sellwood, W., & Jones, C. (2006). A cognitive behavioural group-based educational programme for psychotic symptoms in a low secure setting: A pilot evaluation. *The British Journal of Forensic Practice, 8*(3), 36–46. http://dx.doi.org/10.1108/14636646200600018

McKain, T. L. (1984). Coping skills training and cognitive-behavioral therapy. In L. I. Sank & C. S. Shaffer (Eds.), *A therapist's manual for cognitive behavior therapy in groups* (pp. 9–23). New York, NY: Plenum Press. http://dx.doi.org/10.1007/978-1-4615-8330-1_2

McMain, S., Sayrs, J. H., Dimeff, L. A., & Linehan, M. M. (2007). Dialectical behavior therapy for individuals with borderline personality disorder and substance dependence. In L. A. Dimeff & K. Koerner (Eds.), *Dialectical behavior therapy in clinical practice: Applications across disorders and settings* (pp. 145–173). New York, NY: Guilford Press.

Meichenbaum, D. (1975). A self-instructional approach to stress management: A proposal for stress inoculation training. In I. Sarason & C. D. Spielberger (Eds.), *Stress and anxiety* (pp. 337–360). New York, NY: Plenum Press.

Meichenbaum, D. (1977). *Cognitive-behavior modifications: An integrated approach.* New York, NY: Plenum Press. http://dx.doi.org/10.1007/978-1-4757-9739-8

Meichenbaum, D. (2017). Stress inoculation training: A preventative and treatment approach. In P. M. Lehrer, R. L. Woolfolk, & W. S. Sime (Eds.), *Principles and practice of stress management* (pp. 120–139). New York, NY: Routledge.

Meichenbaum, D., & Asarnow, J. (1979). Cognitive-behavior modification and metacognition development: Implications for the classroom. In P. C. Kendall & S. D. Hollon (Eds.), *Cognitive-behavioral interventions: Theory, research and procedures* (pp. 11–36). San Diego, CA: Academic Press.

Meichenbaum, D. H., & Goodman, J. (1971). Training impulsive children to talk to themselves: A means of developing self-control. *Journal of Abnormal Psychology, 77*, 115–126. http://dx.doi.org/10.1037/h0030773

Miller, A. L., Wyman, S. E., Huppert, J. D., Glassman, S. L., & Rathus, J. H. (2000). Analysis of behavioral skills utilized by suicidal adolescents receiving dialectical behavior therapy. *Cognitive and Behavioral Practice, 7*, 183–187. http://dx.doi.org/10.1016/S1077-7229(00)80029-2

Misurell, J. R., & Springer, C. (2013). Developing culturally responsive evidence-based practice: A game-based group therapy program for child sexual abuse (CSA). *Journal of Child and Family Studies, 22*, 137–149. http://dx.doi.org/10.1007/s10826-011-9560-2

Monti, P., Abrams, D., Kadden, R., & Cooney, N. (1989). *Treating alcohol dependence.* New York, NY: Guilford Press.

Moore, L. M., Carr, A., & Hartnett, D. (2017). Does group CBT for depression do what it says on the tin? A systemic review and meta-analysis of group CBT for depressed adults (2000–2016). *Journal of Contemporary Psychotherapy, 47*, 141–152. http://dx.doi.org/10.1007/s10879-016-9351-6

Moorey, S. (1989). Drug abusers. In J. Scott, J. M. G. Williams, & A. T. Beck (Eds.), *Cognitive therapy in clinical practice* (pp. 157–182). New York, NY: Routledge. http://dx.doi.org/10.4324/9780203359365_chapter_seven

Muñoz, R. F., & Mendelson, T. (2005). Toward evidence-based interventions for diverse populations: The San Francisco General Hospital prevention and treatment manuals. *Journal of Consulting and Clinical Psychology, 73*, 790–799. http://dx.doi.org/10.1037/0022-006X.73.5.790

Nelson-Gray, R. O., Keane, S. P., Hurst, R. M., Mitchell, J. T., Warburton, J. B., Chok, J. T., & Cobb, A. R. (2006). A modified DBT skills training program for oppositional defiant adolescents: Promising preliminary findings. *Behaviour Research and Therapy, 44*, 1811–1820. http://dx.doi.org/10.1016/j.brat.2006.01.004

Nenadić, I., Lamberth, S., & Reiss, N. (2017). Group schema therapy for personality disorders: A pilot study for implementation in acute psychiatric inpatient settings. *Psychiatry Research, 253*, 9–12. http://dx.doi.org/10.1016/j.psychres.2017.01.093

Ness, M. L., & Oei, T. P. S. (2005). The effectiveness of an inpatient group cognitive behavioral therapy program for alcohol dependence. *The American Journal on Addictions, 14*, 139–154. http://dx.doi.org/10.1080/10550490590924773

Neuhaus, E. C., Christopher, M., Jacob, K., Guillaumot, J., & Burns, J. P. (2007). Short-term cognitive behavioral partial hospital treatment: A pilot study. *Journal of Psychiatric Practice, 13,* 298–307. http://dx.doi.org/10.1097/01.pra.0000290668.10107.f3

Newton, E., Landau, S., Smith, P., Monks, P., Shergill, S., & Wykes, T. (2005). Early psychological intervention for auditory hallucinations: An exploratory study of young people's voices groups. *Journal of Nervous and Mental Disease, 193,* 58–61. http://dx.doi.org/10.1097/01.nmd.0000149220.91667.fa

Nielsen, M. (2015). CBT group treatment for depression. *The Cognitive Behaviour Therapist, 8,* 1–11.

Nottingham, E. J., & Neimeyer, R. A. (1992). Evaluation of a comprehensive inpatient rational-emotive therapy program: Some preliminary data. *Journal of Rational-Emotive and Cognitive-Behavior Therapy, 10,* 57–81. http://dx.doi.org/10.1007/BF01061383

Oliver, J., & Baumgart, E. P. (1985). The Dysfunctional Attitude Scale: Psychometric properties and relation to depression in an unselected adult population. *Cognitive Therapy and Research, 9,* 161–167. http://dx.doi.org/10.1007/BF01204847

Organista, K. C., & Muñoz, R. F. (1996). Cognitive behavioral therapy with Latinos. *Cognitive and Behavioral Practice, 3,* 255–270. http://dx.doi.org/10.1016/S1077-7229(96)80017-4

Owen, M., Sellwood, W., Kan, S., Murray, J., & Sarsam, M. (2015). Group CBT for psychosis: A longitudinal, controlled trial with inpatients. *Behaviour Research and Therapy, 65,* 76–85. http://dx.doi.org/10.1016/j.brat.2014.12.008

Page, A. C., & Hooke, G. R. (2003). Outcomes for depressed and anxious inpatients discharged before or after group cognitive behavior therapy: A naturalistic comparison. *Journal of Nervous and Mental Disease, 191,* 653–659. http://dx.doi.org/10.1097/01.nmd.0000092174.38770.e9

Perris, C. (1988a). The foundations of cognitive psychotherapy and its standing in relation to other psychotherapies. In C. Perris, I. M. Blackburn, & H. Perris (Eds.), *Cognitive psychotherapy* (pp. 1–43). New York, NY: Springer. http://dx.doi.org/10.1007/978-3-642-73393-2_1

Perris, C. (1988b). Intensive cognitive-behavioural psychotherapy with patients suffering from schizophrenic psychotic or post-psychotic syndromes: Theoretical and practical aspects. In C. Perris, I. M. Blackburn, & H. Perris (Eds.), *Cognitive psychotherapy* (pp. 324–375). New York, NY: Springer. http://dx.doi.org/10.1007/978-3-642-73393-2_15

Pinkham, A. E., Gloege, A. T., Flanagan, S., & Penn, D. L. (2004). Group cognitive-behavioral therapy for auditory hallucinations: A pilot study. *Cognitive and Behavioral Practice, 11,* 93–98. http://dx.doi.org/10.1016/S1077-7229(04)80011-7

Raune, D., & Daddi, I. (2011). Pilot study of group cognitive behaviour therapy for heterogeneous acute psychiatric inpatients: Treatment in a sole-standalone session allowing patients to choose the therapeutic target. *Behavioural and Cognitive Psychotherapy, 39,* 359–365. http://dx.doi.org/10.1017/S1352465810000834

Reddy, M. S., & Vijay, M. S. (2017). Empirical reality of dialectical behavioral therapy in borderline personality. *Indian Journal of Psychological Medicine, 39,* 105–108. http://dx.doi.org/10.4103/IJPSYM.IJPSYM_132_17

Rehm, L. P. (1977). A self-control model of depression. *Behavior Therapy, 8,* 787–804. http://dx.doi.org/10.1016/S0005-7894(77)80150-0

Reiss, N., Lieb, K., Arntz, A., Shaw, I. A., & Farrell, J. (2014). Responding to the treatment challenge of patients with severe BPD: Results of three pilot studies of inpatient schema therapy. *Behavioural and Cognitive Psychotherapy, 42,* 355–367. http://dx.doi.org/10.1017/S1352465813000027

Rendle, A., & Wilson, H. (2009). Running an emotional coping skills group based on dialectical behaviour therapy. In I. Clarke, & H. Wilson (Eds.), *Cognitive behaviour therapy for acute inpatient mental health units: Working with clients, staff and the milieu* (pp. 173–181). New York, NY: Routledge.

Roper, L., Dickson, J. M., Tinwell, C., Booth, P. G., & McGuire, J. (2010). Maladaptive cognitive schemas in alcohol dependence: Changes associated with a brief residential abstinence program. *Cognitive Therapy and Research, 34,* 207–215. http://dx.doi.org/10.1007/s10608-009-9252-z

Rose, C. (2002). Talking gender in the group. *Group Analysis, 35,* 525–539. http://dx.doi.org/10.1177/05333160260620788

Rosebert, C., & Hall, C. (2008). Training acute inpatient ward staff to use CBT techniques. In I. Clarke & H. Wilson (Eds.), *Cognitive behaviour therapy for acute inpatient mental health units: Working with clients, staff and the milieu* (pp. 143–158). New York, NY: Routledge.

Rosen, B., Katzoff, A., Carrillo, C., & Klein, D. F. (1976). Clinical effectiveness of "short" vs "long" psychiatric hospitalization: I. Inpatient results. *Archives of General Psychiatry, 33,* 1316–1322. http://dx.doi.org/10.1001/archpsyc.1976.01770110044003

Rosner, R., Lumbeck, G., & Geissner, E. (2011). Effectiveness of an inpatient group therapy for comorbid complicated grief disorder. *Psychotherapy Research, 21,* 210–218. http://dx.doi.org/10.1080/10503307.2010.545839

Rosselló, J., & Bernal, G. (1996). Adapting cognitive-behavioral and interpersonal treatments for depressed Puerto Rican adolescents. In E. D. Hibbs & P. S. Jensen (Eds.), *Psychosocial treatments for child and adolescent disorders: Empirically based strategies for clinical practice* (pp. 157–185). Washington, DC: American Psychological Association. http://dx.doi.org/10.1037/10196-007

Rosselló, J. M., & Jiménez-Chafey, M. I. (2006). Cognitive-behavioral group therapy for depression in adolescents with diabetes: A pilot study. *Revista Interamericana de Psicología, 40,* 219–226.

Russell, M., & Doucette, D. (2012). Latino acculturative stress implications, psychotherapeutic processes, and group therapy. *Graduate Journal of Counseling Psychology, 3*(1). Retrieved from https://epublications.marquette.edu/gjcp/vol3/iss1/9

Salkovskis, P. M. (1989). Obsessions and compulsions. In J. Scott, J. Mark, G. Williams, & A. T. Beck (Eds.), *Cognitive therapy in clinical practice* (pp. 50–77). New York, NY: Routledge. http://dx.doi.org/10.4324/9780203359365_chapter_three

Salvendy, J. T. (1999). Ethnocultural considerations in group psychotherapy. *International Journal of Group Psychotherapy, 49,* 429–464.

Sambrook, S. (2009). Working with crisis: The role of the clinical psychologist in a psychiatric intensive care unit. In I. Clarke & H. Wilson (Eds.), *Cognitive behaviour therapy for acute inpatient mental health units: Working with clients, staff and the milieu* (pp. 129–142). New York, NY: Routledge.

Sank, L. I., & Shaffer, C. S. (1984). *A therapist's manual for cognitive behavior therapy in groups.* New York, NY: Plenum Press. http://dx.doi.org/10.1007/978-1-4615-8330-1

Satterfield, J. M. (1998). Cognitive behavioral group therapy for depressed, low-income minority clients: Retention and treatment enhancement. *Cognitive and Behavioral Practice, 5,* 65–80. http://dx.doi.org/10.1016/S1077-7229(98)80021-7

Schaap, G. M., Chakhssi, F., & Westerhof, G. J. (2016). Inpatient schema therapy for nonresponsive patients with personality pathology: Changes in symptomatic distress, schemas, schema modes, coping styles, experienced parenting styles, and mental well-being. *Psychotherapy, 53,* 402–412. http://dx.doi.org/10.1037/pst0000056

Schachter, R. (2011). *Using the group in cognitive group therapy.* Retrieved from https://adaa.org/sites/default/files/Schachter%20168.pdf

Schrodt, G. R., & Wright, J. (1987). Inpatient treatment of adolescents. In A. Freeman & V. Greenwood (Eds.), *Cognitive therapy: Applications in psychiatric and medical settings* (pp. 69–82). New York, NY: Human Sciences Press.

Shaw, B. F., & Wilson-Smith, D. (1988). Training therapists in cognitive-behavioral therapy. In C. Perris, I. M. Blackburn, & H. Perris (Eds.), *Cognitive psychotherapy: Theory and practice* (pp. 140–159). New York, NY: Springer. http://dx.doi.org/10.1007/978-3-642-73393-2_7

Shin, S.-K., & Lukens, E. P. (2002). Effects of psychoeducation for Korean Americans with chronic mental illness. *Psychiatric Services, 53,* 1125–1131. http://dx.doi.org/10.1176/appi.ps.53.9.1125

Shorey, R. C., Stuart, G. L., Anderson, S., & Strong, D. R. (2013). Changes in early maladaptive schemas after residential treatment for substance use. *Journal of Clinical Psychology, 69,* 912–922. http://dx.doi.org/10.1002/jclp.21968

Simpson, E. B., Pistorello, J., Begin, A., Costello, E., Levinson, J., Mulberry, S., . . . Stevens, M. (1998). Focus on women: Use of dialectical behavior therapy in a partial hospital program for women with borderline personality disorder. *Psychiatric Services, 49,* 669–673. http://dx.doi.org/10.1176/ps.49.5.669

Simpson, S. G., Morrow, E., van Vreeswijk, M., & Reid, C. (2010). Group schema therapy for eating disorders: A pilot study. *Frontiers in Psychology, 1,* 182. Advance online publication. http://dx.doi.org/10.3389/fpsyg.2010.00182

Spencer, K. G., & Vencill, J. A. (2017). Body beyond: A pleasure-based, sex-positive group therapy curriculum for transfeminine adults. *Psychology of Sexual Orientation and Gender Diversity, 4,* 392–402. http://dx.doi.org/10.1037/sgd0000248

Spivack, G., Platt, J. J., & Shure, M. B. (1976). *The problem-solving approach to adjustment.* San Francisco, CA: Jossey-Bass.

Springer, T., Lohr, N. E., Buchtel, H. A., & Silk, K. R. (1995). A preliminary report of short-term cognitive-behavioral group therapy for inpatients with personality disorders. *The Journal of Psychotherapy Practice & Research, 5,* 57–71.

Stacciarini, J.-M. R., O'Keeffe, M., & Mathews, M. (2007). Group therapy as treatment for depressed Latino women: A review of the literature. *Issues in Mental Health Nursing, 28,* 473–488. http://dx.doi.org/10.1080/01612840701344431

Steer, R. A., & Beck, A. T. (1997). Beck Anxiety Inventory. In C. P. Zalaquett & R. J. Wood (Eds.), *Evaluating stress: A book of resources* (pp. 23–40). Lanham, MD: Scarecrow Education.

Steil, R., Dyer, A., Priebe, K., Kleindienst, N., & Bohus, M. (2011). Dialectical behavior therapy for posttraumatic stress disorder related to childhood sexual abuse: A pilot study of an intensive residential treatment program. *Journal of Traumatic Stress, 24,* 102–106. http://dx.doi.org/10.1002/jts.20617

Strong, J., Gilbert, J., Cassidy, S., & Bennett, S. (1995). Expert clinicians' and students' views on clinical reasoning in occupational therapy. *British Journal of Occupational Therapy, 58,* 119–123. http://dx.doi.org/10.1177/030802269505800309

Stuart, S., & Bowers, W. (1995). Cognitive therapy with inpatients: Review and meta-analysis. *Journal of Cognitive Psychotherapy, 9,* 85–92.

Swenson, C. (1989). Kernberg and Linehan: Two approaches to the borderline patient. *Journal of Personality Disorders, 3,* 26–35. http://dx.doi.org/10.1521/pedi.1989.3.1.26

Swenson, C. R., Sanderson, C., Dulit, R. A., & Linehan, M. M. (2001). The application of dialectical behavior therapy for patients with borderline personality disorder on inpatient units. *Psychiatric Quarterly, 72,* 307–324. http://dx.doi.org/10.1023/A:1010337231127

Swenson, C. R., Witterholt, S., & Bohus, M. (2007). Dialectical behavior therapy on inpatient units. In L. A. Dimeff & K. Koerner (Eds.), *Dialectical behavior therapy in clinical practice: Applications across disorders and settings* (pp. 69–111). New York, NY: Guilford Press.

Tchanturia, K., Doris, E., & Fleming, C. (2014). Effectiveness of cognitive remediation and emotion skills training (CREST) for anorexia nervosa in group format: A naturalistic pilot study. *European Eating Disorders Review, 22,* 200–205. http://dx.doi.org/10.1002/erv.2287

Van Noppen, B. L., Pato, M. T., Marsland, R., & Rasmussen, S. A. (1998). A time-limited behavioral group for treatment of obsessive-compulsive disorder. *Journal of Psychotherapy Practice and Research, 7,* 272–280.

van Vreeswijk, M., Broersen, J., Bloo, J., & Haeyen, S. (2012). Techniques within schema therapy. In M. van Vreeswijk, J. Broersen, & M. Nadort (Eds.), *The Wiley-Blackwell Handbook of Schema Therapy: Theory, Research, and Practice* (pp. 185–195). West Sussex, England: Wiley.

van Vreeswijk, M. F., Spinhoven, P., Eurelings-Bontekoe, E. H. M., & Broersen, J. (2014). Changes in symptom severity, schemas and modes in heterogeneous psychiatric patient groups following short-term schema cognitive-behavioural group therapy: A naturalistic pre-treatment and post-treatment design in an outpatient clinic: Changes in symptom severity, schemas and modes. *Clinical Psychology & Psychotherapy, 21*, 29–38. http://dx.doi.org/10.1002/cpp.1813

Veltro, F., Vendittelli, N., Oricchio, I., Addona, F., Avino, C., Figliolia, G., & Morosini, P. (2008). Effectiveness and efficiency of cognitive-behavioral group therapy for inpatients: 4-year follow-up study. *Journal of Psychiatric Practice, 14*, 281–288. http://dx.doi.org/10.1097/01.pra.0000336755.57684.45

Verheul, R., Van Den Bosch, L. M., Koeter, M. W., De Ridder, M. A., Stijnen, T., & Van Den Brink, W. (2003). Dialectical behaviour therapy for women with borderline personality disorder: 12-month, randomised clinical trial in The Netherlands. *The British Journal of Psychiatry, 182*, 135–140. http://dx.doi.org/10.1192/bjp.182.2.135

Wessler, R. L., & Hankin, S. (1988). Rational-emotive therapy and related cognitively oriented psychotherapies. In S. Long (Ed.), *Six group therapies* (pp. 159–215). New York, NY: Plenum Press. http://dx.doi.org/10.1007/978-1-4899-2100-0_4

Wessler, R. L., & Hankin-Wessler, S. (1989). Cognitive group therapy. In A. Freeman, K. M. Simon, L. E. Beutler, & H. Arkowitz (Eds.), *Comprehensive handbook of cognitive therapy* (pp. 559–581). New York, NY: Plenum Press. http://dx.doi.org/10.1007/978-1-4757-9779-4_28

Williams, J. M. G., & Moorey, S. (1989). The wider application of cognitive therapy: The end of the beginning. In J. Scott, J. M. G. Williams, & A. T. Beck (Eds.), *Cognitive therapy in clinical practice: An illustrative casebook* (pp. 227–250). New York, NY: Routledge. http://dx.doi.org/10.4324/9780203359365_chapter_ten

Wise, E. H., & Haynes, S. N. (1983). Cognitive treatment of test anxiety: Rational restructuring versus attentional training. *Cognitive Therapy and Research, 7*, 69–77. http://dx.doi.org/10.1007/BF01173425

Wiseman, C. V. (2002). Short-term group CBT versus psycho-education on an inpatient eating disorder unit. *Eating Disorders, 10*, 313–320. http://dx.doi.org/10.1080/10640260214504

Wiseman, C. V., Sunday, S. R., Klapper, F., Klein, M., & Halmi, K. A. (2002). Short-term group CBT versus psycho-education on an inpatient eating disorder unit. *Eating Disorders, 10*, 313–320. http://dx.doi.org/10.1080/10640260214504

Wisniewski, L., Safer, D., & Chen, E. (2007). Dialectical behavior therapy and eating disorders. In L. A. Dimeff & K. Koerner (Eds.), *Dialectical behavior therapy in clinical practice: Applications across disorders and settings* (pp. 174–221). New York, NY: Guilford Press.

Witt-Browder, A. S. (2000). Clients in partial hospitalization settings. In J. R. White, A. S. Freeman, J. R. White, & A. S. Freeman (Eds.), *Cognitive-behavioral group therapy: For specific problems and populations* (pp. 361–384). Washington, DC: American Psychological Association. http://dx.doi.org/10.1037/10352-014

Wolpe, J. (1973). *The practice of behavior therapy* (2nd ed.). New York, NY: Pergamon Press.

Wright, J. H., Thase, M. E., Beck, A. T., & Ludgate, J. W. (Eds.). (1993). *Cognitive therapy with inpatients: Developing a cognitive milieu.* New York, NY: Guilford Press.

Wykes, T., Parr, A. M., & Landau, S. (1999). Group treatment of auditory hallucinations: Exploratory study of effectiveness. *The British Journal of Psychiatry, 175,* 180–185. http://dx.doi.org/10.1192/bjp.175.2.180

Yen, S., Johnson, J., Costello, E., & Simpson, E. B. (2009). A 5-day dialectical behavior therapy partial hospital program for women with borderline personality disorder: Predictors of outcome from a 3-month follow-up study. *Journal of Psychiatric Practice, 15,* 173–182. http://dx.doi.org/10.1097/01.pra.0000351877.45260.70

Yost, E. B., Beutler, L. E., Corbishley, M. A., & Allender, J. R. (1986). *Group cognitive therapy: A treatment approach for depressed older adults.* New York, NY: Pergamon Press.

Young, J. E. (2005). Schema-focused cognitive therapy and the case of Ms. S. *Journal of Psychotherapy Integration, 15,* 115–126. http://dx.doi.org/10.1037/1053-0479.15.1.115

Young, J. E., Klosko, J. S., & Weishaar, M. E. (2003). *Schema therapy: A practitioner's guide.* New York, NY: Guilford Press.

Zerhusen, J. D., Boyle, K., & Wilson, W. (1991). Out of the darkness: Group cognitive therapy for depressed elderly. *Journal of Psychosocial Nursing and Mental Health Services, 29*(9), 16–21.

6

ACCEPTANCE AND COMMITMENT THERAPY–GROUP

Acceptance and commitment therapy (ACT) is an approach embedded in *functional contextualism*, a philosophy that is aligned with the philosophical movement of pragmatism. This school of thought undergirds the assumptions that are made about how humans function, through what processes they change, and what criterion is used as the standard for truth within the approach. Functional contextualism is defined by four essential elements (Hayes, 2004; Hayes, Strosahl, & Wilson, 1999). The first is the theory's focus on a whole human event, and the second is the examination of events in the contexts in which they occur. For contextualists, acts cannot be understood apart from their contexts.[1] These two features are highly confluent with the ethos of group psychotherapy. Complex behaviors of individual members are understood in terms of their interpersonal context. However, for ACT, *context*, as we later discuss, also refers to the individual's way of looking at

---

[1]For further explication of contextualism, the reader is encouraged to consult Hayes, Hayes, and Reese (1988).

http://dx.doi.org/10.1037/0000113-007
Group Psychotherapy in Inpatient, Partial Hospital, and Residential Care Settings, by V. Brabender and A. Fallon

his or her group experience. The third feature of the theory is epistemological: How does the theory define *truth* within the model? Consistent with a functional bent, truth is understood in terms of the extent to which a statement works rather than its conformity to some external reality. This criterion establishes a clear link between ACT and behavior analysis and is a consistent theme in Skinner's writings (Hayes, Hayes, & Reese, 1988). The implication of this feature of ACT for how a psychotherapy group is conducted is that group members would be continually directed to examine whether particular behaviors work for them in the group and beyond. However, *working* must be relevant to some standard, and it is here that Hayes (Hayes et al., 1999) introduced the fourth element of goals and values. Whether a particular behavior works is evaluated by whether it moves an individual toward a goal and is consistent with the person's values. In group psychotherapy, in some manner, the goal that serves as the standard against which to evaluate behaviors has an interpersonal focus. ACT strives to help individuals recognize their values and goals and evaluate their behavior regarding them.

Excellent resources are available for clinicians interested in ACT, and we encourage them to consult those to master this approach. In this chapter, our goal is to explicate ACT regarding its application to the psychotherapy group. Overall, the ACT literature that addresses its use in a group does so incidentally, although exceptions exist. For example, Westrup and Wright (2017) recently wrote a text on ACT and group treatment. Manuals are available for the group treatment of anger (Foret & Eaton, 2014), health anxiety (Eilenberg, Kronstand, Fink, & Frostholm, 2014), interpersonal problems (McKay, Lev, Skeen, & Saavedra, 2012), and psychosis (Wright et al., 2014). We know from the corpus of research on group psychotherapy (e.g., Burlingame, Whitcomb, & Woodland, 2013) that this modality produces the most favorable aspects when the therapist addresses facets of the group climate, such as level of cohesion or degree of conflict. What we aim to do in this chapter is explicate how the therapist can capitalize on the group aspect of Acceptance and Commitment Therapy–Group (ACT-G)—that is, how he or she can draw on some of the special phenomena that characterize the psychotherapy group. However, we recognize that our effort represents only a beginning, which we hope whets the appetites of others interested in ACT-G to develop the integration of group psychology and ACT further.

BASIC SUPPOSITIONS ABOUT HUMAN PSYCHOLOGY

Approaches to psychotherapy are founded on implicit or explicit suppositions about how psychological problems emerge. ACT explicitly sees human suffering as rooted in language and reasoning. For human beings, language has primacy over many other ways of understanding the world and, therefore, is unsurprisingly implicated in human difficulties. The very processes, ACT theorists have noted, that give rise to some of the most prodigious human accomplishments are the ones that beget pain in human beings, patients, and therapists alike. To specify these processes, Hayes and colleagues (1999) introduced relational frame theory, which characterizes how an individual relates to contextual cues. Through the power of language, human beings, in particular, relate to stimuli as classes and possess the capability of drawing connections between stimuli within a given class or stimuli of different classes. Using the language of operant conditioning, Törneke, Luciano, and Salas (2008) observed,

> Early during the normal development of language abilities, humans learn to relate stimuli arbitrarily, which soon becomes a generalized operant response (Healy, Barnes-Holmes, & Smeets, 2000). Through multiple exemplar training, the contextual cues for relating (e.g., same as, opposite of, more than, better than, part of) *are abstracted and then arbitrarily applied to new stimuli.* That is, the child will soon be able to relate stimuli which do not share any formal property, and thereby, stimuli which have never been actually related in his learning history will become functionally effective. (p. 143, emphasis added)

Hence, this capacity enables human beings to be governed by rules in the absence of conditioning to all stimuli within a given class. Hayes et al. (1999) identified three properties that characterize how stimuli within classes are related to one another. The first property is *mutual entailment,* or bidirectionality, such that how A is connected to B in a given context will necessitate how B is connected to A. In such a manner, a stimulus equivalence is established between A and B. Accordingly, if Jaclyn speaks more in the group session than Katie, then Katie speaks less than Jaclyn. *Combinatorial entailment* is somewhat more complex. It specifies that in a context, if A is related to B on a dimension, and B is related to C on that same dimension, A and C necessarily must be related (or entailed) in a preordained way on that dimension (i.e., without being established in direct experience). By way of example, if Mindy (A) is more confrontational than Bernice (B), and Bernice is more confrontational than Andy (C), Mindy will be regarded as more confrontational than Andy in the absence of a direct, experiential comparison. The third property is the *tendency to transform stimulus properties,* such that if the dimensions of x and y are related, then differences on dimension y can be derived from differences on dimension x. Suppose that in a given context, the level of member warmth (x) is positively related to the degree of self-disclosure (y). Then, if Mindy is warmer than Bernice, Mindy will also be expected to exhibit greater self-disclosure in the group than Bernice. Notice that the relationships humans are able to establish are derivative rather than exclusively based on direct experience. Once A and B are brought into relationship with one another, the cognitive activity does not end there. B is placed within the associative network in which A resides such that one connection (that between A and B) leads to a plethora of connections (that between B and all that is connected to A).

When an individual responds to cues within a context by framing the cues using the aforementioned properties, the individual is framing those cues relationally. Stated otherwise, the person is implementing a *relational frame*. What cues are relationally framed depends on the individual's unique conditioning history. Although the notion of relational frames might seem remote from everyday experience, the empirically demonstrated capacity of human beings to impose these frames accounts for important psychological phenomena. On the positive side, the fact that human beings do not need to make connections in the absence of direct conditioning enables human thinking to be efficient and flexible. On the negative side, bidirectionality leads to words becoming associated with the painful experiences they describe. The use of language—ubiquitous and constant in humans—entails that verbalizations used to describe or understand events will be fraught with whatever pain occurred in those events from a person's past. The more cognitive processing occurs, the more unpleasant the internal experience becomes. Exacerbating this effect of bidirectionality (and the other properties) is the effort to control negatively toned inner experiences through various means, an effort that is promoted by most psychotherapies. The processing of experiences to eliminate their impact merely leads to the expansion of the negative tone through the associative network attached to the event that first provoked an unpleasant reaction. This expansion is particularly likely when the individual operates from a *literalist context* wherein the individual merges the symbol for an event with the experience the event describes. For example,

> Jamie tells her group member Cora, "You are a loser," and Cora feels dejected. Cora establishes a stimulus equivalence between herself and being a loser. These concepts (Cora and loser) are now fused. The emotions and thoughts that Cora has from experiences associated with *loser* are now associated with herself. Cora most easily establishes a stimulus equivalence between herself and the notion of loser when she regards her experiences from a literal vantage. However, a change in context can alter how she regards Jamie's communication. If she is able to embrace a nonliteral context in which she sees both Jamie's communication and any reactions stirred up by it as momentary events, she can avoid integrating this negative segment into her view of herself.

WHY PSYCHOLOGICAL PROBLEMS
ARISE FOR HUMAN BEINGS

Psychopathology, within an ACT framework, is not the set of symptoms that ordinarily become targets of treatment but rather the individual's relationship to his or her symptoms. To expand on this idea, Hayes and colleagues (1999) helpfully developed the acronym FEAR to account for why human beings have the troubles they do. Although human troubles can reach a level of intensity such that we refer to them as *psychopathology*, the FEAR concepts are useful in elucidating much of human suffering, including that deemed to be in the normal range. In thinking about the elements of FEAR, we consider how they might manifest in the group situation.

F in the acronym stands for *fusion with one's thoughts*, and it refers to the phenomenon of an individual taking on a literal perspective that leads him or her to see inner, private experiences as real (Hayes et al., 1999). In our example of Cora, we saw that she regarded the label *loser* literally by seeing it as describing some reality in herself. However, members in a group situation do not have to be directly addressed to engage in cognitive fusion:

> Violet listened as a new member of an inpatient group talked about his suspicions of his neighbors. In his narrative, he described their ethnicity and a number of negative characteristics they exhibited. After the session, Violet contacted the therapist, saying she did not wish to attend anymore because the group was making her feel bad about herself. She revealed that she shared the ethnicity of the individuals the new member found objectionable. Violet said it was upsetting to her to think she has the characteristics this member mentioned. Violet did not know whether the member thought she had these characteristics. She established an equivalence with these individuals and believed the description of them held some relevance to her. That is, she took his comments as having objective reality in relation to herself and was, accordingly, deflated. Psychotherapy groups in which members are invited to offer feedback to one another provide plentiful opportunities for fusion to occur.

E stands for *evaluation of experience*. Hayes et al. (1999) made the point that once momentary affects, sensations, and cognitions are regarded as thing-like, the question that immediately asserts itself is, Is this thing good or bad? If it is bad, a motive is created to eliminate it. If it is good, the question arises as to whether it is good enough, an easy step to take given that human beings can use language to imagine the ideal form of a quality (Hayes, 2002a). When judged against an ideal, most individuals are likely to find themselves lacking.

A corresponds to *avoidance of one's experience* or experiential avoidance, a process wherein an individual attempts to eliminate unpleasant thoughts or feelings. For example, we could see experiential avoidance in Violet's decision to leave her psychotherapy group. The means human beings adopt to avoid bothersome internal events are variable, but they share a common effect of increasing or intensifying the thoughts and feelings that are the targets of the avoidance efforts. Violet, for example, by avoiding the group, will have made a statement to herself that this member's views on people of her ethnicity are extremely important, even authoritative, and should be evocative of her emotional reactions and self-impressions. To avoid something, it must be a focus, and once it is a focus, it cannot truly be avoided. Robust empirical support exists for the notion that experiential avoidance is implicated in a great variety of psychological problems (see Hayes, 2004, for a review).

R refers to *reason-giving for one's behavior* or the human propensity to develop explanations for behavior that undermines the individual's well-being. The fusion of internal states provides the means for identifying factors that are seen as causally connected to behaviors that are not working for an individual. For example, a member may say she did not participate in the group because she was depressed during the session. As Hayes et al. (1999) noted, this explanation might well be compelling to others who could even show sympathy toward the reason-giver and thereby support the tendency to offer reasons. In fact, her nonparticipation might be due to a variety of factors, one of which might or might not be her internal state during the session. However, positing this factor as a causal link to her inactivity in the group—whether true or not—does not serve her goal of deriving benefit from the group modality. After all, the group member might have a variety of private events during the group. By focusing on uncontrollable reactions, the group member is hindering herself from homing in on the zone in which her control resides. In this way, her reason-giving is fostering, at best, stasis, not advancement. At worst, reason-giving entails an intensive focus on the negative states that the individual regards as aversive.

ACCEPTANCE AND COMMITMENT THERAPY–GROUP TREATMENT

The ACT acronym stands for the basic activities that are pursued in the treatment, *accept* your thoughts and feelings and be present, *choose* a valued action, and *take action*, en route to achieving greater mental health (Harris, 2009). ACT conceptualizes mental health as living a vital life in consonance with one's values while accepting those internal experiences that accompany the state of being alive and that pursuing one's values begets. Six elements constitute the basic activities of ACT.

Acceptance

The first element, *acceptance*, involves the client's[2] assumption of a stance of "creative hopelessness." At first blush, it might seem strange that a treatment promotes hopelessness. However, the hopelessness pertains to the viability of the methods that clients use to diminish or eliminate pain. Experiential avoidance and reason-giving and the literal use of language that bolsters both, as noted previously, only amplify pain. Hopelessness does not pertain to the person him- or herself or that person's future—that is, the capacity to have a life that the client values. The specifier *creative* is important in that it points to the openness the client must adopt to embrace more workable solutions once the hopeless strategies are abandoned. For group psychotherapy participants, the presence of other members can be an asset in members' achieving creative hopelessness. Although all members of the group are likely to use experiential avoidance and reasons to attempt to control private events, they will do so in different ways, even if they happen to share symptom patterns such as depression and anxiety. Sometimes, members can more easily see others' experiential avoidance than their own, but in recognizing this effort in another, they lower the threshold for self-awareness.

In group psychotherapy, the therapist can support the development of a norm of members applying *workability* as the standard for assessing members' behaviors and approaches to their experiences. As members recognize each other's ways of coping with group events (internal and external), the therapist can raise the question of how these practices advance their relationships with one another and serve their goals and values.

Successful ACT work leads to acceptance of one's current state without any expectation that that state will change. Acceptance is transformed into willingness when the client is helped to divest him- or herself of the quest to control interior experience and to allow the self to have whatever bodily sensations, feelings, cognitions, impulses, and so on, might come to the fore. Willingness exercises are used according to the kinds of experiences that evoke the avoidance. For example, trauma survivors will engage in exercises that entail emotional exposure to elements of the traumatic events. Pain patients will be helped to distance the transcendent self from the pain by asking the patient to "physicalize painful experiences" (Hayes, 2002b, p. 61) by specifying the color, shape, size, and so on, of the pain. In groups in which members have symptom heterogeneity (transdiagnostic groups), such tailoring might have to give way to more broadly applicable techniques.

---

[2]In our other chapters, we primarily use the term *patient* to refer to individuals receiving treatment in the three settings of interest in this text. However, *patient* is so at odds with the ethos of ACT, that in this context, we use the term *client*.

The therapist assists group members in moving away from the literal use of language through the use of metaphors. Language creates a problem in that it supports reifying experiences in a fashion that progressively removes a person from direct experiences. For example, in helping members to see the futility and unworkability of experiential avoidance, the therapist presents the concept of the Chinese finger trap, which tightens more strongly around the bearer's finger the more the bearer tries to pull away from it. Metaphors can often make otherwise incomprehensible concepts understandable. Upon their introduction, the therapist can also hearken back to them to remind the members of a concept that might have been forgotten. Most important, however, metaphors "can be actively constructed to foster the transformation of stimulus functions of critical aspects of the client's environment" (Monestès & Villatte, 2011, p. 1). If the therapist were to use words, say to dispense the advice "express your feelings," the client would likely construct a type of rule from it that pertains to social consequences, also known as a *ply* (e.g., "If I express my feelings, I will secure my therapist's approval"). The problem with the rule is that it is applied across contexts and in ways that can be detrimental to the person. The greater the number of rules the individual acquires, the more rigid the person becomes. Providing a metaphor is different from providing a rule in that the metaphor entails offering a new perspective on a person's experience. It encourages the person to examine experience to see whether the relationship among the elements in the metaphor is paralleled by the relationship of elements in one's experience. For example, on being presented with the Chinese finger trap metaphor, the person is likely to ask, "Hmmm, is it true that if I try harder and harder to avoid a feeling, its grip on me merely tightens?" The metaphor, therefore, immerses the individual fully in the here and now as opposed to nonfigurative language that often removes the person further from his or her experience.

For these reasons, ACT is a metaphor-rich treatment, and Hayes and colleagues (e.g., Hayes & Wilson, 1994) have provided a plethora of useful metaphors for the ACT practitioner. Therapists should individualize metaphors for the individual member and the specific group. However, individuals can develop their own metaphors that might have great personal resonance. In some cases, an individual's metaphors might be so compelling to the group as a whole that the group adopts it. The metaphor, then, becomes part of the group's identity and contributes to cohesion among members. Group treatment has the advantage that all members bring their imaginal resources to crafting metaphors and, as various members elaborate on them, they achieve greater salience and potency (Duffy, 2006; Gans, 1991).

Once clients know in a general way that what they have done has not worked, they come to appreciate that the effort to control private events through experiential avoidance—an effort strongly supported by living in an environment of other language users—is what leads to unfavorable outcomes for the person. Gradually, the client is guided in recognizing that the effort to control might work in some situations (e.g., in dealing with the physical environment or when the material avoided is not important) but not in others (e.g., feelings attached to important issues). During this step and the next, individuals are likely to have fuller access to many feelings they ordinarily seek to escape. The group aspect is helpful in that members can recognize that these feelings are shared. They are supported in recognizing that having feelings is a large part of what makes one human.

Contact With the Present Moment

This element engages *mindfulness*, the state of being fully within the present and aware of events in one's internal and external environments. Willingness permits contact with the present moment. When experiential avoidance does not have a hold on a person's inner life, that person is freed to attend to immediate events without judgment (Hayes, 2002b; Masterpasqua, 2016). This stance is likely to deepen members' connections with one another in the psychotherapy group. When members can listen to one another without judgment, the effort to control one another based on judgment diminishes. Being attentive to what is there within another creates a basis for empathy. Without judgment, the enterprise of giving feedback is fortified in that members look at one another's behavior in terms of whether particular behaviors possess workability (i.e., help the individual move toward his or her goals) rather than whether they are inherently good or bad.

To assist group members in making contact with the present moment, a variety of exercises, some of which are derived from the Buddhist tradition, can be used. Examples of such exercises appear in Table 6.1.

Defusion

Earlier in this chapter, the tendency of individuals to fuse thoughts with reality was described through the example of Cora. Because Cora had the thought that she is a loser, she conjectured that she must be a loser. All forms of ACT, including ACT-G, seek to reverse this process. That is, participants are encouraged to recognize that they can have a different type of relationship with their thoughts, one in which they recognize that a thought is just that. Hence, Cora would come to see that *loser* is a name she calls herself from time to time. She would be supported in recognizing that *loser* is not more than a word. "Being present" would support this transition because Cora would realize that her immediate experience is not of herself being a loser but of herself having a particular thought. Such a shift would enable her

TABLE 6.1

Examples of Acceptance and Commitment Therapy Exercises

Name of exercise	Description of activity	Purpose
Rules of the game exercise (Hayes, Strosahl, & Wilson, 1999)	The member identifies the basic rules that he or she summons to provide a blueprint for living. Particularly noted are rules such as "No pain, no gain" that motivate the client to control his or her experiences.	The recognition and exploration of these rules helps the client to see how arbitrary notions are given great power in how the individual regards him- or herself.
Contents on cards exercises (Hayes et al., 1999)	All of the variations on this type of exercise require the client to write unwanted thoughts and emotions on cards. In one variation, the therapist tells the client not to allow the cards to touch his or her lap. The therapist flips each card in turn toward the client. The client bats it away. The therapist then tells the client to allow the card to fall where it will. The therapist repeats the same action.	The client learns that it is a choice what to do with psychological contents. That is, the client can either struggle to avoid them or simply let them be (i.e., to appear as they will).
Argyle socks exercise (Hayes et al., 1999)	The therapist directs the client to accept momentarily the belief that he or she regards it as essential that college boys wear argyle socks. They consider whether the client could act in a way that is consistent with this belief. The client is encouraged to identify a number of acts that would be consistent with this belief. It is then pointed out to the client that he or she need not be in possession of a particular emotional state to pursue actions consistent with values.	Here the client learns that once the client has recognized a value, he or she is not dependent on a particular internal state to translate the value into action. They also appreciate that external action rather than internal events, is a domain under their control.
Exposing the "worst self" (McKay, Lev, & Skeen, 2012; Ciarrochi & Bailey, 2008)	Clients identify an event in which they behaved with their worst self (i.e., engaged in behaviors that they sorely regretted). The individual is then directed to recognize that it is his or her observer self that is witnessing these behaviors.	The individual is helped in accessing the transcendent self that stays constant amidst changing internal experiences. The individual is helped to differentiate the "worst self" from the actual self. This exercise seeks to alter the individual's relationship with private events.

TABLE 6.1

Examples of Acceptance and Commitment Therapy Exercises   (*Continued*)

Name of exercise	Description of activity	Purpose
Evaluations versus descriptions (McKay, Lev, Skeen, & Saavedra, 2012)	Members divide into pairs. One person is asked to describe an event. The other person listens, but every time the narrator makes a judgment, the listener says "evaluation." Members of the pair switch roles.	Members begin to differentiate between descriptions and evaluations. In recognizing that evaluations occur on an ongoing basis simply as part of how the human mind works, they gradually see that evaluations are constructions of the mind and not inherent in external reality.

to have a measure of distance from her thoughts, making them less believable, even if they remained as frequent.

Self in Context/Transcendent Self

Self in context forms a couplet with *contact with the present moment*, a pairing that Hayes (2017) described as "showing up" (p. 10). This element entails an important discrimination that can lessen the urgency to engage in experiential avoidance. The therapist makes a distinction between the self and the various psychological contents—feelings and thoughts—that the individual experiences. In doing so, the therapist helps the client to *defuse* the negative content from the self, thereby rendering it less consuming. Consider the following interaction:

Group member: I am such a bad person; I feel ashamed.

Therapist: So, you find yourself thinking the sentence, "I am a bad person." Of course, that is just a thought and the shame is just a feeling. Neither are you. It is *you* who can notice that you can think thoughts or have feelings. But they are not you any more than the socks that you wore to group today are you.

Here again, the operation of the therapeutic factor of *universality* (Yalom & Leszcz, 2005), the awareness that members are not alone with their experiences, helps drive this separation between the transcendent self and momentary psychological content. Many events that occur within and outside the group engender the same feelings in members. They can see that the feelings are common ones—even in the moment as group events occur—and pass as new events occur and other feelings predominate. As members become aware of commonalities, cohesion in the group builds, which further fuels members' work (see Burlingame, McClendon, & Alonso's, 2011, meta-analysis of 40 studies on the positive effects of group cohesion).

As with other core processes, ACT provides metaphors that underscore the distinction between self-as-context and self-as-content. For example, the image of a chessboard is summoned with the board itself being the conscious, transcendent self and the individual pieces being the elements that constitute inner experience at any moment (Walser & Hayes, 2006). The elements naturally cluster together in teams that then stand in opposition to one another. Through this imagery, the client is helped to recognize that if he or she focuses on the pieces, he or she will be consigned to waging battle on one set of pieces or another. How the battle unfolds determines how the person feels about the self. However, if the client focuses on the board itself, the pieces can do what they will without fundamentally shaking the client's sense of self.

Additional examples of ACT metaphors appear in Table 6.2. Often, once metaphors are introduced, the clients themselves will use them throughout the therapy as touchstones. Clients also frequently revise and refine metaphors to fit their preferred imagery and situations. The therapist should encourage this customization of metaphors (Hayes et al., 1999).

Values

This ACT element entails members' discovering values and goals consistent with those values. Hayes et al. (1999) emphasized that "all ACT techniques are eventually subordinated to helping the client live in accord with his or her chosen values" (p. 205). Group applications of ACT are no exception. However, to do so, the therapist must assist the client in (a) distinguishing between values and goals and (b) engaging in a values clarification process. The therapist supports members in seeing that whereas *values* are broad aspirational principles, *goals* are concrete, specific aims that should be in the service of the person's principles. Whereas values can never be accomplished, goals can. For example, a group member might value establishing satisfying, intimate relationships, with the more specific goal of being competent in expressing her needs to others.

The values clarification process entails directing members' attention to value domains: marriage, couples, and intimate relations; family relations; friendships and social relations; career and employment; education and personal growth and development; recreation and leisure; spirituality; citizenship; and health and physical well-being. This process entails the completion

TABLE 6.2
Examples of Acceptance and Commitment Metaphors

Name of metaphor and source	Description	Purpose
Tug of war with a monster (Hayes, Strosahl, & Wilson, 1999)	The client is asked to imagine having a tug-of-war with a powerful monster. The monster is in a bottomless pit in which the client risks being pulled. The harder the client pulls, the harder the monster pulls and the closer the client gets to the edge. The client is urged to recognize that the task is not to win the tug-of-war but to drop the war.	Promotes creative hopelessness by fostering in the client a willingness to have various psychological experiences. That is, the client sees that the task is not to emerge victorious over thoughts and feelings but simply to allow them to be.
Swamp (Hayes, Strosahl, & Wilson, 1999)	The client fantasizes about taking a trip to a beautiful destination. En route, the client encounters a swamp. Wading through the swamp is unpleasant. Steps can be slow and effortful. Small fish might bite at the traveler's ankles. The smells from the swamp might be repellent. The traveler must decide whether to turn or continue toward the destination.	Underscores that the inevitable obstacles faced as human beings move in the direction of their goals requires the reaffirmation of goals. Also, it conveys that individuals grapple with obstacles not because they wish to do so but, rather, because doing so is necessary to pursue a given direction.
High school sweetheart (Hayes, Strosahl, & Wilson, 1999)	The client is taken back to the loss of a sweetheart in high school through rejection. The client is then asked to think about two scenarios—one in which the individual allowed him- or herself to feel the hurt and then open up again versus one in which hurt was avoided and the individual remained closed, leading the hurt to turn to trauma.	Helps clients see that self-protection from a single hurt can beget further deprivation.
Skiing (Hayes, Strosahl, & Wilson, 1999)	The client is presented with the situation of a skier who is at the top of a mountain and is encountered by a person flying a helicopter who asks the skier where he or she is going. He or she says to the bottom of the mountain at which point the pilot grabs the skier and, in a gesture of supposed helpfulness, flies him or her to the bottom of the mountain. The skier takes the lift to the top of the hill, and the same sequence repeats itself.	This metaphor conveys an important ACT maxim that "Outcome is the process through which process becomes the outcome" (Hayes, Strosahl, & Wilson, 1999, p. 221). The client can grasp through this metaphor that the ski lodge (the goal) is important only because it provides a direction for the skiing (the process).

(continues)

TABLE 6.2
Examples of Acceptance and Commitment Metaphors   *(Continued)*

Name of metaphor and source	Description	Purpose
Gardening	Here the situation is that of the gardener who, while cultivating soil in one spot, plants a garden. However, she or he then detects another spot that seems more inviting for her or his efforts. She or he leaves the original spot and moves to the next spot. Each time the gardener invests in one spot, her or his efforts are interrupted by another alluring prospect.	The gardener never realizes the potential of any one realm by moving from spot to spot. She or he is unable to build on her work and whatever produce is yielded is likely to be short term. However, remaining in a spot and truly cultivating invariably involves noticing its flaws and accepting the feelings attached to them. Pursuing values (the garden) involves accepting the range of experiences that values-driven action evokes.

Note. ACT = acceptance and commitment therapy.

of homework assignments. Specifically, the client completes two measures. First, the Values Narrative Form (Hayes et al., 1999) entails the client providing a valued direction narrative for each of the aforementioned domains. Second, the Values Assessment Rating Form entails the client rating each domain on (a) the importance it has for the individual, (b) the individual's success in living it over the past month, and (c) the relative priority the individual places on working on it at present. In sharing the homework material and exploring its implications further in the session, members are called on to share personal material perhaps never communicated to anyone else previously because they pertain to often-secret dreams and wishes.[3,4] Fortunately, the group has had an opportunity to develop a reasonable level of trust at the point this step occurs. A challenge of this step is that the individual nature of goals and values can easily create a problem in ensuring that all members receive sufficient attention. A go-around format might most easily enable the therapist to support each member's work at this juncture.

---

[3]In fact, in group psychotherapy, the future perspective tends to be given short shrift. However, psychodrama (Moreno, 1946) represents an exception.
[4]For more chronic patients, this is especially true because often others engage with these individuals in relation to their problems rather than their aspirations.

As Westrup and Wright (2017) helpfully pointed out, group psychotherapy can be helpful in the values clarification process. Although it is true that each person's values are very much his or her own, it nonetheless is the case that members can draw inspiration from others who are going through this process. For example, one member hearing another talk about the importance the latter places on being an excellent parent might at that moment recognize that she, too, embraces that value.

Committed Action

The sixth step is members' developing a capacity for committed or values-based action—that is, action that is aligned with their goals and values. Without action, goals and values are hollow. Members are helped to see that committed action will often produce distress of various sorts. Commitment is a willingness to accept this distress to live congruently with one's values. Members also are helped in seeing that a commitment to action is not made in one moment but, rather, must be renewed again and again, particularly following what the individual might regard as a failure (e.g., an episode of loss of sobriety following the individual's committing to sobriety). Buttressing the movement toward goals is the capacity to identify barriers that might present themselves, one of which is the refusal to accept inner experiences that such movement stimulates. However, other obstacles are likely to arise, and the therapist helps members to see how they can mobilize all the core processes to respond to those obstacles productively. For example, contact with the present moment enables members to see possible solutions in their inner or outer environments that might not otherwise be apparent.

All six core processes contribute to the overarching aim of ACT, fostering *psychological flexibility*, which Hayes (n.d.) defined as "the ability to contact the present moment more fully as a conscious human being, and to change and persist in behavior when doing so serves valued ends" (p. 1). Illustrating the interrelationships between the change processes and the psychological flexibility to which they contribute is the hexaflex, seen in Figure 6.1. Psychological flexibility is associated with a variety of positive outcomes such as mental health, the capacity to learn new skills, job performance (Bond & Flaxman, 2006), and diminished daily emotional exhaustion (Biron & van Veldhoven, 2012). It has been demonstrated to enhance pain tolerance (Feldner et al., 2006) and moderate the effects of somatization and health anxiety on core areas of quality of life (Leonidou, Panayiotou, Bati, & Karekla, 2016). As Levin, Herbert, and Forman (2017) pointed out, one limitation of the psychological flexibility research is that this concept is measured almost exclusively with self-report measures.

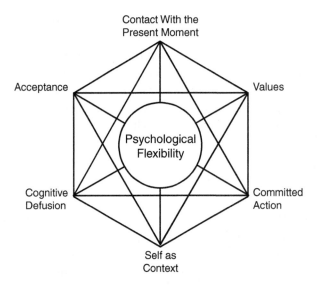

Figure 6.1. Hexaflex. Copyright 2017 by Steven C. Hayes. Reprinted with permission.

TECHNICAL CONSIDERATIONS

Role of the Leader

Stance of the Leader

In ACT, the stance of the leader is as an egalitarian collaborator who, like the group member, participates in the human condition and has fundamentally the same struggles. Hayes et al. (1999) described the need for the therapist to show "radical respect" (p. 274) for the client, meaning that the therapist recognizes the client's entitlement to embrace a set of values of his or her choice and craft a lifestyle that is uniquely his or her own.

This approach necessitates that therapists take pains not to present themselves as someone who has arrived at a fundamentally different level than that of the group member. The group psychotherapist who is actively applying ACT to his or her life—a person who is striving to achieve a high level of psychological flexibility—is in the best position to convey this common bond with group members authentically (Westrup & Wright, 2017). The leader is transparent about his or her reactions in the group—a feature that promotes members' openness. This position does not require the therapist to be highly self-disclosing about personal struggles. One tool that the group psychotherapist has is the use of interventions at different levels of analysis. Although at times it will be necessary for the ACT-G therapist to make individual interventions, particularly when exploring values, at other times, the therapist can make interventions at the level of the group (e.g., "At this moment in the group, we are feeling . . ."). Such an intervention conveys a sense that the members and therapist have a bond of humanity that makes certain emotions part of what constitutes living.

Leadership Activities

According to Wright et al. (2014), group applications of ACT are useful because "the group format enables group members to learn from one another, receive reinforcement from peers, and benefit from positive peer pressure and support" (p. 18). The therapist's role is to help members realize the potential of this modality. One of the first tasks of the therapist is to ensure that members are in a state of readiness to work in the group, an objective that can be accomplished through the pretraining. Wright et al. recommended an individual pretraining session because the values-focus often lends itself to an initial individual conversation. However, often, inpatient, residential, and day hospital settings do not permit this kind of individualized attention, particularly given the need to place members in groups soon after admission. We have found that the small group interview can accomplish this purpose. In this pretraining session, members are apprised of the goals of the group and member behaviors that support the goals. Hayes et al. (1999) emphasized the importance of the informed consent in which the client is encouraged to refrain from expecting immediate gains but rather to persist in the process throughout its twists and turns. Although this recommendation is useful in many types of therapy, it is particularly important for this approach because, during the course of the treatment, the client will be facing that which had been previously avoided, an occurrence that might lead the client to regard him- or herself as backsliding.

In conducting the sessions themselves, the therapists take the group members through a series of experiential exercises, metaphors, and paradoxical interventions. Although the introduction of concepts is necessary at various points, the therapist is not primarily engaged in providing psychoeducation but rather group facilitation by initiating and processing exercises (Ossman, Wilson, Storaasli, & McNeill, 2006) for each step of ACT. For example, therapists use the observer exercise to help the members identify a transcendent self that exists apart from whatever psychological content is occupying consciousness at the moment (Hayes, 2002b). In this exercise, once members have had an opportunity to center themselves, they are asked to focus on a memory from their relatively recent past, such as one occurring in the prior summer. Once members have an image in mind of a moment during that time, they are asked to remember all the inner experiences associated with that moment. They are then encouraged to notice how these contents are separate from the self's engaging in the act of noticing these contents. This process is then repeated with other memories until members have a firm basis of seeing that self that lasts across time. Recognizing the self as distinct from content supports members in meeting the content directly rather than resorting to avoidance strategies.

Content of the Session

Often, the ACT-G session begins with a mindfulness exercise. For example, McKay, Lev, Skeen, and Saavedra (2012) recommended beginning each session with 5 minutes of mindful focusing or the five senses exercise. *Mindful focusing* involves having group members notice their breath as it proceeds from their noses to their diaphragms and then to recognize private events while labeling them *thought*, *emotion*, or *sensation*. The therapist encourages them "not to hold onto any experience. Just label each one and let it go" (p. 43). Members continue with this quiet attention to internal events for 2 minutes. The *five senses exercise* entails members focusing in turn on each of their five senses. In other formats, such as Foret and Eaton's (2014) anger group, the mindfulness or present moment exercises are different in each session.

Once ACT-G gets underway, group members typically have homework on which to report. As members share their experiences, the therapist can highlight particular concepts and encourage members to do the same and to relate metaphors that illumine aspects of each member's work. In the middle of the session, the therapist can introduce new concepts, which are brought to life through relevant exercises. The therapist can draw on examples from members' lives that they have introduced in the context of sharing their experiences with homework assignments. Foret and Eaton made the important point that the therapist should not only conduct the exercises but also engage group members in an exploration of their experience with each exercise. They counseled that, in doing so, the therapist should ask questions that help members to tune into their experiences more fully rather than evaluate them or even understand fully the concept the exercise was illumining.

In midsession, therapists might draw on techniques that are particularly suited to the needs of the members. Wright et al. (2014) advocated that, with members who are psychotic, it is especially helpful to have members test out two or more of their distorted beliefs in a behavioral experiment to develop cognitive flexibility. Here, members learn to adopt an experimental attitude toward their ideas. For example, one psychotic patient who was convinced that his thoughts were being broadcast by a satellite was encouraged to test out various implications of his ideas. The point was not so much to dissuade him from his views—a move that could be consistent with experiential avoidance—but to assess their functionality.

TABLE 6.3
Acceptance and Commitment Therapy

Elements of the model	Characteristics of the model
View of psychological problems	Psychological problems are rooted in psychological inflexibility, especially experiential avoidance and cognitive defusion.
Goals of model	ACT seeks to increase psychological flexibility, which in turn enables the individual to lead a value-centered life rather than one focused on the avoidance of negative experiences.
Methods of action	A pragmatic analysis is made of member's current coping strategy (experiential avoidance) creating a space (creative hopelessness) to move toward a new stance (acceptance) that enables the member to achieve clarity about values and begin to work toward them.
Intervention techniques	Six components feed into psychological flexibility, and each component is served by a host of interventions. Common interventions are systematic questioning, exercises, metaphor use, and paradoxical interventions.
Adaptation of the model to a brief time frame	The therapist identifies one or more of the six core components of the model and provides members with some psychoeducation and experiential exposure to them.
Use of group process	• Members use universality to recognize that suffering is endemic to human experience. • In identifying one another's experiential avoidance strategies, they might better be able to recognize their own. • Through identification they can recognize values and goal that might not have been evident.

Note. ACT = acceptance and commitment therapy.

The session typically ends with homework assignments that flow from the new topic introduced. A summary of ACT-G appears in Table 6.3.

CLINICAL ILLUSTRATION OF AN ACCEPTANCE AND COMMITMENT THERAPY–GROUP APPROACH

A dual diagnosis substance abuse group met in a day hospital facility. The group consisted of nine members—six men and three women—and a male and female cotherapist. This closed-ended group was slated to meet for 10 sessions. In the current session, number eight, the therapists were helping members explore how they could act in a way consistent with their goals and values even while experiencing distressing thoughts and feelings.

Group Members

Aidan is a 30-year-old man who is HIV positive and living with his grandmother who has difficulties with mobility.

Olivia is a 22-year-old woman who abused alcohol and cocaine. She also struggled with anger management issues. She had recently been fired as a grade school teacher because of her absenteeism.

Lincoln is a 45-year-old man who has been in and out of rehabilitation for 20 years and is extremely depressed and hopeless. For expositional ease, the other six members will not be described.

At the beginning of the session, following a brief mindfulness exercise, the therapists focused on members' homework assignments that involved following through on their plans for action that are consistent with goals and values, despite encountering obstacles. Like all members, Aidan had completed the Values Assessment Rating Form (Hayes et al., 1999) in which he affirmed the value of having close relationships with his family members. He also completed the Goals, Actions, Barriers Form (Hayes et al., 1999) in which he established the goal of being present several hours a day to care for his grandmother's physical and social needs. His committed action was to anticipate his grandmother's needs before he left the house for other activities. He also chose the value of having strong, caring relationships within the LGBT community and committing himself to social justice ends. His intended action was to attend a fund-raising meeting.

> *Lincoln:* You look morose today.
>
> *Aidan:* I couldn't get any sleep. First, I couldn't get any sleep because I had to rush to the ER. A neighbor had to take my grandmother there because I was at an AIDS fundraiser. And then I was up in the night because I felt so guilty that I hadn't been present when she had difficulty breathing.
>
> *Olivia:* You can't be with her 24/7.
>
> *Aidan:* I know that, but it's torture to think of her home helpless. After I left here yesterday, I spent a couple of hours with her and got her all set up, or I thought I did. But then she had a spell.
>
> *Olivia:* I have to ask you this: Did you drink something when you had the insomnia? Or take some pills or something?
>
> *Aidan:* Oh, I thought of it. And I'm glad I didn't because I might have missed coming in today. But I did something else I shouldn't. I played this video game to distract me from feel-

ing upset about the whole thing, so I actually got to sleep later than I would have if I had just . . . (*trails off*).

Therapist: Just . . . what?

Aidan: What we talked about. If I had just tried not to fight what I was feeling. In fact, I ended up getting up so late that I couldn't look after my grandmother like I should have this morning.

Therapist: I think there a couple of important things going on here. What do members see?

Lincoln: The guilt was keeping him awake. He didn't drink, and that was good. But he still tried to avoid the guilt, and that made even more trouble for him.

Olivia: I do the same thing—when I feel guilty, I just want to find a way to get rid of it. It never works, not for long anyway.

Lincoln: Or with any feeling—like the way I wanted to drop out of the program altogether yesterday because I was angry at the director, but had I left, I would have been angry for a long, long time because I've been doing pretty well here.

[*Other members of the group identify what they are inclined to do when guilt and other disturbing feelings surface.*]

Therapist: It sounds as though members can all relate to the urge to get rid of the guilt. But can anyone think of a metaphor that can help us with that?

In an earlier group session, the *two scales metaphor* was introduced. It was presented to group members early in treatment as the therapists explored with them the alternatives of controlling their feelings or controlling their lives. The reader can find this metaphor and many others in the ACT treatment manual by Hayes et al. (1999). Essentially, it involves describing to the client two scales, one of which is salient and the other far less so. The salient scale corresponds to the client's painful experience—in this case, guilt. The other scale is the client's willingness to experience his or her inner life. The client is told that both scales go from 1 to 10, and when one scale, Guilt, is high but Willingness is at a 0, it is as if the handle is locked and unable to be moved to a lower position. The distinction is made that whereas the Guilt scale cannot be controlled, the Willingness scale can. When the Willingness scale is high, the guilt might be high or low but is capable of fluctuating. Because the group had been captivated by this metaphor when it was originally presented, the therapist engaged with them in exploring its application to a number of members and their distinctive patterns of internal experiences. Then, Aidan made an observation.

Aidan: I feel that I've been able to accept feelings that I have not been able to accept before. But that guilt gets to me. When I walked into the hospital, I knew what the staff were thinking, "Selfish! He's a selfish person. He should have been with her." They just gave me that look.

Therapist: Let's see how the group can be helpful to Aidan here.

[*The therapist's judgment was that this element of Aidan's experience was one that related to deliteralization strategies that were presented earlier in treatment, but ones that required reinforcement.*]

Lincoln: Well, I don't think Aidan can read their minds, but even if he could, the word *selfish* is just a word. It doesn't mean that that is who Aidan is. It's like that exercise we did with the people on the bus.

[*Lincoln is referencing the passengers on the bus metaphor, also described in Hayes et al. (1999).*]

Therapist: Can you or someone else remind us of that?

Aidan: Well, it's like these mean passengers are in the back of the bus. And you get them to stay in the back, but they tell you where you can go. Then, you stop and try to get rid of them. But they don't go because they're strong and you can't overpower them.

Therapist: That's right. What else?

Olivia: You do what they want. And they are in your face. And you get them to go to the back, but the deal is that for them to go to the back you have to do what they want. And you worry because they've gotten stronger and could do something awful to you. But they don't do anything awful—the worst is that you have to look at them in all of their ugliness.

Aidan: I don't remember that they are ugly.

Olivia: That's how I think about it.

Therapist: So, what's the tie-in?

Aidan: I think it's like the staff calling me selfish—I mean, they didn't say that—but I was sure they were thinking it. And that word *selfish* is scary for me because that's what my father said when I came out. He said I was hurting my mother and being selfish. So, I think of myself that way.

Olivia:	But it's not really you; it's just a thought that goes through your mind, just like the guilt is a feeling that goes through your mind. If you can say—look at me having this thought, having this feeling—well, I think you would just fall back asleep.
Therapist:	And even if Aidan didn't, he could have engaged in valued action.
Aidan:	I thought about it—I had some e-mails to get out for a committee I'm on.
Therapist:	Exactly! But there's something else, too. When we engage in value-driven action, we are always going to invite those people on the bus that we don't want but show up. As we've been saying, it's unavoidable. Aidan's experience provides us with an illustration. His going to the hospital was a values-driven action. But in doing so, he confronted the looks of the nurses, and those looks evoked negative reactions in him. We don't really know what they were thinking but what if they were thinking something negative about Aidan—people do have negative thoughts about one another, right? So, to pursue actions consistent with his goals and values, Aidan needs to be willing to take on some negative reactions. All of you were assigned to take committed action in relation to an important goal. Who would like to go next in sharing how it went?
Olivia:	I feel mine turned out sort of like Aidan's. When I called my sister to repair our relationship, she accused me of wanting money from her. I can't blame her. That's what I wanted in the past. I wish she had given me time to say what I wanted to say.
Lincoln:	Did you get really mad?
Olivia:	Strangely, no. Maybe it's because she didn't call me any horrible name. But maybe, too, it's because I knew when I made that call, it might make me upset. I had that image of the passengers on the bus the moment I called. I told myself to be willing to accept whatever I was going to feel. And I did feel awful. But I didn't explode. If I had exploded, I think I would have accepted that, too.
Aidan:	So, what now?
Olivia:	I thought I would write her a letter. Lay it all out. Give her time to mull it over.
Lincoln:	I'll bet that works better.

Therapist: Part of willingness is continuing on the path even when you hit an obstacle and knowing new obstacles will occur. And in any future action, success is not seen in the outcome—how Olivia's sister responds—but in the process of continuing on the chosen path. Lincoln, perhaps we'll find some of these same themes in your experiences with your homework. Are you ready to share?

Comment on the Session

This group is run in a manner that allows for a great deal of spontaneous interaction to occur among the group members. When a group process develops, the format becomes a medium having its own strengths beyond what individual therapy can provide. A benefit of a group approach is that members are less likely to learn new verbal rules for regulating behavior. Although the group is broadly supportive of Olivia's willingness to accept her reactions stimulated by her sister's reaction, the support—existing on a peer level—is less likely to translate into a verbal reward than it would be were this feedback to come exclusively from a figure of authority. Another benefit is that members have an opportunity to practice what Hayes et al. (1999) called "the observer perspective" (p. 270). While easily identifying with one another, members can look at each other's experiences with a measure of distance. That is, they can regard one another's experiences with the kind of perspective one has in looking at paintings at an art gallery (Hayes et al., 1999). Through this practice, they, at least in principle, are better able to adopt this perspective regarding their content.

The fact that members can do as much as they can on their own is connected to the longevity of the group. Members have had the opportunity to explore most of the central tenets of ACT. As can be seen, they now share a common frame of reference that they take the initiative in applying.

STATUS OF THE RESEARCH

Research Resources

Wachtel (2010) argued that a limitation of empirically supported treatments is that, too often, they are directed toward symptomatic change. Such change reflects in a limited way the kinds of changes people seek in going into psychotherapy. ACT distinguishes itself from many other behaviorally oriented approaches in seeking as primary changes aspects of human functioning other than symptom status. Evaluating ACT, therefore, requires that measures are used other than those reflecting symptoms. Fortunately, this approach provides both the researcher and clinician with a storehouse of resources for pursuing ACT. These resources consist of tools to measure process and mediation factors and tools to measure outcome. Specific outcome measures are necessary because ACT seeks to increase a person's potential for valued living, and the traditional self-report measures of symptoms are not adequate for this task. Some of the major measures used have been demonstrated to be sensitive to changes that occur over participation in ACT. An example of such a tool is the Acceptance and Action Questionnaire (Bond et al., 2011). This instrument, which asks the participant to rate 49 items on a 7-point Likert scale, measures psychological flexibility or the person's capacity to accept internal experiences and move toward goals despite those experiences. It is available in many languages. An example of a measure that can capture information about a mediating mechanism as well as outcome is the Cognitive Fusion Questionnaire (Gillanders et al., 2014). Although a desired outcome of ACT is to lessen cognitive fusion, such a diminishment is also expected to produce other positive changes, such as the capacity to pursue valued action. Psychometric study of this scale has suggested that it possesses good construct validity.

A comprehensive list of resources is available through the Association of Contextual Behavioral Science (https://contextualscience.org/). Because ACT is applied in many different contexts, a great array of tools has been developed for different populations, including instruments suitable for application with children and adolescents.

Outcome Findings

This treatment approach has spawned a great deal of research interest, in large part because the developers of this model were themselves interested in its rigorous evaluation. A sufficient mass of studies has been generated to enable the conduct of meta-analyses on different problem areas. To the best of our knowledge, meta-analyses are not available for group applications in inpatient, day hospital, and residential treatment centers. We, therefore, are reliant on individual investigations of the usefulness of ACT-G in these settings. ACT research is distinguished from that of many other approaches by the consistent focus on studying whether the mechanisms that are hypothesized to produce favorable change do indeed mediate the positive change that occurs.

Meta-Analytic Findings

Meta-analyses have found that ACT produces moderate size effects when it is compared with either treatment as usual (TAU) or wait list groups.

Powers, Zum Vörde Sive Vörding, and Emmelkamp (2009) found an effect size (ES) of .42 when ACT was compared with a control group. In this same investigation, a comparison of ACT with a wait-list group or a psychological placebo yielded an ES of .68 and with TAU, .42. Khoury et al. (2013), investigating studies comparing ACT with wait list groups, obtained an ES of .53; pre–post comparisons yielded an ES of .55. These ESs are in the small to moderate range.

Lower ESs result from comparisons between ACT and active treatment. Ruiz (2012) looked at 16 studies in which ACT was compared with cognitive behavior therapy (CBT). The resultant ES was .40, with ACT producing more favorable primary outcomes than CBT. Khoury et al. did not find ACT to produce results different from CBT, behavior therapies, or psychopharmacologic treatments. Similarly, Powers et al. (2009) and Öst (2014) found that ACT did not have an advantage over established treatments such as CBT.

Some meta-analyses on ACT studies have been performed in relation to particular diagnostic groups. For example, Öst (2014), using particularly rigorous study selection criteria, assessed 60 randomized controlled trials of study outcomes of patients with a wide range of disorders. Across studies, a small ES of .42 was obtained. On the basis of a series of meta-analyses for studies on specific conditions, Öst concluded that ACT is "probably efficacious for chronic pain and tinnitus, possibly efficacious for depression, psychotic symptoms, OCD, mixed anxiety, drug abuse, and stress at work, and experimental for the remaining disorders" (p. 1). Öst provided a number of methodological suggestions for future research on ACT.

One particularly relevant finding is a meta-analysis of group versus individual applications. Ruiz (2012) found that although the format of treatment did not show a differential effect, the ESs were higher for group delivery (ES = .50) as opposed to individual delivery (ES = .31). These patterns are consistent with the general finding from a recent meta-analytic study that when identical treatments are compared, no differences occur for individual versus group therapies in outcome, treatment acceptance, dropout, and remission rates (Burlingame et al., 2016).

According to the Society of Clinical Psychology of the American Psychological Association (2018), modest research support has been achieved for the use of ACT with depression, psychosis, mixed anxiety disorders, and obsessive–compulsive disorder. Strong research support exists for chronic pain disorder.

Overall, ACT produces outcomes that exceed those of placebo or wait list conditions. Its effects appear to be at least as favorable as other standard treatments. However, further work has to be done to establish the conditions under which it holds an advantage over other treatments. In doing such research, the investigator should seek to move beyond traditional measures of symptom relief to include the kinds of outcomes sought by ACT, such as the individual's quality of life and capacity to find meaning in it.

Group Treatment in Inpatient Hospital Programs, Partial Hospital Programs, and Residential Treatment Center Programs

ACT groups have been studied in outpatient settings with favorable outcomes (e.g., Bohlmeijer, Fledderus, Rokx, & Pieterse, 2011; Gratz & Gunderson, 2006; Lillis, Hayes, Bunting, & Masuda, 2009; Zettle, Rains, & Hayes, 2011). However, the number of studies that focus specifically on group treatment within inpatient hospital programs, partial hospital programs, and residential treatment center programs is quite small. McKay, Lev, and Skeen (2012) reported on a study done by Lev in which 44 male clients who were in a partial hospital recovery program for substance abuse were randomly assigned to TAU or TAU plus a 10-week ACT group designed to treat interpersonal problems. TAU consisted of 12-step study, relaxation, anger management, and other interventions common to a substance abuse program. Investigators measured interpersonal functioning before and after treatment using the Inventory of Interpersonal Problems (IIP-64; Horowitz, Alden, Wiggins, & Pincus, 2000). A t-test comparing pre and post IIP-64 score differences for ACT plus TAU versus TAU yielded an ES of 1.23, a large effect. The group that received the ACT protocol exhibited greater favorable change than the group receiving TAU only.

Juarascio et al. (2013) compared the outcomes of eating-disordered individuals in a residential treatment center program receiving TAU versus TAU plus ACT-G. The investigators pointed out that, ordinarily, the treatment of this population yields rather modest outcomes. They found that those receiving ACT in addition to TAU "trended toward less global eating pathology, shape concerns, and weight concerns post-treatment, as well as greater willingness to consume a distressing food" (p. 21). They also showed enhanced psychological flexibility, a major aim of ACT.

Support for the Mediational Mechanism

One respect in which ACT is exceptional is in the strength of commitment of ACT researchers to assess the extent to which the outcomes produced by ACT are due to mechanisms that are postulated to produce them. Overall, the research is consistent with the notion that the elements of ACT, such as lessening experiential avoidance, are responsible for producing favorable outcomes (Ruiz, 2012). For example, Gaudiano, Herbert, and Hayes (2010) found that inpatients receiving ACT showed a diminishment in hallucination distress. Importantly, they found that this shift was mediated by the believability of the hallucinations, a finding consistent with ACT theory. The mediating mechanism was the believability of the hallucinations on hallucination distress. In the previously cited study, Juarascio et al. (2013) found that willingness to experience negative contents while still engaging in valued behaviors mediated changes in eating attitudes and behavior.

DEMANDS OF THE MODEL

Clinical Mission

ACT-G need not require a theoretically homogeneous treatment community. Still, it is likely to be used to better advantage in the group situation if staff in the program have a grasp and acceptance of the principles of ACT. Otherwise, they could work at cross-purposes with the treatment. For example, staff might encourage patients to engage in experiential avoidance even though the modes of avoidance might differ from the more destructive ones patients embraced in the past. If the entire milieu embraces ACT, the opportunities for group members to practice application of ACT concepts increases greatly and the potential for members of the community to receive contradictory messages diminishes markedly.

Size of the Group

ACT groups seem to range from eight to 10 members (McKay, Lev, & Skeen, 2012). For symptomatically homogeneous groups, members might share some common experiential avoidance strategies, thereby lessening the time to address this step. Nonetheless, each member will have aspects of avoidance that are unique. Working on values, goals, and action steps is necessarily individualized. The group should not be so large that members are denied the opportunity to engage in an individual exploration of these topics with the group's help.

Composition of the Group

This model appears to be suitable for persons with a wide range of diagnoses and level of functioning. It has been found to be effective with depression and anxiety (Bohlmeijer et al., 2011; Forman, Herbert, Moitra, Yeomans, & Geller, 2007), psychotic symptoms such as delusions (Bach & Hayes, 2002; Gaudiano & Herbert, 2006; Martins, Castilho, Santos, &

Gumley, 2016), pain management, (Wetherell et al., 2011), symptoms of borderline personality disorder (Morton, Snowdon, Gopold, & Guymer, 2012), eating disorders (Juarascio et al., 2013), panic disorder (Gloster et al., 2017), functional somatic disorders (Kallesøe et al., 2016), neurological disorders (Hill et al., 2017), and impulsivity (Morrison, 2017).

In using ACT-G with different patient populations, the therapist must take care to make appropriate adaptations. For example, Jacobsen, Morris, Johns, and Hodkinson (2011) reported on their efforts to use mindfulness groups with a psychotic inpatient population. They reported that during the sessions, the therapist must invite the group members to engage in the exercises; assuming members' participation as one might with a higher functioning population is likely to increase the threat potential of the group in members' perceptions. Using this encouraging but not mandating approach, Jacobsen et al. were able to engage most of the members in the mindfulness activities. Likewise, Butler et al. (2016, p. 12) talked about the importance of tailoring the mindfulness exercises that often launch the session to prevent psychotic individuals from entering the states of deep concentration that can precipitate auditory hallucinations. These authors provided elaboration on the modifications that are necessary or desirable at each stage of the ACT-G for this patient population. They noted that the passengers on the bus metaphor is a particularly helpful tool with this population and demonstrate its use in a video (https://contextualconsulting.co.uk/insights/passengers-on-the-bus-metaphor-acting-out-in-a-group).

Temporal Variables

Optimally, groups are closed ended because steps build on one another. The empirical literature suggests, though, that few sessions are needed for members to achieve some benefits from treatment. For example, Bach and Hayes (2002), using only four individual ACT sessions with psychotic patients, reduced the rate of rehospitalization over a 4-month period by 50%. McCracken, Sato, and Taylor (2013) showed positive changes (lower depression and disability, higher pain acceptance) in ACT-G for chronic pain patients in only four sessions. Johns et al. (2016) obtained favorable findings (e.g., positive mood changes) in an outpatient psychotic patient population over four sessions. However, the design was preexperimental (pretest–posttest).

Therapist Variables

ACT can be applied successfully with fairly neophyte therapists. For example, Eisenbeck, Scheitz, and Szekeres (2016) investigated the administration of an ACT versus TAU group protocol by professionals who were well trained in prison interventions but relatively new to ACT. Participants were randomly assigned to the ACT-G or TAU-G. The TAU-G involved sessions on coping techniques, effects of drug use, and other psychoeducation topics relevant to this population. The investigators found that the ACT group exceeded the TAU group in fostering values-based behaviors, including at a 3-month follow-up. Participation in neither group effected a shift in symptoms or psychological flexibility. Psychological flexibility is a primary goal of ACT, whereas symptomatic change, often not expected by this model, sometimes occurs. The important point was that the therapists, relatively new to ACT, were able to apply it in a manner that led to a positive change that was consistent with the model.

ACT-G can and has been delivered by solo therapists or a cotherapy team. The latter has the usual advantage that different therapists can attend to different aspects of the group. For example, one therapist can work with the member who at a given moment, is the focus of the group; the other therapist can help other members identify with the spotlighted member's work.

SUMMARY

ACT, one of the newest models to emerge on the group psychotherapy landscape, is a contextual therapy and part of the third wave of behaviorism (Hayes, 2004), with Skinner's behaviorism and CBT being the first two waves. ACT fosters psychological flexibility through the cultivation of six core processes: acceptance, contact with the present moment, defusion, self in context (or transcendent sense of self), values, and committed action. ACT is rooted in a strong empirical tradition, and the amount of outcome research that has been generated on it in a relatively brief period is impressive. Still, the research is not sufficiently robust to allow us to know in what venues and with what patient populations it is most successful. However, findings on ACT groups taking place in larger therapeutic programs are promising. A feature that particularly recommends ACT-G for application in inpatient settings is its amenability to a brief time frame. It also appears to be suitable for the range of functioning that the therapist often encounters in inpatient, partial, and residential settings. To maximally realize the potential of this model, a major challenge for the group psychotherapist is to find ways to tap group process. This chapter, in addition to covering the basics of ACT-G, has endeavored to identify interventions by which the therapist can foster a group climate that is going to be most conducive to members deriving benefit from the group.

REFERENCES

Bach, P., & Hayes, S. C. (2002). The use of acceptance and commitment therapy to prevent the rehospitalization of psychotic patients: A randomized controlled trial. *Journal of Consulting and Clinical Psychology, 70,* 1129–1139. http://dx.doi.org/10.1037/0022-006X.70.5.1129

Biron, M., & van Veldhoven, M. (2012). Emotional labour in service work: Psychological flexibility and emotion regulation. *Human Relations, 65,* 1259–1282. http://dx.doi.org/10.1177/0018726712447832

Bohlmeijer, E. T., Fledderus, M., Rokx, T. A. J. J., & Pieterse, M. E. (2011). Efficacy of an early intervention based on acceptance and commitment therapy for adults with depressive symptomatology: Evaluation in a randomized controlled trial. *Behaviour Research and Therapy, 49,* 62–67. http://dx.doi.org/10.1016/j.brat.2010.10.003

Bond, F. W., & Flaxman, P. E. (2006). The ability of psychological flexibility and job control to predict learning, job performance, and mental health. *Journal of Organizational Behavior Management, 26,* 113–130. http://dx.doi.org/10.1300/J075v26n01_05

Bond, F. W., Hayes, S. C., Baer, R. A., Carpenter, K. M., Guenole, N., Orcutt, H. K., . . . Zettle, R. D. (2011). Preliminary psychometric properties of the Acceptance and Action Questionnaire-II: A revised measure of psychological inflexibility and experiential avoidance. *Behavior Therapy, 42,* 676–688. http://dx.doi.org/10.1016/j.beth.2011.03.007

Burlingame, G. M., McClendon, D. T., & Alonso, J. (2011). Cohesion in group therapy. *Psychotherapy, 48,* 34–42. http://dx.doi.org/10.1037/a0022063

Burlingame, G. M., Seebeck, J. D., Janis, R. A., Whitcomb, K. E., Barkowski, S., Rosendahl, J., & Strauss, B. (2016). Outcome differences between individual and group formats when identical and nonidentical treatments, patients, and doses are compared: A 25-year meta-analytic perspective. *Psychotherapy: Theory, Research, & Practice, 53,* 446–461. http://dx.doi.org/10.1037/pst0000090

Burlingame, G. M., Whitcomb, K., & Woodland, S. (2013). Process and outcome in group counseling and psychotherapy. In J. L. DeLucia-Waack, C. R. Kalodner, & M. Riva (Eds.), *Handbook of group counseling and psychotherapy* (pp. 55–67). Thousand Oaks, CA: Sage.

Butler, L., Johns, L. C., Byrne, M., Joseph, C., O'Donoghue, E., Jolley, S., . . . Oliver, J. E. (2016). Running acceptance and commitment therapy groups for psychosis in community settings. *Journal of Contextual Behavioral Science, 5,* 33–38. http://dx.doi.org/10.1016/j.jcbs.2015.12.001

Ciarrochi, J., & Bailey, A. (2008). *A CBT-practitioner's guide to ACT: How to bridge the gap between cognitive behavioral therapy and acceptance and commitment therapy.* Oakland, CA: New Harbinger.

Duffy, T. K. (2006). White gloves and cracked vases: How metaphors help group workers construct new perspectives and responses. *Social Work With Groups, 28,* 247–257. http://dx.doi.org/10.1300/J009v28n03_16

Eilenberg, T., Kronstand, L., Fink, P., & Frostholm, L. (2014). Acceptance and commitment group therapy for health anxiety—Results from a pilot study. *Journal of Anxiety Disorders, 27,* 461–468.

Eisenbeck, N., Scheitz, K., & Szekeres, B. (2016). A brief acceptance and commitment therapy-based intervention among violence-prone male inmates delivered by novice therapists. *Psychology, Society, and Education, 8,* 187–199. http://dx.doi.org/10.25115/psye.v8i3.173

Feldner, M. T., Hekmat, H., Zvolensky, M. J., Vowles, K. E., Secrist, Z., & Leen-Feldner, E. W. (2006). The role of experiential avoidance in acute pain tolerance: A laboratory test. *Journal of Behavior Therapy and Experimental Psychiatry, 37,* 146–158. http://dx.doi.org/10.1016/j.jbtep.2005.03.002

Foret, M., & Eaton, P. (2014). *ACT for anger group.* Retrieved from https://contextualscience.org/act_for_anger_group

Forman, E. M., Herbert, J. D., Moitra, E., Yeomans, P. D., & Geller, P. A. (2007). A randomized controlled effectiveness trial of acceptance and commitment therapy and cognitive therapy for anxiety and depression. *Behavior Modification, 31,* 772–799. http://dx.doi.org/10.1177/0145445507302202

Gans, J. S. (1991). The leader's use of metaphor in group psychotherapy. *International Journal of Group Psychotherapy, 41,* 127–143. http://dx.doi.org/10.1080/00207284.1991.11490640

Gaudiano, B. A., & Herbert, J. D. (2006). Acute treatment of inpatients with psychotic symptoms using Acceptance and Commitment Therapy: Pilot results. *Behaviour Research and Therapy, 44,* 415–437. http://dx.doi.org/10.1016/j.brat.2005.02.007

Gaudiano, B. A., Herbert, J. D., & Hayes, S. C. (2010). Is it the symptom or the relation to it? Investigating potential mediators of change in acceptance and commitment therapy for psychosis. *Behavior Therapy, 41,* 543–554. http://dx.doi.org/10.1016/j.beth.2010.03.001

Gillanders, D. T., Bolderston, H., Bond, F. W., Dempster, M., Flaxman, P. E., Campbell, L., . . . Remington, B. (2014). The development and initial validation of the cognitive fusion questionnaire. *Behavior Therapy, 45,* 83–101. http://dx.doi.org/10.1016/j.beth.2013.09.001

Gloster, A. T., Klotsche, J., Ciarrochi, J., Eifert, G., Sonntag, R., Wittchen, H. U., & Hoyer, J. (2017). Increasing valued behaviors precedes reduction in suffering: Findings from a randomized controlled trial using ACT. *Behaviour Research and Therapy, 91,* 64–71. http://dx.doi.org/10.1016/j.brat.2017.01.013

Gratz, K. L., & Gunderson, J. G. (2006). Preliminary data on an acceptance-based emotion regulation group intervention for deliberate self-harm among women with borderline personality disorder. *Behavior Therapy, 37,* 25–35. http://dx.doi.org/10.1016/j.beth.2005.03.002

Harris, R. (2009). *ACT made simple: An easy to read primer on acceptance and commitment therapy.* Oakland, CA: New Harbinger.

Hayes, S. C. (2002a). Acceptance, mindfulness, and science. *Clinical Psychology: Science and Practice, 9*, 101–106. http://dx.doi.org/10.1093/clipsy.9.1.101

Hayes, S. C. (2002b). Buddhism and acceptance and commitment therapy. *Cognitive and Behavioral Practice, 9*, 58–66. http://dx.doi.org/10.1016/S1077-7229(02)80041-4

Hayes, S. C. (2004). Acceptance and commitment therapy, relational frame theory, and the third wave of behavioral and cognitive therapies. *Behavior Therapy, 35*, 639–665. Medline http://dx.doi.org/10.1016/S0005-7894(04)80013-3

Hayes, S. C. (2017). *Introduction to the hexaflex.* Retrieved from https://contextualscience.org/introduction_to_the_hexaflex

Hayes, S. C. (n.d.). *The six core processes of ACT.* Retrieved from http://www.contextualscience.org/print/book/export/html/842

Hayes, S. C., Hayes, L. J., & Reese, H. W. (1988). Finding the philosophical core: A review of Stephen C. Pepper's *World Hypotheses: A Study in Evidence. Journal of the Experimental Analysis of Behavior, 50*, 97–111. http://dx.doi.org/10.1901/jeab.1988.50-97

Hayes, S. C., Strosahl, K. D., & Wilson, K. G. (1999). *Acceptance and commitment therapy: An experiential approach to behavior change.* New York, NY: Guilford Press.

Hayes, S. C., & Wilson, K. G. (1994). Acceptance and commitment therapy: Altering the verbal support for experiential avoidance. *The Behavior Analyst, 17*, 289–303. http://dx.doi.org/10.1007/BF03392677

Healy, O., Barnes-Holmes, D., & Smeets, P. M. (2000). Derived relational responding as generalized operant behavior. *Journal of the Experimental Analysis of Behavior, 74*, 207–227. http://dx.doi.org/10.1901/jeab.2000.74-207

Hill, G., Hynd, N., Wheeler, M., Tarran-Jones, A., Carrabine, H., & Evans, S. (2017). Living well with neurological conditions: Evaluation of an ACT-informed group intervention for psychological adjustment in outpatients with neurological problems. *The Neuropsychologist, 3*, 58–63.

Horowitz, L. M., Alden, L. E., Wiggins, J. S., & Pincus, A. L. (2000). *Inventory of Interpersonal Problems (IIP-32/IIP-64).* London, England: Psychological Corporation.

Jacobsen, P., Morris, E., Johns, L., & Hodkinson, K. (2011). Mindfulness groups for psychosis: Key issues for implementation on an inpatient unit. *Behavioural and Cognitive Psychotherapy, 39*, 349–353. http://dx.doi.org/10.1017/S1352465810000639

Johns, L. C., Oliver, J. E., Khondoker, M., Byrne, M., Jolley, S., Wykes, T., . . . Morris, E. M. (2016). The feasibility and acceptability of a brief Acceptance and Commitment Therapy (ACT) group intervention for people with psychosis: The 'ACT for life' study. *Journal of Behavior Therapy and Experimental Psychiatry, 50*, 257–263. http://dx.doi.org/10.1016/j.jbtep.2015.10.001

Juarascio, A., Shaw, J., Forman, E., Timko, C. A., Herbert, J., Butryn, M., . . . Lowe, M. (2013). Acceptance and commitment therapy as a novel treatment for eating disorders: An initial test of efficacy and mediation. *Behavior Modification, 37,* 459–489. http://dx.doi.org/10.1177/0145445513478633

Kallesøe, K. H., Schröder, A., Wicksell, R. K., Fink, P., Ørnbøl, E., & Rask, C. U. (2016). Comparing group-based acceptance and commitment therapy (ACT) with enhanced usual care for adolescents with functional somatic syndromes: A study protocol for a randomised trial. *BMJ Open, 6,* e012743. http://dx.doi.org/10.1136/bmjopen-2016-012743

Khoury, B., Lecomte, T., Fortin, G., Masse, M., Therien, P., Bouchard, V., . . . Hofmann, S. G. (2013). Mindfulness-based therapy: A comprehensive meta-analysis. *Clinical Psychology Review, 33,* 763–771. http://dx.doi.org/10.1016/j.cpr.2013.05.005

Leonidou, C., Panayiotou, G., Bati, A., & Karekla, M. (2016). Coping with psychosomatic symptoms: The buffering role of psychological flexibility and impact on quality of life. *Journal of Health Psychology.* Advance online publication. http://dx.doi.org/10.1177/1359105316666657

Levin, M. E., Herbert, J. D., & Forman, E. M. (2017). Acceptance and commitment therapy: A critical review to guide clinical decision making. In D. McKay, J. Abramowitz, & E. A. Storch (Eds.), *Treatments for psychological problems and syndromes* (pp. 413–432). New York, NY: Wiley. http://dx.doi.org/10.1002/9781118877142.ch27

Lillis, J., Hayes, S. C., Bunting, K., & Masuda, A. (2009). Teaching acceptance and mindfulness to improve the lives of the obese: A preliminary test of a theoretical model. *Annals of Behavioral Medicine, 37,* 58–69. http://dx.doi.org/10.1007/s12160-009-9083-x

Martins, M. J., Castilho, P., Santos, V., & Gumley, A. (2016). Schizophrenia: An exploration of an acceptance, mindfulness, and compassion-based group intervention. *Australian Psychologist, 51,* 1–10. http://dx.doi.org/10.1111/ap.12210

Masterpasqua, F. (2016). Mindfulness mentalizing humanism: A transtheoretical convergence. *Journal of Psychotherapy Integration, 26,* 5–10. http://dx.doi.org/10.1037/a0039635

McCracken, L. M., Sato, A., & Taylor, G. J. (2013). A trial of a brief group-based form of acceptance and commitment therapy (ACT) for chronic pain in general practice: Pilot outcome and process results. *The Journal of Pain, 14,* 1398–1406. http://dx.doi.org/10.1016/j.jpain.2013.06.011

McKay, M., Lev, A., & Skeen, M. (Eds.). (2012). *Acceptance and commitment therapy for interpersonal problems: Using mindfulness, acceptance, and schema awareness to change interpersonal behaviors.* Oakland, CA: New Harbinger.

McKay, M., Lev, A., Skeen, M., & Saavedra, K. (2012). Group protocol (Appendix C). In M. McKay, A. Lev, & M. Skeen (Eds.), *Acceptance and commitment therapy for interpersonal problems: Using mindfulness, acceptance, and schema awareness to change interpersonal behaviors* (pp. 131–189). Oakland, CA: New Harbinger.

Monestès, J.-L., & Villatte, M. (2011). Metaphors in ACT: Understanding how they work: Using them—Creating your own. *ACT Digest: Echoes from Acceptance and Commitment Therapy*. Paris, France: Elsevier-Masson. Retrieved from https://contextualscience.org/files/ACT_Digest_Special_Issue_n%C3%82%C2%B02.pdf

Moreno, J. L. (1946). Psychodrama and group psychotherapy. *Sociometry, 9*, 249–253. http://dx.doi.org/10.2307/2785011

Morrison, K. L. (2017). *Effects of acceptance and commitment therapy on impulsive decision making.* Salt Lake City: Utah State University.

Morton, J., Snowdon, S., Gopold, M., & Guymer, E. (2012). Acceptance and commitment therapy group treatment for symptoms of borderline personality disorder: A public sector pilot study. *Cognitive and Behavioral Practice, 19*, 527–544. http://dx.doi.org/10.1016/j.cbpra.2012.03.005

Ossman, W. A., Wilson, K. G., Storaasli, R. D., & McNeill, J. R. (2006). A preliminary investigation of the use of acceptance and commitment therapy in group treatment for social phobia. *International Journal of Psychology & Psychological Therapy, 6*, 397–416.

Öst, L. G. (2014). The efficacy of Acceptance and Commitment Therapy: An updated systematic review and meta-analysis. *Behaviour Research and Therapy, 61*, 105–121. http://dx.doi.org/10.1016/j.brat.2014.07.018

Powers, M. B., Zum Vörde Sive Vörding, M. B., & Emmelkamp, P. M. (2009). Acceptance and commitment therapy: A meta-analytic review. *Psychotherapy and Psychosomatics, 78*, 73–80. http://dx.doi.org/10.1159/000190790

Ruiz, F. J. (2012). Acceptance and commitment therapy versus traditional cognitive behavioral therapy: A systematic review and meta-analysis of current empirical evidence. *International Journal of Psychology & Psychological Therapy, 12*, 333–357.

Society of Clinical Psychology of the American Psychological Association. (2018). *Psychological treatments.* Retrieved from https://www.div12.org/treatments/

Törneke, N., Luciano, C., & Salas, S. V. (2008). Rule-governed behavior and psychological problems. *International Journal of Psychology & Psychological Therapy, 8*, 141–156.

Wachtel, P. (2010). Beyond "ESTs": Problematic assumptions in the pursuit of evidence-based practice. *Psychoanalytic Psychology, 27*, 251–272. http://dx.doi.org/10.1037/a0020532

Walser, R. D., & Hayes, S. C. (2006). Acceptance and commitment therapy in the treatment of posttraumatic stress disorder. *Cognitive-Behavioral Therapies for Trauma, 2*, 146–172.

Westrup, D., & Wright, M. J. (2017). *Learning ACT for group treatment: An acceptance and commitment therapy skills training manual for therapists.* Oakland, CA: New Harbinger.

Wetherell, J. L., Afari, N., Rutledge, T., Sorrell, J. T., Stoddard, J. A., Petkus, A. J., . . . Atkinson, J. H. (2011). A randomized, controlled trial of acceptance and commitment therapy and cognitive-behavioral therapy for chronic pain. *Pain, 152,* 2098–2107. http://dx.doi.org/10.1016/j.pain.2011.05.016

Wright, N. P., Turkington, D., Kelly, O. P., Davies, D., Jacobs, A. M., & Hopton, J. (2014). *Treating psychosis: A clinician's guide to integrating acceptance & commitment therapy, compassion-focused therapy & mindfulness approaches within the cognitive behavioral therapy tradition.* Oakland, CA: New Harbinger.

Yalom, I. D., & Leszcz, M. (2005). *Theory and practice of group psychotherapy.* New York, NY: Basic Books.

Zettle, R. D., Rains, J. C., & Hayes, S. C. (2011). Processes of change in acceptance and commitment therapy and cognitive therapy for depression: A mediation reanalysis of Zettle and Rains. *Behavior Modification, 35,* 265–283. http://dx.doi.org/10.1177/0145445511398344

7

THE PROBLEM-SOLVING MODEL

The capacity to resolve effectively the plethora of situational problems that abound in every individual's life is highly associated with healthy functioning. Everyday problems can be classified as impersonal (e.g., mathematical), intrapsychic (e.g., anxiety), or interpersonal (e.g., conflict with friends). The skills required to solve each kind of problem are essential to one's ability to manage life. Yet, the individual processes needed in resolving each kind of problem appear to be somewhat different (Meichenbaum & Goodman, 1971; Spivack, Platt, & Shure, 1976). The contrast is most apparent between the impersonal problem, which is predominantly an intellectual activity, and the interpersonal, in which the interaction between self and others has emotional components (e.g., getting divorced or changing jobs). The assessment, potential consequences, and solution often involve an appreciation of mutuality that includes empathy with the other's perspective and comprehension of and skill in interpersonal

http://dx.doi.org/10.1037/0000113-008
Group Psychotherapy in Inpatient, Partial Hospital, and Residential Care Settings, by V. Brabender and A. Fallon

exchange. Often, the kinds of problems affecting individuals overlap, for example, when intrapsychic problems such as impulsivity or anxiety may affect interpersonal conflict.

Psychiatric patients—whether they are children, adolescents, or adults—exhibit deficits in interpersonal problem-solving abilities when compared with their healthier compeers. Almost all the models of group psychotherapy presented in this book attempt to aid patients in buttressing their interpersonal problem-solving capacities, albeit sometimes indirectly. Models range in promoting problem solving—at one extreme exposing, redefining, or resolving unconscious conflict surrounding a problem, and, at the other, improving ability to perceive and implement the basic social skills of interpersonal exchange. Interpersonal problem solving is also a major feature of all the cognitive and cognitive behavior therapies (E. Coché, 1987). The problem-solving model presented in this chapter focuses on (a) identifying one's approach style to a problem, and (b) teaching effective, rational problem-solving steps in a direct, straightforward manner. This framework emphasizes the significance of cognitive and affective processes that mediate the individual's ability to perceive and think through the alternatives and consequences of an interpersonal problem before taking action as a way to improve psychological functioning.

THEORETICAL UNDERPINNINGS

The ability to think rationally, flexibly, and creatively and then to implement an effective problem-solving strategy is an important part of environmental adaptation. Success in this domain ensures survival, contributes to feelings of competence, and promotes psychological health. The seminal research of Spivack (1984) and his colleagues supports the link between interpersonal problem-solving abilities and emotional health.[1] Some of the skills required to negotiate interpersonal exchanges and to solve problems that arise from these exchanges are acquired by 4 years of age (Raeff & Benson, 2003; Shure & Spivack, 1982; Shure, Spivack, & Jaeger, 1971) and continue to be important for successful functioning throughout the life span.

---

[1]Additional evidence such as the positive relation of interpersonal problem solving to the number of close friendships and degree of family support (Hansen, St. Lawrence, & Christoff, 1985) buttress the link between interpersonal problem-solving ability and emotional health. Interpersonal problem solving appears to be positively correlated with social competence (Platt & Spivack, 1972b). Social skill competence, a related area, is positively correlated with intrapsychic foundations (e.g., Bellack, Morrison, Wixted, & Mueser, 1990). The development of each of these skills has been articulated elsewhere in considerable detail (Spivack et al., 1976).

The Relation of Problem-Solving Capabilities to Psychiatric Illness

The importance of interpersonal problem solving in adaptive functioning has been elaborated in the relational/problem-solving model of stress (D'Zurilla & Nezu, 2007; Nezu, Nezu, & D'Zurilla, 2012). This model articulates the relationship between stressful events, problem solving, and mental health/psychopathology. The foundation of the model suggests that certain genetic types and early life stress create or exacerbate biological vulnerabilities that affect an individual's reaction to stress later in life (i.e., increased stress sensitivity).[2] Children learn to cope with life's challenges and develop problem-solving strategies from family and important others. The quality of the child's coping (i.e., mastering an active and systematic approach to problems rather than an avoidant one) serves to moderate the negative effects of stress in an ongoing manner. Poor problem-solving skills increase the likelihood of additional tribulations (e.g., chronic lack of resources) and increase the probability of the occurrence of more serious life events (e.g., trauma), which in turn, intensifies stress, psychologically and physiologically. Coupled with early neurobiological vulnerabilities, increased stress predisposes the individual to develop psychological symptoms. In this model, problem-solving skills can increase coping capacities and thus function as a buffer to the effects of stress (Bell & D'Zurilla, 2009a).

Empirical support is solid for a relationship between inadequate interpersonal problem solving and psychopathology for children (e.g., Rubin & Rose-Krasnor, 1992; Shure, 1997; Shure & Spivack, 1972, 1982), adolescents (Davila, Hammen, Burge, Paley, & Daley, 1995; Im-Bolter, Cohen, & Farnia, 2013; Levenson & Neuringer, 1971; Platt, Spivack, Altman, Altman, & Peizer, 1974) and adults (Dammann et al., 2016; Platt & Spivack, 1972a, 1972b, 1974; Thoma, Friedmann, & Suchan, 2013) regardless of social class or intellectual functioning. Similarly, individuals with symptoms of psychosis, depression, anxiety, suicidal ideation and behaviors, and substance abuse have significant problem-solving deficiencies. (See Chang, D'Zurilla, & Sanna, 2004, and Nezu, Wilkins, & Nezu, 2004, for a review of this work.)

Problem-solving models assume that the capacity to think about interpersonal exchange may make a significant contribution to an individual's actual psychological and social adjustment (Spivack, 1984). The nexus of the problem-solving model is that by direct intervention, the group experience can alter thinking, which leads to a change in problem-solving capabilities (Platt & Spivack, 1975). Early studies found that individual formal

---

[2]For example, individuals with "short" variants of the serotonin transporter gene *5-HTT* have been found to have fewer problem-solving strategies (Wilhelm et al., 2007).

instruction and extensive training specifically in problem formulation and the production of alternative solutions enhance people's abilities to subsequently generate effective alternative solutions to real-life problems (Nezu, 1980, 1986). Direct training in the decision-making processes also improved individuals' capacities to make better decisions (Nezu, 1980). Thus, specific and formal training in skills that allow the individual to solve everyday problems more effectively facilitates interpersonal effectiveness.

Together, the aforementioned lines of research compellingly establish the relevance of problem-solving training to the treatment of psychological disorders. The relation of such training to treating such disorders is based specifically on the following assumptions: (a) individuals with psychiatric disorders have deficiencies in problem-solving skills; (b) the capability to think about problem solving may contribute to a person's actual adjustment; and (c) training in this skill can specifically and directly enhance a person's ability to solve current and future problems, improve daily functioning, increase self-esteem, and ameliorate some psychological symptoms (Goldfried & Davison, 1976; Platt & Spivack, 1975; Spivack, 1984).[3]

The Locus of Deficient Problem-Solving Skills in the Psychiatric Population

The particular focus of treatment and the design of adequate problem-solving training require attention to the specific nature of the patients' deficiencies. Psychiatric patients do not differ from healthy individuals on all the skills required for adequate problem solving. For example, on tasks measuring problem recognition and causal thinking, adolescent psychiatric patients did not differ significantly from their healthy counterparts (Platt, Spivack, Altman, et al., 1974). Severity of illness, age at first break, diagnosis, and symptomatology may influence the development of problem-solving skills (Nezu et al., 2012).

The major differences between psychiatric patients and their emotionally healthy counterparts seem to be primarily in the areas of attitude toward problem solving and the generation, evaluation, and implementation of possible solutions. These differences are both qualitative and quantitative. When compared with healthy individuals, psychiatric patients generated fewer total solutions and a diminished proportion of effective solutions

---

[3]Although the empirical support for the thesis that interpersonal problem solving plays an important role in healthy functioning is substantial (and that good problem-solving skills are positively correlated with emotional well-being), no causal effect has been established. Whether improvement of problem-solving skills impacts the neurobiological sensitivity is also an unanswered question (Nezu, Nezu, & D'Zurilla, 2012).

(Nezu, 1986; Platt, Scura, & Hannon, 1973; Platt & Spivack, 1972a, 1972b; Shure & Spivack, 1972).

With respect to evaluation, psychiatric patients were as competent to place these solutions in a hierarchy of effectiveness as were healthy individuals (Platt, Siegel, & Spivack, 1975; Richard & Dodge, 1982).[4] However, the psychiatric patients were not able to generate alternative consequences of a given act or solution (e.g., being able to generate "If I express my anger about what she did, she might see I mean business" or "She might not listen to me because I made her feel bad" or "She might cut off our friendship"). This type of thinking is a significant component of social adjustment from a very early age (Shure & Spivack, 1982) and differentiates impulsive children from nonimpulsive children (Spivack & Shure, 1974). Healthy individuals were more likely to include the element of introspection in the decision-making process before resolving the problem with an action. In contrast, psychiatric patients tended to give more responses that reflected taking immediate, impulsive, concrete, and physically aggressive action and were less likely to spontaneously generate consequences of hypothetical transgressions or good deeds (Platt & Spivack, 1974; Spivack & Levine, 1963; Shure & Spivack, 1972).

The subsequent process of implementation consists of articulating the sequence of the means of solving a problem. This process involves recognizing obstacles and appreciating that goal achievement may take time. It becomes significant in social adjustment sometime during grade school and remains important for adequate social adjustment throughout the life span (Shure & Spivack, 1972). In several studies, psychiatric patients were not able to create and elaborate this sequence and rationale to the same extent as were their healthy counterparts (Gotlib & Asarnow, 1979; Platt et al., 1975; Shure & Spivack, 1982). Psychiatric patients were not as skilled in perceiving the multiple tiny steps that are required to carry out a solution to a problem. Marsha Linehan recognized this and formally incorporated skill development of this "chaining process" into her dialectical behavioral training (see Chapter 5, this volume).

Depression and suicidality have been studied with regard to problem-solving abilities. Individuals with significant depression seek less information, make use of fewer available resources, have difficulty in resolving ambiguous circumstances, and make poorer overall decisions (Leykin, Roberts, & DeRubeis, 2011). In contrast, suicidal patients solve problems actively and impulsively, but they are inflexible in shifting response sets, are rigid in their conceptualizations of the problem, generate a limited number of viable

---

[4]This was not true of adolescent psychiatric patients. They have more difficulty evaluating the effectiveness of alternative solutions than do their healthy counterparts (Platt et al., 1974).

alternative solutions, and narrowly and impulsively focus on the goals rather than evaluate ways to achieve them (Cohen-Sandler, 1982; Grover, Green, Pettit, Monteith, Garza, & Venta, 2009; Levenson & Neuringer, 1971; Linehan & Wagner, 1990).

These deficiencies in both adolescents and adults cannot be accounted for by lack of general intelligence (Siegel, Platt, & Peizer, 1976) or originality of thinking (Gotlib & Asarnow, 1979) and are independent of social background or social class (Platt & Spivack, 1974). Regardless of level of education, social background, or sophistication, healthy individuals from widely differing cultural backgrounds agree on what constitutes a hierarchy of effective and socially appropriate ways of solving problems (e.g., Bellack, Sayers, Mueser, & Bennett, 1994; Leff et al., 2006, 2009; McGuire, 2005). These studies clearly suggest that successful therapeutic intervention with psychiatric patients must focus on the development and practice of problem-solving skills related to the generation (both amount and kind) of potential solutions (Platt & Spivack, 1975).

Mechanisms of Change

Skill at interpersonal problem solving affects social adjustment. Yet, even within the problem-solving model authors differ on what are the crucially operative mechanisms. Some view interpersonal problem solving as fundamentally involving social judgments and cognitive processes (i.e., social cognition) and thus view problem-solving training as cognitive or cognitive behavior therapy (Wessler & Hankin-Wessler, 1989). Other contributors, viewing problem solving within a psychodynamic framework, believe the critical mechanism of change to be in the regulation of self-esteem (e.g., Spivack et al., 1976). Good problem solving makes people more interpersonally effective and thereby less prone to social failures. This greater effectiveness enhances self-esteem, which in turn immunizes an individual from the development or exacerbation of symptoms. Still others view problem-solving training as primarily a behavioral process (overt or covert) in that, although the development of the skills is important, solving problems through the behavioral implementation of a decision is emphasized (Goldfried & Davison, 1976).

The most recent theoretical perspective on problem solving views it as a metacognitive process that fuels motivation to solve problems and fosters the development of a set of cognitive and behavioral skills. Together, these skills and processes buffer the stresses of everyday challenges and major negative life events and reduce the negative emotions generated (D'Zurilla & Nezu, 2010). By teaching individuals to cope better with stressful situations, problem-solving training can attenuate neurobiological vulnerabilities, increase resilience, and prevent health and mental health difficulties. In this model, problem solving mediates the relationship between stressful minor circumstances and major circumstances. In addition, poor problem-solving skills impacts the frequency of problematic interpersonal situations.

GOALS OF TREATMENT

Problem-solving training can be conceptualized as helping the individual develop a learning set that increases the probability that he or she will cope more effectively with a wide range of situations (Goldfried & Davison, 1976). The major goals are threefold: (a) to help the individual develop an optimistic attitude toward the possibility that problems have solutions, (b) to acquire a specific method of problem solving, and (c) to reduce tendencies to avoid or act impulsively and prematurely toward solution attainment.

The first goal is to help patients view the myriad of problems they face as solvable challenges that involve time and further thought. When the setting allows for a longer term approach, patients can be assessed individually (either formally or informally), and their specific maladaptive approaches to problems can be identified. In shorter term settings, the importance of problem orientation (e.g., optimism) and the labeling of specific dysfunctional ones can be labeled in the group setting. Those who continue to view themselves as unable to cope with problems successfully and consider problems to be unsolvable have more negative outcomes (Bell & D'Zurilla, 2009a; Malouff, Thorsteinsson, & Schutte, 2007).

The second goal focuses on acquiring a specific method of problem solving—learning to formulate problems, to generate solutions, and to identify the most viable alternatives. Problem-solving training increases the availability of alternative solutions and improves the patient's likelihood of selecting the most effective response from among these alternatives (D'Zurilla & Goldfried, 1971). The goal of training is not to focus on specific solutions to individual situations but instead to teach a general coping strategy so that patients are in a better position to manage more effectively a wide variety of social circumstances (Kanfer & Busemeyer, 1982). Immediate reduction of symptoms is not a major goal of this model. However, the acquisition of problem-solving skills is expected to enrich the range of coping responses available to an individual and will lead to fewer failures in adaption to problematic situations. Although sometimes no appropriate solution or course of action is immediately apparent, the extent to which the patient expects that he or she will be able to manage difficulties increases the likelihood of eventual success in obtaining an acceptable resolution. Increased confidence in problem-solving ability is associated with improved problem-solving and decision-making skills (Kanfer & Busemeyer, 1982). Success with problem solving can reduce helplessness and hopelessness as an orientation toward the problem-solving process and can engender optimism. On a longer term basis, a decreased perceived vulnerability to failure renders individuals more resistant to the acquisition or exacerbation of symptoms.

Problem-solving therapy can be delivered in an individual or group setting, but it has been shown to have greater benefit when patients participate in the group (Cuijpers, van Straten, & Warmerdam, 2007). Although the focus in this training is on the individual rather than either the group or developing relationships among group members, the group setting uniquely offers a supportive ambience that allows members to observe and comment on social interactions within the group (Wessler & Hankin-Wessler, 1989). The group setting provides an opportunity for group members to observe firsthand the interactions that particular members report to be problematic and vicariously learn about their own problems by observing other members' attempts to apply the model. Group members offer a greater array of solutions than a therapy dyad might be able to generate and can provide other perspectives when solutions are evaluated. Members will also add enthusiasm in the role-play implementation process. Hope and an optimistic attitude can be fostered when group members see that they are not alone in their struggles. In an open-ended group, as members become more senior and more proficient in problem-solving strategies, they display a more nuanced and sophisticated examination of the problems from which newer members can observe and learn.

TECHNICAL CONSIDERATIONS

The problem-solving model has been extremely well articulated. Several available manuals and procedural articles are available for the interested clinician (E. Coché, 1987; Goldfried & Davison, 1976; Nezu et al., 2012; Platt & Spivack, 1975; Tannenbaum, 1991). These specify in detail each of the steps involved in the acquisition of problem-solving skills, a step-by-step therapeutic procedure for acquiring them (often including the specific scenarios), and the tasks and techniques required of the leader.

Group Composition and Patient Selection

The most important variable in composition is the homogeneity of cognitive development. The model functions less effectively when members are at radically different levels of cognitive functioning (e.g., J. Coché & Coché, 1986). Child, adolescent, adult, and geriatric patients have been able to improve their problem-solving skills with this training when groups are homogenous with respect to these broad age groups (Arean et al., 1993; Hussian, 1987). Groups range in size from four to 12 voluntary participants. Younger, more acute, and physically and verbally active patients function better with few patients in the group.

A wide variety of psychological disorders appear to benefit from the training, including patients with unipolar and bipolar depression (Grey, 2007; Nezu & Perri, 1989), eating disorders (Bannan, 2010); suicidal symptoms (Bannan, 2010; Joiner, Voelz, & Rudd, 2001), borderline personality disorder (Dammann et al., 2016), antisocial tendencies (Biggam & Power, 2002), and alcohol and drug abuse (Carey, Carey, & Meisler, 1990). Patients recovering from acute psychotic episodes, as well as chronic schizophrenics, also appear to profit from participation (Barbieri, Boggian, Falloon, Lamonaca, & the Centro Diurno 5, 2006; Liberman, Eckman, & Marder, 2001; Radcliffe & Bird, 2016; Tarrier, Beckett, Harwood, Baker, Yusupoff, & Ugarteburu, 1993).

Although both diagnostically heterogeneous and homogeneous groups improve with problem-solving training, many clinicians prefer some heterogeneity because patients offer a greater array of problems. This variability both gives members more practice in applying the problem-solving steps and cultivates their awareness that what is important are the skills they develop, not the specific solutions that they acquire.

The inclusion requirements are (a) a reasonable degree of intellectual capability and verbal facility, although efficacy has been demonstrated with intellectually deficient adults (Loumidis & Hill, 1997; Nezu, Nezu, & Arean, 1991); (b) an ability to effect some change on the environment; (c) and the ability to inhibit immediate responding (Hussian, 1987). Patients with serious memory disturbances (e.g., those receiving electroconvulsive treatment or having serious brain pathology) are excluded (E. Coché, 1987). The moderate degree of memory loss that is commonly found in geriatric populations in psychiatric and assisted living facilities does not preclude effective training as long as modifications are made (Arean et al., 1993). For example, use of a large visible blackboard might be essential for geriatric groups to aid members' compromised memories. Patients whose disruptive or otherwise antisocial behaviors undermine the group's progress are also excluded (e.g., some antisocial personality disorders and manic patients).

This model provides an excellent first group experience. Participation in problem-solving groups with a creative and engaging leader can be an enjoyable experience. Patients can usually be convinced that the group is worthwhile, because the need for problem-solving skills and patients' deficits can be easily demonstrated. Members get tremendous satisfaction from being presented with a task that they can actually accomplish within the session. The highly structured experience allows a relatively anxiety-free adaptation to a group format, which, in turn, catalyzes interest in outpatient group treatment (E. Coché, 1987).

Time Frame for Efficacy

Generally, more sessions yield better outcomes (Malouff et al., 2007). When our book *Models of Inpatient Group Psychotherapy* (1993) was published, 30-day hospital stays were not uncommon. For mixed-diagnostic acute care inpatient populations, E. Coché (1987) recommended an eight-session closed-ended group over a 2-week period with no preset topics of discussion. A shorter series of sessions for such patients was less effective, and patients who participated in less than seven sessions did not derive the desired benefits from the training. Although adolescent inpatient units and facilities for chronic patients might still be able to accommodate the eight-session closed-ended group, such a lengthy stay at an adult acute care facility is a rarity.

This problem-solving model, however, has enormous malleability in its form and content. The appropriate time frame for efficacy depends upon developmental stage (child, adolescent, or adult), setting (short-term, long-term, inpatient hospital program [IHP], partial hospital program [PHP], or residential treatment center [RTC]), diagnosis, level of acuity and severity, and intellectual functioning. Usually a range of 8 to 20 sessions can provide significant benefit. A more holistic approach (recommended by Nezu et al., 2012) requires more time than the specific skills-based problem-solving training. More sessions are required for severe psychiatric symptoms, chronic brain injury, and developmental disabilities. The spacing of sessions is open to the requirement of the setting. Session placement can range from daily or twice daily for short-term PHPs up to once weekly over the course of several months for a longer term, open-ended RTC. Some benefit likely can be gained even when patients attend only a few sessions if the expectation of goals to be accomplished is limited (Grey, 2007; Radcliffe & Bird, 2016). For example, a single session can focus on one aspect of the training (e.g., learning to brainstorm, or learning to view problems as challenges). In facilities where patients have frequent but short admissions for stabilization, exposure to other aspects of the training and reinforcement of the skills might occur in subsequent sessions and admissions.

If the content of the sessions (e.g., problems with drugs, self-discipline, parents) is prespecified, a shorter series of five sessions has been shown to be efficacious (Edelstein, Couture, Cray, Dickens, & Lusebrink, 1980; Hussian & Lawrence, 1981). The length of the session usually varies from 60 to 90 minutes, but it can be as brief as 30 minutes or as long as 3 hours (e.g., Linehan & Wagner, 1990), depending on the composition of the group and members' abilities to focus on the material (Nezu et al., 2012).

Role of the Leader

The therapist's central functions are to provide and maintain the structure and boundaries of the group, to teach and navigate the group through the necessary steps of the problem-solving model, and periodically to remind group members of their goal to learn *how* to solve problems. The therapist educates members about each of the basic steps of the model and stresses the importance of methodically, tenaciously, and consistently following the procedure without deviation. The therapist can impart the basic tenets of the approach by lecturing, distributing handouts, modeling, providing direct feedback on members' behaviors in the group, acting as a coach, developing homework assignments, and creating new experiences for group members directly by role playing and indirectly by providing a good group experience (Nezu et al., 2012).

The therapist takes an active role in each session, whether lecturing, coaching, or remaining silent (Brabender, 2002). If the group does not follow the prescribed order of steps or does not adequately complete a task, the therapist intervenes. This requirement at times creates a demand on the leader to interrupt an ongoing process to prevent the group from skipping a step while not discouraging members' participation.

A moderate level of directiveness is ideal, with the avoidance of extremes. The therapist should never be so directive that he or she fails to communicate caring for the group members (Brabender, 2002). Moreover, the leader should avoid insisting on brief, precise verbalizations in which less time is spent on each step and a considerable number of problems are dealt with in each session. With this extremely task-oriented focus, important curative elements of group technique (e.g., cohesiveness) likely receive inadequate attention. In addition, some creative solutions are likely to arise only if the atmosphere is relaxed (E. Coché, 1987). Also undesirable is the leader allowing group members to talk as long as they wish on any particular problem, permitting tangents and digressions. This style creates a group atmosphere that builds cohesiveness, fosters a pleasant experience, but misses the point of problem-solving training.

Frequently, members present vague problems that must be fine-tuned and more specific to be workable. Clinical acumen is required to refocus or rephrase problems so that they have the potential to be resolved. For example, in working with borderline patients, Linehan reframed suicidal and other dysfunctional behaviors as part of the members' learned problem-solving repertoire used to manage or ameliorate psychic distress (Linehan & Wagner, 1990). A therapist working with chronic or acute psychotic individuals might encounter a member who presents a problem that reveals psychotic thinking. The leader can reformulate this problem so the group can address it.

For instance a paranoid thought that people are talking about a patient can be refocused as a self-esteem problem or a perceptual difference problem.

The therapist must organize and prioritize problems in a way that is manageable for the group. Variation exists in the method of establishing priorities. For example, if a member drops out, the leader can choose to disregard this event and continue, treat the event as a group problem and allow the group to work on it, or speak with the individual member. The therapist must also decide in what way a problem is to be addressed. For example, when a member requests help with a problem but then rejects all possible solutions given, this individual can be viewed as having a specific deficiency in problem-solving ability, namely a tendency to reject solutions before thoroughly examining their potential usefulness. If this member can own and recognize this "yes–but" tendency as a problem, it can be worked on in the group as well. One general approach to such a member is to request that the member withhold all criticism during the solution-generating step. If criticism occurs in the evaluating step, the therapist can invite other group members to comment on their success with a particular solution or advise members that any one solution may not work equally well for all.

The second task of the therapist is the management of the group process (Wessler & Hankin-Wessler, 1989). Problem-solving training views the individual as the focus of change; however, group dynamics (norms, boundaries, cohesiveness, patterns of communication, and emerging leadership roles) are important because they can enhance or detract from members' learning to solve problems and translate newly developed skills into appropriate action. For example, the practice of giving here-and-now group problems preference over problems dealing with issues outside the group effectively covers most problems that arise within the group. The therapist encourages the group to "own" a given problem and to work toward its resolution by generating and then evaluating alternative solutions. This process may arouse anxiety, which is diminished by the therapist's conveyance and nurturance of an attitude that difficulties can be mastered when approached with the right frame of reference and with the sense of accomplishment that this technique engenders.

The therapist is also responsible for regulating the emotionally expressive interactions among members (Wessler & Hankin-Wessler, 1989). Even though problem-solving groups are primarily task oriented, emotional reactions are not uncommon. It is also important that the therapist titrate the level of emotional expressivity and not permit antitherapeutic statements and actions by group members to influence other members in a detrimental way. Management of each session also requires that the therapist ensure that no one or two members dominate or disrupt the session. When such circumstances arise (e.g., when a member deals with social anxiety by incessant talking), the therapist has a number of alternatives. One is to intervene outside the session by discussing the problem individually with the monopolizer; this intervention can reduce the frequency of the behavior without causing additional anxiety. A second tack is to consider it a group problem, which the group can address, a strategy that may be effective as long as the group is not too intimidated by the monopolizer and if the latter is willing to listen nondefensively to the group's comments. This strategy is likely to work only after members have been together for a while and have a high level of trust in the process and therapist. A third method involves the therapist's placing him- or herself strategically next to the monopolizer where it is easier with hand and body gestures to influence the monopolizer's frequent interruptions. Whatever strategy is used, it is important to highlight the healthy aspects of the high verbal activity level (e.g., that the member is also displaying an interest in the group, often manifesting a good deal of concern for other members by trying to help them, but is working too hard in the group).

Sometimes members present problems in an effort to induce the group leader to take some kind of action, usually to repair something in their environment, rather than work toward a solution themselves. Members wish immediate action but desire to retain a passive role in the process. In such a situation, the therapist must stress that the goal of the group is to teach members how to solve problems themselves rather than have others solve problems for them (Kanfer & Busemeyer, 1982). In the therapeutic process, it is necessary for the therapist to help the member "own" the problem. In most cases, the problem can be redefined so that the member can accept and then work on the problem.

Leaders can either work alone or in cotherapy teams. The neophyte group therapist or relatively untrained personnel who may have limited theoretical knowledge about psychopathology or group dynamics can easily learn the basic procedure. Nonpsychology personnel (Rosenblum, 1983), graduate students, and even patient "graduates" have successfully functioned as leaders or coleaders (E. Coché, 1987). The more structured and preset the agenda and content, the less experience is required.

Setup and Content of the Problem-Solving Session

The problems addressed and the session format can be customized to the patients' needs and the setting constraints. There are three model formats, all of which address problems with the patient's problem approach, and teach and practice problem-solving skills. The first, described by Nezu, Nezu, and D'Zurilla, is most fully articulated in their training manual (Nezu et al., 2012). A series of modules follows a preset format in which problem-solving skills are assessed, issues of problem style and orientation are addressed, and planful problem-solving skills are taught with discussion, handouts, and practice.

One or more sessions are devoted to each aspect of problem-solving, with eight to 20 sessions being the recommended minimum for more impaired populations. The eight areas of suggested coverage are (a) assessment and treatment planning, which includes evaluative positive and negative orientations to problem solving and three problem-solving styles of planful, impulsive, and avoidant; (b) introductory sessions with presentation of the relationship of problem-solving abilities to how it impacts current reactions to current problems, the negative effects of stressful events, how the body and brain reacts to ongoing stresses, and how the skills taught can improve coping ability and increase resilience; (c) teaching strategies of visualization, externalization, and simplification to deal with the problem of cognitive overload; (d) strategies to deal with emotional dysregulation and ineffective problem solving, which involves teaching strategies to reinforce the STOP, SLOW DOWN, THINK, and ACT framework (e.g., discussions of identifying triggers and skills such as relaxation are taught); (e) promoting positive thinking and overcoming negative thinking and low motivation; (f) planful problem-solving (discussed in the content below); (g) guided practice of the entire problem-solving model; and (h) termination.

The second format, also involving a preset structure, has preselected hypothetical problem modules germane to the particular patient population (Bedell & Michael, 1988). For example, chronic institutionalized psychiatric patients may participate in a 5-week problem-solving program that discusses problem areas such as banking, budgeting, medication, health, telephone usage, meal planning, transportation, and community resources (Edelstein et al., 1980). Geriatric patients in a nursing home may have problem scenarios that include such topics as loss of freedom, fears of unending institutionalization, and staff difficulties (Hussian, 1987; Mellinger, 1989). The step-by-step problem-solving model is taught with attention to dysfunctional attitudes and behavior being infused into the discussion. A variant of this model is to focus on a specific type of problem such as suicidal behavior and relationship issues, rather than on hypothetical situations (Pollack, 1991). In such a situation, members bring in their own problems relevant to the identified theme. This variation can also be used when a dramatic shift in environment or role status is anticipated, such as discharge from the program.

In the third format, only the problem-solving progression is fixed, with the content determined by the concerns of members. E. Coché (1987) advocated giving preference to in-house problems over external or non-institutional problems, the rationale being that greater saliency provides more immediate positive reinforcement. For example, problems with staff members (e.g., "I am angry at my doctor, but I can't tell her") are given priority over an inability to express one's thoughts and dissatisfactions to one's boss at work. In contrast, Hussian (1987) stressed the exploration of extra-institutional problems, believing that this focus helps patients to generalize from the therapy setting to real-life events. How the therapist frames the problem is crucial. Members have a natural interest in specific solutions. By focusing on particular problems, the therapist may give the content of the problems and solutions greater salience, thereby distracting members from the all-important task of acquiring the principles of problem solving.

The atmosphere of the group can range from a traditional group format with chairs in a circle to an instructional format around a table with a blackboard, notebooks, and self-monitoring cards. Because group members must absorb a significant number of steps and didactic information, several techniques have been developed to facilitate this task. The use of a wall-poster display of the problem-solving steps can help members both remember the procedure and reveal whether the group is skipping any of the steps, a technique especially helpful to patients with cognitive organization and memory limitations.

All problems and solutions are logged on paper, in a composition book, on a blackboard, or in large newsprint. The advantage of the blackboard or newsprint is the immediate availability to aid memory and encourage creative combinations. Recording in a composition book allows for review many sessions later. A problem is recorded after the group has gained clarity on it. All solutions are recorded even if ideas are only a variation of a prior solution. A copy of the problem and solutions can be given to the author of the problem when the group has completed its work that day on the problem.

Problem-Solving Steps

Assessment and Preparation

A 30- to 60-minute individual screening and preparation session with the leader is advocated (J. Coché & Coché, 1986). The interview functions as a role induction in which prospective group members are taught appropriate member behaviors to enhance their ability to derive benefit from the group. Resistance to being a member of a group is explored. When time permits, a much more in-depth evaluation of the patient's problem-solving attitudes and skills is recommended. The Social Problem-Solving Inventory—Revised, short version, is a 25-item scale with Likert ratings, which takes 10 minutes to complete and can be distributed and returned prior to the screening (Nezu et al., 2012). This instrument assesses positive and negative problem orientation, rational problem-solving skill, impulsivity, and avoidance. During preparation, the therapist has the patient generate an example of a problem in order to assess the patient's ability to identify problems and emotional reactions to them, to implement a solution, and to assess outcome. The therapist should provide feedback to the patient concerning areas of strength and weakness in problem-solving capacities and help the patient apply this to the example he or she presented. Many patients are not aware when problems emerge and cannot make a connection between the development of a problem and their nonconscious emotional reactions. This discussion begins to sensitize them to their problems and this process.

Although a private screening and assessment session may be ideal, we have introduced this preparation as part of the first group meeting or patient's first group session. We have found staff assessment and recommendations to the group to be sufficient to determine suitability for the group, particularly if we periodically educate staff about criteria and invite them to observe the group. The Social Problem-Solving Inventory can be completed as part of the admission packet or introduced later on the unit by nursing and returned to the leader prior to the first group. In addition, prospective members are given a preparation handout that explains the workings of the group. (See Brabender & Fallon, 1993, for an example.)

The evaluative styles and approach to problem solving are presented in Table 7.1.

Orientation to the Problem-Solving Group

The group begins with a basic orientation each time membership changes. This step includes a rationale for the kind of treatment provided by the group and information on how the group proceeds. The extensiveness of the orientation depends on whether pre–group preparation has occurred, the general proclivities of the therapist, and the constraints of the setting. The orientation can include an in-depth introduction to all of the central concepts and principles of problem-solving therapy. For example, in addition to a basic outline of the procedure, the therapist may develop the notion of the

TABLE 7.1
Evaluating Style and Approach to Problem Solving

Approach to problems	Positive	Optimistic that problems can be solved and that individual has the capacity to do so
	Negative	Views problems as unsolvable or problems solvable, but the individual is unable to do so
Problem-solving style	Planful	Methodically reviews the problem and options and implements solution
	Impulsive	Quickly and without evaluation reacts to the problem
	Avoidant	Denies the existence or significance of the problem

importance of being assertive and exerting control over events in one's life (i.e., positive problem orientation). The therapist might also talk about the importance of identifying problems when they occur and about how deficient problem-solving skills are an interpersonal handicap that may lead to depression, withdrawal, and learned helplessness (Hussian & Lawrence, 1981). If the group is open-ended, members should be encouraged to informally present many of these concepts, as it helps them internalize the connections.

If the exigencies of the clinical setting preclude the use of a large portion of the group's session for orientation, the therapist might simply explain that deficient problem-solving skills are an interpersonal handicap, that people get frustrated when they are unable to solve impersonal as well as interpersonal problems, and that the purpose of the group is to help members become experienced in interpersonal problem solving (E. Coché, 1987). Viewing problems as a solvable challenge enhances the patient's willingness to engage wholeheartedly in the problem solving of everyday life and thus in the group (Nezu et al., 2012). Once members begin to practice the problem-solving strategy and are successful in coping effectively with actual problem situations, these optimistic expectations will be strengthened. The importance of recognizing problem situations when they occur and resisting the tendency to either avoid the problem or react automatically without thoroughly considering issues also should be stressed at the beginning, as well as throughout the group, as necessary for patient populations that are impulsive or avoidant.

Whether the problems are preset or determined by the members, a step-by-step problem-solving procedure is followed: preliminary problem description, clarification of the problem, generation of alternatives, evaluation of the alternatives, role playing, implementation of the decision, and verification of the correctness of the decision and concomitant correction of actions.[5] Each step is repeated each time a new problem is presented. The emphasis and time spent on each step may vary for different patient populations. For example, geriatric patients may require more prompting, concrete examples, and emphasis on the noncritical generation of alternative solutions than may

---

[5]These problem-solving steps are not intended as a model of human problem solving. The model presented uses a static model, which conceptualizes the individual as confronted with a set of unchanging goals and alternative solutions. The individual chooses an alternative and carries it out, and that particular problem is terminated. Examples of these problems are committing suicide or having an abortion, as the opportunity to modify or correct one's course of action is limited (Kanfer & Busemeyer, 1982). In contrast, in the dynamic problem-solving model, the individual objectives may change over time and it may be necessary to search for new solutions in response to feedback received. For example, the goal of developing a new relationship is one that may continuously be improved. Also in everyday life, an individual may move from one stage to another and back again. With more complex problems, one may also work simultaneously on several subproblems, each at a different stage of development. Therefore, the sequential approach as presented here should be viewed as a heuristic and efficacious way for organizing therapeutic procedures (Goldfried & Davison, 1976).

younger patients (Hussian, 1987). Impulsive adolescents may require a longer period to anticipate long-term negative consequences. The number of problems that the leader anticipates discussing each session will also influence the extent to which each step is emphasized.

If members are expected to bring in their own problems, an introduction to encourage members to identify problematic situations from their experiences—past, present, and expected future—may be needed. At the one extreme, patients may not be aware of when a problem occurs. These members need to learn to identify their problems and their unique emotional reactions and triggers. If skills are lacking to manage the cognitive overload in multitasking, exercises in sessions or for homework may improve this aspect (see Nezu et al., 2012). Patients may also consciously avoid facing problems because they are not optimistic about their skills to solve problems or have unrealistic expectations about possible outcomes or the time it takes. Other group members can help with realistic appraisals or expectations. At the other extreme are individuals prone to difficulties modulating their distress (e.g., even minor problems are perceived as overwhelmingly stressful). To assist patients in identifying specific problem areas, the therapist might explain the signal value of distress (i.e., that disturbing emotions, whatever their nature, often signal a problem that requires the person's attention; Linehan, 1987). Members can be encouraged to observe their own behaviors between sessions and to keep a daily record of problematic situations that produce emotional reactions. The emotional reaction can be a signal for the member to look for the events (cognitive and external) that may precipitate these feelings (D'Zurilla & Goldfried, 1971). Higher functioning or more seasoned group members can model this connection for the less verbal, less organized members (E. Coché, 1987).

Presentation of a Problem

If the problems have been set prior to the session, then the leader reads the problem either to the group or to one particular member who can then ask others for help (Hussian & Lawrence, 1981). The advantages of using a hypothetical problem are that it does not require patients to detect problematic events, eases the acceptance of having problems, prevents a single member from dominating the sessions, and allows the group to work on common problem areas sooner than they might using members' spontaneously offered problems.

If members generate problems, the leader requests volunteers to present a problem. Often, the first few sessions focus on problems pertaining to life in that setting—conflicts with staff or other patients (E. Coché, 1987; e.g., "My roommate leaves her dirty clothes on the floor; what should I do?"). As the group progresses, members are more likely to take responsibility for such problems and confront more threatening material. Occasionally, a member starts with a very personal problem such as, "My husband doesn't want to have sex with me because he says I am not attractive; what should I do?" This high level of disclosure can either foster group openness or make members uncomfortable and cause them to avoid further discussion of personal issues.

Problem Clarification and Information Gathering During the Session

This step is often the most challenging because the reality of a problem may be different from the individual's perception of it. Members frequently are not able to present their problems in a clear, concise manner. A problem may need to be restated to provide the kind of information that is likely to maximize the outcome in the subsequent step (D'Zurilla & Goldfried, 1971). Problem refinement is accomplished by defining all relevant aspects of the situation. The particular thrust of the focus on content (and level of inquiry) depends on the theoretical inclination of the therapist and members' sophistication and insight. For example, problem clarification can proceed as a psychodynamic inquiry, primarily exploring feelings, thoughts, and conflicts that make the situation problematic. Alternatively, the inquiry can proceed at a more behavioral level in which the problem is defined by specifying the major issues concerning who, what, where, and when in brief, concrete, and measurable terms (Bedell & Michael, 1988). For either type of inquiry, identifying the member's primary goals and the barriers that make the situation troublesome is important (D'Zurilla & Goldfried, 1971). Both external situational events and internal events (e.g., thoughts and feelings) are important for a thorough description of the problem (Goldfried & Davison, 1976). Group members are encouraged to ask specific questions that seek greater clarity to the problem. The gathering of relevant additional information is an essential skill in problem solving. Reinforcing appropriate information seeking also clarifies members' understanding of the situation, teaches them to resist impulsively providing obviously inappropriate suggestions, and conveys that everyone may see the situation differently.

The tendency of members to tell their "life stories" often poses a problem. A lengthy soliloquy may represent a misunderstanding of the model and a resistance to a technique that avoids focusing on past experiences. Some kinds of patient groups may require the therapist to approximate how much to reveal (e.g., "In three to four sentences tell us . . ."). If a member's level of detail is not necessary to generate adequate solutions, then it is important for the therapist to intervene by asking the presenting member if the information is relevant to solving the problem, encouraging the group to proceed to the next step, or querying the group as a whole as to whether the information is sufficient to solve the problem (E. Coché, 1987).

Generating Solutions

After the problem has been sufficiently clarified, the therapist facilitates the generation of solutions. This step is at the core of problem-solving group training given that patients are particularly deficient in their abilities to produce alternative solutions to a problem. During this step, the major task is to generate a range of possible solutions among which some may be effective (Goldfried & Davison, 1976).[6] Imagination and creative combination are welcomed, and criticism is disallowed. Quantity is emphasized over quality, as brainstorming is more likely to generate effective responses than is requesting that individuals produce only high-quality responses (D'Zurilla & Goldfried, 1971).

Members of the group generate as many possible solutions as they can without making any judgments regarding risk, possibility of success, practical aspects, or systemwide ramifications (Hussian, 1987). When beginning this step with each new problem, the therapist should explain the brainstorming method, emphasizing postponement of all criticism until the group has moved to the next step (E. Coché, 1987). Restating the disallowance of criticism is necessary because patients have a proclivity, quickly and readily, to judge solutions. The leader must repeatedly and in different ways reinforce that all solutions are welcome, whether they are bizarre, psychotic, humorous, completely impractical, or potentially damaging. For instance, the leader may say, "This is great—we've come up with 11 different solutions. Who can think of a way to combine two of them?" The written log reinforces that each solution is important and helps members to explore other possible alternatives.

The therapist actively aids members to see potential solutions in their comments but refrains from making specific suggestions so that the group does not develop a dependency on the therapist, which could seriously handicap members' abilities to develop problem-solving skills. The therapist need not fear that the final decision will be damaging or criminal. Data on individuals with sociopathic tendencies suggest that these tendencies decrease after problem-solving training (E. Coché & Douglas, 1977). Solutions need to be relevant to the specific problem presented so that their quality can eventually be evaluated (Goldfried & Davison, 1976). To achieve specificity, the group may first need to generate many broad suggestions and then be encouraged for more specific alternatives. It may be necessary to return to the previous step to obtain more information in order to develop more specific solutions before moving to the evaluation step.

---

[6]This step originated from Osborn's (1963) method of brainstorming, a procedure designed to facilitate idea finding in group sessions.

Evaluation and Decision Making

Once the generation of all solutions has been exhausted, the leader makes a very clear transition to the next phase by announcing that it is time to examine the ideas and determine which ones are feasible. The leader or another group member reads the problem and solutions from the log. Group members can be asked for opinions about which solutions are most likely to be successful and which are least likely. Or the therapist can ask the problem presenter for a perspective that evaluates several pros and cons of one or several solutions. Therapists who use this model usually have their own favorite methods of giving the discussion a focus, attempting to determine the utility of a decision in light of the values of the individual who presented the problem, and preventing that member from getting into a "yes–but" interchange. J. Coché and Coché (1986) focused on the "weighing" of solutions (i.e., which ideas are most likely to be successful and what will be the cost if one solution is chosen rather than another). Cost can be defined in terms of money, hard work, pain, hurt feelings, disturbed relationships, loss of prestige, and other similar concepts. The weighing of solutions is an important skill that implies that most solutions are not without a price; concomitantly, the lesson aids members to avoid a complete rejection of others' solutions. Weighing is an extremely useful step for adolescents with sociopathic or impulsive tendencies because it enables them to learn that immediate solutions to problems often require some significant long-term cost (e.g., stealing has immediate rewards but long-term potential for negative consequences such as prison).

A different means to various solutions was developed by Hussian (1987), who utilized a scale (–2 to +2) that group members rated the dimensions of personal benefits, benefits for others, short-term advantages and disadvantages, and long-term positive and negative consequences. The four sets of scores that accompany each presented solution are tallied, and the most viable solutions are chosen. Whether one elects to use a numerical approach or not, the utility of a decision should be assessed keeping in mind not only the individual's particular values but also the values of significant others who often label and influence what is effective in a particular environment (D'Zurilla & Goldfried, 1971). Sometimes during this phase a new alternative emerges. The suggestion is acknowledged and entered into the log, and its feasibility is discussed in a manner similar to that of the other solutions.

One problem that may arise during this period is when a member is too interested in foisting his or her favorite solution onto the group. The leader may need to carefully remind the group that not all solutions work for all people. The therapist too must guard against his or her own eagerness that the member who presented the problem come up with the right solution. For example, a member may decide that the best solution to dealing with feelings toward a disliked staff member is to avoid the staff member. Certainly, it would be appropriate for the therapist to question possible consequences of this action. Often other members will be able to voice the same concern. However, after sufficient discussion, the member has autonomy to choose a solution that maximizes positive consequences given their current interpersonal skill set.

The group then discusses specific implementation of the chosen solution. Strategies of implementation are often considered a separate step and skill set (Nezu et al., 2012). Successful implementation is dependent upon interpersonal abilities and may require the acquisition of new skills (e.g., strategies to cope with intense anxiety). When options for implementation are numerous, they are generated and weighted in the same manner as evaluation of solutions. Alternatively, ideas of implementation may be considered as a new (or subsequent) problem for the group after others have had the chance to work on their problems. This latter position has the beneficial effect of teaching members that many problems cannot be resolved by going through the procedure just once but may require two or more rounds (E. Coché, 1987).

Role Playing

Cognitive and behavioral rehearsal (role playing) can give members the psychological preparation to withstand challenges and obstacles that they are likely to encounter in everyday life. This step is optional, although with geriatric patients (Hussian, 1987) and more severely disturbed patients (Douglas & Mueser, 1990) it is usually necessary. The leader typically decides whether the presented problem and perhaps one or more of the proposed solutions lends itself to role playing in the group. Although members might resist role playing when it is first introduced, their willingness to participate can be increased by an explanation of the advantages of participation and by a willingness of the leader to participate as well. Usually, the presenting member takes his or her own role and enacts the chosen solution. This experience allows the member to practice a behavior never used before and gives him or her a feeling of mastery before the real-life situation occurs. Sometimes the presenting member plays the role of the opponent with whom an issue is to be addressed. This exercise gives the member an alternative perspective and can provide ideas for additional strategies in dealing with other people (E. Coché, 1987). If the leader takes the presenting member's role, he or she can model particular behaviors that the member may adopt.

Verification and Reporting Back to the Group

After the member agrees to act on a solution, he or she is invited, but not required, to report back to the group in subsequent sessions on its effectiveness.

This procedure encourages members to observe the consequences of their actions and to match outcomes against their expected predictions. It also highlights the real-life quality of the work done in the group sessions. In addition, it rewards other members for producing solutions and stimulates them to produce more (E. Coché, 1987). Sometimes a participant will report that a chosen solution was not successfully implemented. The group can accept this information as a challenge to generate a revised problem, and the steps begin anew.

The six problem-solving steps are presented in Table 7.2.

The essential features of the problem-solving model appear in Table 7.3.

CLINICAL ILLUSTRATION OF THE PROBLEM-SOLVING APPROACH

This illustration takes place in a PHP where patients attend an hour-long, open-ended group 3 days a week for 1 to 6 months. New members enter at the beginning of the week. There are two therapists: a senior permanent staff leader and a student who manages the flip-chart log and participates as a leader when comfortable. Patients are assessed for problem-solving skills and prepared for the group experience in a one-on-one session with a group therapist.

TABLE 7.2
Problem-Solving Skill Steps

Step	Reminders
Present a problem.	Seek a volunteer to present a problem that can be solved or preselect one relevant to the population.
Clarify the problem.	Help members ask questions to obtain relevant information needed to solve the problem.
Generate solutions.	Encourage any and all solutions. Don't allow criticisms.
Evaluate the solutions.	Assess the pros and cons for both the long term and the short term. Weigh the pros and cons for the individual and for others.
Develop strategies for implementation.	Generate ways to implement the solution. Role play the chosen strategy. Encourage the individual to try out the solution.
Verify the solution to the problem.	Encourage the member to report on the success of the solution and implementation; if it is not completely successful, it can be formulated as a new problem.

Note. Adapted from *Models of Inpatient Group Psychotherapy* (p. 440), by V. Brabender and A. Fallon, 1993, Washington, DC: American Psychological Association. Copyright 1993 by the American Psychological Association.

TABLE 7.3
TABLE 7.3
Problem-Solving Approach

Elements of the model	Characteristics of the model
View of psychological problems	Good problem solving enables better coping with stressful situations. Poor problem solving further increases the likelihood of problematic interpersonal situations.
Goals of model	Enhance an individual's ability to approach problems positively and to develop the skills needed to develop a plan to problem solve and implement it.
Methods of action	Repeatedly expose the individual to problems in daily functioning and with other members, which helps him or her learn a specific method of healthy problem solving.
Therapeutic techniques	• Identify the approach toward problem solving and foster positive beliefs that problems can be managed. • Teach patients to identify and clarify their problems in living. • Encourage generation of multiple solutions and discourage judgment. • Help patients develop plans for evaluating and implementing the best solutions. • Support implementation and encourage reporting successes or failures to the group.
Adaptation of the model to a brief time frame	When the member's tenure is brief (1 to 3 days), place emphasis on (a) obtaining appropriate recommendations from unit staff, (b) increasing the number of sessions per day, (c) adding new group members only once per week, (d) providing orientation to the group at the beginning of the session, and (e) using preselected problems already identified to be common for that particular population.
Use of group process	Use attention to the group process to reinforce how the individual's specific problem can unfold. Group process can become the problem focus.

Group Members

Janie is a 45-year-old African American woman who exhibits ongoing paranoid ideation. She has been hospitalized more than a dozen times since the age of 18, usually after being found wandering in dangerous neighborhoods at all hours of the night. During hospitalizations her paranoid thoughts recede with antipsychotic medication and a structured environment. The PHP is an effort to reduce hospitalizations. Upon entering the group several months ago, she had a positive attitude toward problem solving but a very impulsive style. She also has had significant deficits in every problem-solving step. She is frequently late to the morning group and enters the group interrupting whoever is talking with a soliloquy of missteps that occurred that morning to get to the program.

Ally is a 30-year-old Hispanic woman who carries diagnoses of schizotypal personality disorder. The staff have reported that at times she appears to be responding to internal stimuli, but she denies hearing voices. Once homeless, she now lives in a group home. Her residence requires that she attend the PHP. This relatively new member is generally quiet, but when she does speak she is easily offended when she feels others are not paying attention to her. She entered the group with limited problem-solving skills and an avoidant style of problem solving.

Chuck is a 60-year-old Russian immigrant who lives by himself. His neighbors reported to the police that he would yell as he threw food out his window. He was evaluated in the emergency department and referred to the PHP, as he was not considered a danger to himself or others. He revealed that he was throwing the food away because someone was entering his apartment and poisoning his food. He has been caught shoplifting food. He often mutters to himself. When it can be heard, he appears to be responding to voices in Russian. He entered the group with a very negative orientation toward problem solving, but he has become more engaged and positive with time. He has a generally avoidant style of problem solving, and he defines problems and solutions with a paranoid frame.

Dan is a 35-year-old single Caucasian man with a history of brief hospitalizations usually after he makes a superficial suicide gesture. He has been employed, although he often quits because he perceives others to have slighted him. At times he is also grandiose in talking about his previous employment and what he believes he can accomplish. He has sometimes been irritable and oppositional in group, but he is often very sensitive to other members' needs. His skill in defining and evaluating others' problems is reasonably well developed; however, he is impaired by a negative attitude toward his abilities and an impulsive style.

Stephy is a 23-year-old African American woman who exhibits a tremendous amount of anxiety. She reports obsessive fears and thoughts about tragedies happening to her mother. She also reports many fears and phobias, toward which she has developed compulsive responses such as counting related to driving and crossing bridges. She has rapid speech and hyperactive body movements. She lives with her mother, who is very critical of her. After several verbal fights with her mother, she cuts herself and then is admitted for short hospital stays. Previously, this very bright member had been enrolled in community college, but she has not been able to complete a single term because hospitalizations disrupt her attendance. She is attending the PHP 3 days a week and taking two college classes on the other 2 days with the hope of breaking this cycle of failure. In sessions, she is very loquacious, often interrupting others. She is also very anxious to please the therapists and frequently gives the socially desirable response. Her attitude tends to be hopeful about developing problem-solving skills, but she is generally overcome by anxiety and fear. She both avoids dealing with problems and is impulsive. Although she has a moderate ability to solve abstract problems, in the group her ideas are usually egocentric and self-referential.

Ingrid (the new member) is a 40-year-old single Caucasian woman diagnosed with bipolar disorder, hospitalized three times in the last 4 years with psychotic depressive delusions. Between episodes, she has worked for a large insurance company managing large databases. She aspires to enter management but has negative, oppositional, and conflictual relationships with coworkers. She has a very negative problem-solving attitude and is impulsive in her actions. Despite her high level of employment, her problem-solving skills are deficient with limited and concrete alternatives to solving problems.

The Session

> [The therapist greets group and introduces Ingrid. Other members introduce themselves.]

Dr. Z: The first thing we should do is get Ingrid up to speed. Let's tell her what we do here in the problem-solving group and why it's important.

> [Therapist invites early participation rather than giving the information, which serves to help group members recognize the importance of the problem-solving group and develop a positive orientation toward problem-solving.]

Stephy: I can start. I've found it helpful in a lot of ways—we just talk about when we have problems in life, we come up with different solutions and listen to each other's ideas.

Ingrid [interrupting]: Does it solve your problems?

Stephy: Yes, I've found it helpful, and I think everyone here has found it helpful in some way.

Chuck: Not all the time.

Dan: Basically, if you have something going on in your life, you bring it up, and then people tell you things to try and fix it. And sometimes it works; usually, it doesn't.

Stephy: But that's what is good. It's hard to solve things on the first try, but we keep bringing up the problems, and I think we can find solutions.

Dr. Z: Yes, good start, everyone. We all have daily hassles and also chronic issues. We all can improve the way we go about solving those daily and serious problems. Sometimes problems may not seem like they can be solved, but as Stephy says, we keep at it and our motto is "Where there is a will there is a way." What happens when we hope they go away and just avoid them?

Ally: They change to worse.

Dr. Z: Right. Daily hassles can make us feel very stressed, if we don't know how to effectively manage them. If, as Ally says, you avoid them, they tend to build up. If you don't have a good method to solve problems or if you try to solve them too quickly, it can make the situation even worse. So it's good to figure out a method to solve problems that we can fall back on. Anybody have anything they want to add?

Stephy: Like for me, just listening to what you're saying makes me feel better, yeah.

          [Janie enters the room and interrupts Stephy.]

Janie: Hi, everyone! Hi, Dr. S, hi, Dr. Z.

Dr. Z: Hi, Janie! Have a seat. We have a new member and we are talking . . .

Janie: Hi, what's your name? I just came here. I forgot my bag and had to go back and missed the bus, and the next one was late. I could not find my jacket, and someone stole it . . .

Dr. Z. [interrupting]:   Well, we're glad you're here. We're in the middle of helping Ingrid learn about our group.

Stephy: We were talking about what we learn in problem-solving group . . .

Chuck [interrupting]:   You're gonna start all over again?

Stephy: I'm just reviewing what we learned. So we were just talking about what we've done in group to help us with problem solving and, you know, how sometimes it's easier said than done.

Janie: I left my food at home. You know, with the bird spit man and the food was . . .

Dr. Z: Maybe we can hold that a minute and just ask Ingrid: Do you have any questions now?

Ingrid: No.

Dr. Z: OK, good. So on your seats are the problem-solving steps [referring to the sheet of problem-solving steps]. We take each step, one at a time, discuss it, and then move onto the next step. [*Asks group members to say what each step is adding at the end.*] Remember, last time we had 16 solutions, and today maybe we will find even more. And remember as we think of solutions [*Group chimes in loudly and in unison, "No criticism"*]. Yes, excellent. Janie, last time you said you wanted to bring up a problem.

Janie: I know! I have all these credit cards, and one of my credit cards, the Victoria's Secret one, has like $2,500 on it, and I've been trying to pay it, and the guy said you just have to pay the minimum, and he told me to open it. But then I had to open another one at Boscov's, so I have one at Boscov's, but he said I can just pay the minimum, but I don't know what happens. It keeps getting bigger every month even though I keep paying the minimum.

Stephy: When did this start?

Janie: I got the Victoria's Secret one 10 years ago, and then I got the Boscov's one the other day because I wanted to get a pair of boots, but I didn't have any money because it was the end of the month.

Dan: Wait! So you're still buying things with another card?

Janie: Well, I like to go shopping sometimes. Usually, at the beginning of the month I have some money, but I don't know what happens; it keeps just getting higher.

Dr. Z: Janie, let me just stop you a minute; we need to figure out exactly the problem. The problem is a big problem for you. I don't know if we can tackle the whole problem today because there are many aspects to the problem. First there is the idea that you have a big credit card debt and, even though you're paying off the minimum, somehow it keeps getting bigger. So I guess the question is, what would you specifically like help with today?

[*Focus the problem on something that can be managed in one session.*]

Janie: Well, I wanna make it so that every month the number on my credit card is less.

Dr. Z: You want to reduce the debt. [*Janie nods.*]

Stephy: But do you know how to reduce the debt? Like, what do you think you can do?

Janie: I don't know—the guy told me just pay minimum and I pay it, but it's not working.

Dan: Well, try not using it to buy new things.

Dr. Z:	Dan, that's a solution, and one we can use, but let's clarify what the problem is.
	[Therapist needs to remind the group to stay with defining and clarifying the problem.]
Dan:	OK, so maybe I'll clarify. Sounds like the problem is that you keep spending money on these cards, and you don't have the money, so you can't even pay it off.
Janie:	I know!
Chuck:	The problem is we don't get enough SSI to begin with. You can't live on that stuff.
Janie:	Yeah, when I first got SSI, it was like $600 a month, and that was 20 years ago, and it's still only $630 a month.
Ingrid:	What do you buy? Like, stuff you need?
Janie:	I don't know. I got these boots and this jacket, because it's cold out and was on sale and I had to go to the store 20 miles away because the one here didn't have it, so they ordered me one to the other store, and I got it there.
Dan:	Why did you need the jacket?
Janie:	Well, it was on sale.
Ingrid:	Is that all you do all day, just go shopping from store to store?
Janie:	Yeah, I go places and do things for my family. I have to shop for my family too and my cousin who's at home. He got paralyzed and can't shop. Sometimes, things get lost because the ghost thieves in my house steal stuff from me and my family.
Stephy:	I don't know; sometimes I feel like we buy things for ourselves and other people are buying it for us too, and then we end up having so much stuff. You're like, what am I gonna do with all this stuff? Do you know what I mean? So that . . .
Dan:	What are you saying about ghosts stealing from you?
Janie:	Yeah, sometimes it's the entity who steals. Like my sister one time said she lost her passport and she said, "We must have a poltergeist because I don't know where it is!" And the poltergeist steals my stuff, too, so sometimes I got this stuff from Donna Karan at TJ Maxx . . .
Dr. Z:	OK, Dr. S., let's get the problem on the chart. Just to clarify, are you spending money while you're here, too?
Janie:	Maybe on the weekends. I told my sister to just pay the minimum every month. She gets my check and takes that amount out of my check.

Dr. Z:	Right now, it's being paid down. But what you're worried about is that the balance is going to get higher when you leave?
Stephy:	That is so stressful. Like, I don't even know how you deal with it honestly because even just listening to you I'm like that sounds so stressful, like how would you even deal with that? Money concerns are so stressful.
Ingrid:	You could just relax.
Dr. Z:	Ingrid, you're starting to give us some ideas for solutions. But let's make sure we have everything we need to solve the problem [*reinforces the step progression*].
Stephy:	Do you trust your sister?
Janie:	Yeah! She's a lawyer.
Dan:	Since you're in this program, I'll bet your debt's coming down, and so the problem might be being solved. I'm just trying to figure out what the bottom-line problem is.
Ingrid:	It's that she keeps buying stuff that she doesn't need or have money for.
Stephy:	But is someone actually taking your clothes? You can't really trust people, honestly. The reality is people steal stuff. Do you think people are stealing your stuff and that's why you have to buy stuff for yourself all the time?
Janie:	Well, it's the poltergeist that's in my house that steals from my whole family.
Chuck:	What's a poltergeist?
Ally:	It's like a ghost.
Dr. Z:	The poltergeist, SSI, we don't have control over that. Let us help Janie figure out what she can do to reduce her problem. Her problem is she keeps spending. When she leaves the program, the debt will build up again, because of some of the reasons that she told us. We're going to have to think of solutions that can help Janie deal with that inclination to buy. Is that the problem?

[*Janie nods, and Dr. S writes the problem on the flip chart.*]

| Stephy: | I can't get over the idea that somebody might be stealing, like you can't trust people. I understand what you're saying—not having control over your own money. I get anxious about people stealing stuff from me, too. You have to fend for yourself. So I understand why that would be upsetting . . . like that's a whole |

other component, but I just feel like that's a factor in this situation, not being able to trust people.

Chuck: Do you have locks? Gotta lock up everything.

Dr. Z: So the issue of trust may be part of the problem. Another part is, do you like to buy?

Janie: Yeah, I go on the bus. I like to go to different places. I can look at the new stuff. I really like shopping at stores like Victoria's Secret and The Limited. Sometimes when I'm on the bus I forget where I am a little bit.

Dan: We're bouncing around the subject, which is you like to shop, you feel a need to shop, and you can't stop doing it—so why not just give your check to someone who can? So are we on "Generating Solutions"?

Dr. Z.: Good catch, Dan. We are not quite there yet if we have not fully clarified the problem. As you said, part of the problem is that Janie likes, feels the need, and feels good about shopping, so we have to figure out some way to deal with that aspect.

Chuck: Why do you feel good?

Ingrid: Is she not supposed to have pleasure in anything?

Ally: Why can't she come up with another hobby?

[*The question of why Janie feels good is not something to which she may have conscious awareness. As the group begins to offer solutions, the therapist makes the decision to transition to the next step.*]

Dr. Z.: So, we've defined and clarified the problem; let's go to the next step—thinking about all solutions. They don't have to be realistic, anything we can think of. Remember—no . . . [*Group chimes in "criticisms"*]. Right! So I think Ally and Dan had two possibilities.

Dan: Give your check to someone who can manage your money, like your sister.

Stephy: I have another one. I think that you could also just stay in the house . . .

Ally: Wait! What about what I said? Find another hobby.

Dr. S: OK, that's a good solution.

Stephy: You're not gonna shop if you just stay in your house; just stay there.

Janie: No, I don't think I can do that . . .

Dr. Z: Janie, remember, we're not at the evaluation step yet. Let's look at all the possibilities first. Stephy, I definitely want to hear yours after Dr. S writes Ally's.

Ally: Find another hobby. I feel like I said that already. [*She walks out.*]

[*Short interchange in which therapists encourage Ally to stay, but she leaves. Dan also protests.*]

Stephy: Anyway, like I was saying, I mean, I feel like sometimes people don't listen to me but, um, I was also trying to mention that you just stay in the house or stay in your room, because if you stay in your room then you won't spend money. I mean, when I stay by myself I don't get into trouble because I stay in my room and then I don't get into trouble that way; then I don't have to feel nervous about things either.

Ingrid: Someone just left because you wouldn't listen to them.

Dr. Z: Ingrid, you commented on Ally leaving. I think Dan also is a little upset and Stephy reacted by filling in. This is another very important issue that we should talk about. It's important for the functioning of our group to talk about it. At the same time, I'm thinking that we're in the middle of working with Janie's problem. Let's continue with the problem. We'll come back to the issue of Ally leaving after we have been through the problem-solving steps.

[*The therapist acknowledges the importance of the group event of a member leaving and the impact on the group and its functioning; however, the therapist gives priority to teaching a method of problem solving over the effect and meaning of the abrupt leaving on the members. Given Ally's psychotic undercore, Ally's reasons for leaving are only partly because she felt ignored. Likely she was finding the group an overwhelming experience. This aspect could not easily be explored with her or the group until she had a much greater sense of security in the group.*]

Janie: I could get more money.

Ingrid: From where?

Dan: You're not allowed to throw out solutions. No criticisms.

Stephy: This poltergeist, who are they?

Chuck: It's not real.

Stephy: Maybe it is real, we don't know that. To her it's real. You don't know everything in the world. There's always options for things.

If we could get down to the bottom of if it is real, then maybe she wouldn't feel like she needs to shop and get debt.

Ingrid: I've never had debt.

Stephy: Can you throw out your credit cards? 'Cause then if you throw out your credit cards at least you won't accumulate more debt.

Janie: I know, 'cause then I can't use them, right?

Chuck: Why do you need this stuff? Can you just make a list of what you actually need?

Dan: Buy less of it.

Janie: I can stay here in the program so I don't buy.

[Dr. S writes each solution on the flip chart.]

Dan: Is that enough solutions?

Dr. Z: We should try to think of as many as possible so that Janie has a lot to choose from.

Chuck: Just use cash and ACCESS card to get food. I ain't got no credit cards.

Stephy: Or maybe you could, like, pray. Like, sometimes I pray; when I was younger I was told that if you pray it can help with your problems.

Janie: One time I found $20.

Dan: Don't you have a rich family that can pay this stuff or your sister?

Janie: She has some money but not a lot of money.

Stephy: But do you trust her? Just wanna make sure.

Dr. Z: You know one thing that strikes me is that we have come up with very specific solutions, but we haven't really figured out what Janie can do to feel good other than shop.

Janie: I go to the library sometimes.

Stephy: But then if she goes to the library, she's leaving her house. The more she puts herself out there, the more trouble she can get in.

Dr. Z: Well, I think what you're all getting into now is figuring out what's the best solution and what isn't. Let's see if there are any more solutions before we go to that step.

Ingrid: Exercise.

Chuck: I don't understand how that helps with shopping.

Dan: She said it's a way to feel good; we know that Janie likes to feel good by shopping, and so she can find something else. It's better than spending a hundred dollars a day.

Janie: I know, because everything's so expensive.

Chuck: If you exercise won't you still have the urge to shop? What helps you deal with urges? I usually just get pissed off.

Stephy: When I get really mad or anxious, I sometimes distract myself. Maybe if there's something that can distract you. I've been told by my therapist that you could draw or color. Like journal, she's also told me to write a story. Anything with arts and crafts, singing, writing a song, writing a poem—you could write a script for a movie, so many things that you could do just to distract yourself when you're feeling nervous.

Janie: Sometimes I watch movies.

Dan: What about, like, eating a snack or something? What do you like to eat?

Janie: I try to eat fish; my doctor said I should eat more vegetables. Like tilapia.

Dr. Z: Great. Janie might do any of these things to feel good also.

Chuck: Who's going to sing when they feel like they're going to shout?

Stephy: I don't think it's ridiculous.

Dr. Z: Remember, no . . .? [*silence, group fills in "criticisms"*]. You know it's so easy for us to get into evaluating things. We want to gather as many solutions as possible. The more, the better. Janie, if you don't shop, what happens, how do you feel?

Janie: I don't know, 'cause I just stay at home and I get bored.

Dr. Z: But are you aware of any kind of feeling inside?

Janie: I just feel bored and, like, I want to go do something, and I don't know what to do. Sometimes I don't want to stay at home because the ghost thieves . . . I don't know what else to do when I go out, so I shop.

Dr. Z: It sounds like you get bored and maybe uncomfortable with your own thoughts at home. Feeling that things are out of your control and may be taken away from you when you are just sitting at home. You use shopping to distract and to feel better. That was an important part of the problem that we need to address.

[*Several members talk at once, offering other suggestions but each wandering into his or her own concerns related to distrust. The con-*

versation becomes somewhat derailed by a discussion of dogs and whether you can trust them or how they could hurt you. The group continues with other solutions offered, such as finding specific people to talk to—mother, nephew, therapist, social worker.]

Stephy: See, nobody's listening!

Dan: When I'm away from home, it feels like I'm missing my dog.

Janie: I know, yeah, I want a dog.

Dan: Yeah, but talking to someone is another solution. But who could you talk to? Your paralyzed nephew?

Dr. Z: Are we able to think of anything else, maybe combine any two?

Ingrid: You're looking for love in the wrong places, in the stores.

Stephy: I understand, I also do stuff that isn't helpful, but that's why my therapist gives me suggestions. Maybe some of these suggestions can help you, too. It's scary out there.

Chuck: You could just steal it instead.

Stephy: Yeah, but if she steals, then the police might come, and you can't trust the police.

Dr. Z: We are not yet to the evaluation step; other combinations?

Stephy: Praying could be combined with anything. I would pray and stay inside the house.

Dan: Give your check to your sister; she could give you enough money so that you could buy something. You won't be spending as much so these two could work.

Ingrid: The boots!

Chuck: But that's like you're a little kid.

[*A discussion among the members ensues as to whether it is a good idea to act like a little kid. The therapist interrupts when it gets derailed further.*]

Dr. Z: Hold that thought, Chuck. Let's move to the next step. Wow! We have 19 or 20 solutions. I really think we should give ourselves a hand. We've come up with more than we have before, and there's a wide variety of solutions. It's time to decide on the best solution for Janie.

Dan: This is definitely the best. You said that it was a good idea, to give your check to your sister plus setting up an allowance to pay debt.

Dr. Z: Let's ask Janie. What are your ideas about which ones would work for you?

Janie:	Well, I don't think that one [*referring to Dan's*], 'cause my sister used to get my check, but I got it back. So I don't want my sister to have it again.
Stephy:	So maybe her sister's doing something that's shady. Did she steal it or anything?
Janie:	No. I think I should not go shopping every day.
Ingrid:	Do you think you're managing your money well? What about the ghosts?
Stephy:	We should investigate the poltergeist thing too, because that might actually be a factor. I'd be nervous about it.
Dr. Z:	These are important aspects. Janie, if you were going to shop less, what do you think you could realistically commit to?
Janie:	Maybe I could just go on days that I don't see my doctors. I see my doctors two days a week.
Dr. Z:	OK . . . that would be like 3 days a week . . . and then you wanted to combine it with something else.
Ingrid:	Money.
Dr. Z:	Combine it with . . . with spending less money? What are your thoughts about how to do that?
Janie:	Maybe instead of going to Ann Taylor, I can go to Ross. It's not as expensive.
Dan:	What do you think about the first solution, which is to give your sister the check?
Ingrid:	You could shop and not buy anything.
Stephy:	Well, you said shopping makes you feel good, right? Would going shopping and not buying things also make you feel good?
Janie:	Maybe . . . I like to go out and look at things, so I could not buy something every time.
Chuck:	So then you put a cap on how much you spend in a week and can't spend anymore.
Stephy:	My therapist says that limits are a good thing.
Dan:	Yeah, but tell me if I'm wrong, once you leave here, the cap is going to change. That's what always happens. I leave here and I don't remember anything.
Chuck:	That's why you have to use cash. Get rid of credit cards.

Stephy: Do you trust yourself to have a cap and follow it? How are you going to feel good, too?

Janie: Yeah! I've never tried it before.

Stephy: Isn't that the point of this problem-solving group? To try new things?

Dr. Z: OK, so let's think about what a cap could be. What's a realistic cap that you could agree to?

Janie: Maybe $100?

Ingrid: No. You only get $600 a month, and it wouldn't make sense.

Chuck: You have to buy food.

Janie: $50, is that OK? I live with my sister, and the minimum on my credit card is $300.

Stephy: This is so stressful. This problem is just too big. You have to stop spending money, you have to start paying off your debt, so many things, maybe it's too big to solve.

Dr. Z: Stephy, you are right that it is a big problem, maybe too big to solve in one day. We cannot expect to solve the problem in one day, but Janie does have to start somewhere with the problem. She has made a good start. She recognizes it is a problem. She wants to do something about it. We need to try small steps. We have the weekend coming up. Janie, you suggested a $50 limit. How about if we go with that? Janie can let us know if she was able to stay within her budget, how it felt if she was. Was she still able to feel good?

[*Janie nods assent.*]

Stephy: Does this plan make you nervous? It makes me nervous!

Dan: It makes me nervous, yeah.

Dr. Z: Why does it make the two of you nervous?

Stephy: When you have these problems and they're so big and you don't know if you can trust things will work out. I just feel like it's so overwhelming; who knows if it's actually going to work. What if this is all for nothing? Can you even trust us? Can you trust the people outside? Exactly, so how do we know this problem will get better?

Chuck: You can't trust anyone!

Dan: You said you can't trust anyone, but for me it is, can you trust yourself to do it? Because I would not. I would leave and be, like, OK, that was good.

Dr. Z [hands the flip-chart problem and solutions pages to Janie]: Janie, we are going to give these to you. Are you willing to try limiting your spending to $50 this weekend? *[Janie nods yes.]* Let us know how it goes. We have about 20 minutes left, and there are two issues floating around. The first is that Ally left and we have feelings about it. Second, I hear this question of "What is the use?" This question gets to the heart of our attitudes toward problem solving. If we think this negative way, it is hard to have much energy and enthusiasm to do the hard work of trying to problem solve. Which problem would you like to deal with first?

Dan: Ally leaving.

Janie: I don't know why she left.

Stephy: Yeah, I don't know why she left. I feel like we wanna help each other, but then it seems like she doesn't have our best interest in mind. . . . Maybe she's leaving because she doesn't care.

[Cotherapist writes problem on flip chart: "Ally left and we don't know why and we have feelings about it and we want to talk about it."]

Ingrid: It was rude! Like I just came here for the time and she just left, who does that?

Chuck: Leaving is better than hitting someone.

Dr. Z: So let's try to think about what the issue is. Did something happen in the group that we could not talk about?

Dan: You guys saw what happened? She was saying something. Someone talked over her. She got angry and left.

Stephy: Exactly! It feels like sometimes people don't even listen. We're here trying to solve these really big problems so that we can feel better and not be so nervous all the time.

Dr. Z: Yes, we are trying to learn a method of how to solve problems. With Janie, we had an unbelievable number of solutions and people had lots of enthusiasm about them. We don't want to lose that. On the other hand, the problem is that everybody needs to be heard, too. And how can we do it in a way so everybody feels like their solution is valuable. The problem seems to be how can we be enthusiastic, ensure that everyone gets to participate and give their solution, but also be able to listen. How to offer solutions and listen, too.

Janie: I think everybody had really good answers; there were lots of answers.

Dan: But when you think something is bad or I don't want to call you out [*to Chuck*], but you said stealing was one, and I wanted to respond with, "Oh, that's not a good idea."

Chuck: Yeah, but that's a solution. I've done it before and it worked.

Dr. Z: Dan you were concerned maybe that Janie might choose that suggestion?

Dan: Right. By listening, you are getting bad advice.

Dr. Z: I understand what you are saying. You are concerned that you want Janie to pick the best solution, but I can tell you from my experience and research that coming up with *all* types of solutions, brainstorming, if they're good, bad, ugly, is better, is going to eventually give you more good solutions to choose from. Evaluating each solution as it is presented prevents people from thinking creatively.

Dan: So maybe that's what the problem was, even thinking that, any solution has to be accepted. And I don't think I was doing that right.

Dr. Z: Dan, I don't think you were alone in that. How do we generate as many different solutions as possible, keep our enthusiasm, but make sure that everyone gets to say their piece?

Stephy: My therapist says to put yourself in there 100% and it might help you feel better.

Dan: But sometimes the way you do that makes other people feel bad. And then they leave. You just talk. You said "whatever," and then Ally left, and she's like my friend, she's cool. And she was frustrated because you were interrupting and saying "my therapist told me this."

Stephy: My therapist said that I should try to be as active as possible and say things, and I was trying to say the things that were on my mind. She told me I should, too. That's why I was talking at the beginning because I felt like maybe that would help with the group, but I guess maybe I was wrong. Maybe I can't trust you guys; I don't know.

Dr. Z: It seems like we are looking for what caused Ally to leave. There were a lot of factors. But Dr. S and I are in charge of the group; it is our responsibility. Maybe you are wondering if you can trust us and why didn't we prevent her from leaving. What are Dr. S and I doing for the group to ensure that everyone has the chance to contribute and to listen as well?

Stephy: I came in with a good attitude, and now I feel like I should just go back to my room.

Dr. Z: I think we have identified the problem and defined it. We are ready to think of solutions. Stephy, what would help you stay with us? That would be generating a solution.

Stephy: Maybe feeling heard in some way.

Janie: Maybe Dr. Z. can tell us when it's our turn to talk?

Stephy: Maybe if people could say positive things if they agree.

[Dr. S. writes down these solutions.]

Stephy: Sometimes, even earlier like when Janie came in and I was trying to catch her up on what we were talking about at the beginning, I was trying to summarize what we were saying so she could get involved, and I felt like everybody was just like ganging up on me.

Dan: Yeah, I get frustrated when someone comes late and we have to stop and start over.

Stephy: Yeah, I was kind of frustrated by that too, and I was just trying to cope with it by updating her on what we were talking about at that moment, and then people got upset and said we were already talking about that, and I felt like I wasn't heard again.

[Dr. S writes, "When members feel frustrated with the group process, they try to cope with it by providing information about what is going on in the group."]

Dr. Z: So I want to go back to this feeling of you [Stephy] not being heard. You're feeling like we cut you off, and maybe I cut you off, too. And that had something to do with your feeling like you weren't heard. Where is the balance? We have to balance between trying to stay on focus with the problem. With lots of people having so many things to say, how could we stay on task but then help everyone feel heard? I'm noticing that we are out of time, so unfortunately we are not going to be able to finish this problem, but we can go back to this because I think this is a really important issue that we can participate and feel heard. So what do you think, guys? I think we had a really good day today. I am looking forward to working on this again on Wednesday.

Comment on the Session

Depending upon the milieu, most problems that low functioning members introduce will be ones originating outside the program, although those generated within the group are at least as effective in providing practice application of the skills. It is most effective when problems are of an interpersonal nature, because the group becomes a social microcosm of the patient's experience in the world. Even utilizing problems originating outside the group, members often witness an interaction with the patient that parallels the patient's presenting interpersonal problem. However, with lower functioning patients, the ones offered are often basic problems in living. Sparse social resources ensconce and exacerbate these issues (e.g., fixed and limited public funding). The problem of credit card overspending that Janie presents, at face value is not interpersonal, but is quite common for a broad spectrum of psychopathology; its origins, manifestations, and solutions will depend upon social status and resources as well as intrapersonal and interpersonal functioning. In general, chosen solutions must address not only the behavioral interaction but also the underlying affective components (i.e., the way in which the problem behavior is immediately and emotionally gratifying), such as why the behavior feels good and what other substitute behaviors could be more adaptive behaviors. Higher functioning patients are able to present some solutions that address the multilayered nature of the problem and the nuances of its impact on complex personality functioning. Solutions for lower functioning patients, though, are often egocentric and concrete, as can be seen by those that are offered to Janie. Because all solutions are accepted, the model can easily accommodate a range of cultural, ethnic, religious, and gender diversity. Allowing the presenter to choose the most effective solution honors possible differences that might otherwise arise in a diverse population.

In a lower functioning group, a great deal of chaos periodically erupts as members talk over one another and offer non sequitur ideas to understand the problem, choose solutions, and evaluate them. As members get to know one another better, their efforts to hide some of their distorted and psychotic thinking diminishes, as can be seen in this vignette. The leader has to be comfortable with and prepared for a certain amount of derailed chatter that patients engage in and find a balance between adherence to the model and spontaneous, burgeoning, freewheeling associations.

As therapists become familiar with a certain clientele, they will find that common themes emerge. The issue of trust is important; with this particular group, it is concretized in the delusion of a poltergeist that is mentioned throughout the session. It would be helpful for it to be addressed, but the delusion itself (in this case, the poltergeist) must be reframed into a problem for which solutions can be generated.

A group-as-a-whole problem can be successfully addressed in a problem-solving group as well. For example, in one group of adolescents on an intermediate residential unit, two of the members formed a subgroup that was flirtatious in nature, eating together, spending free time together, and speaking only to each other in group. Other members of the group felt left out and envious. The problem was addressed when several members expressed their anger toward the subgroup for their lack of interest in other members' problems. In generating solutions, a therapist who has an understanding of the effects of subgrouping on group climate is in a better position to help the group anticipate these effects and arrive at a realistic solution.

We contend that negative events that potentially impact the group's functioning must be addressed in the group. When such an event occurs, therapists must decide whether to focus on the unfolding event and abandon the problem at hand or table it until the current problem has been fully processed. For reasons outlined in the transcript, the therapists took the latter path. There was much more that could have been done with Janie's problem in terms of implementation and role playing, but the therapists, mindful of time, felt that the issue of a member's unexpected departure needed to be acknowledged and aired. As Janie agreed to implement a spending limit, the issue of trust reemerges.

The example here illustrates how an upsetting event in the group (i.e., Ally's leaving) can be transformed into a group problem to be addressed within the problem-solving framework. Adherence to the model, using either an individual or a group problem, promotes learning the method of problem solving. As therapists create the space to discuss it, the issue of trust reemerges. The therapist attempts to reframe this as a balancing of listening versus enthusiastically contributing and allows the group to make a choice between discussing this issue or Ally's leaving. As members verbalize their thoughts, the problems with their interactional abilities become salient. As they voice their frustrations of a member arriving late, their inability to tolerate their own and others' negative affect and feedback, and their defensiveness about their own contributions becomes apparent.

When discussing Ally's leaving, members start to turn on each other as they begin to perceive that Ally may have felt unheard, that Stephy had interrupted her, and the group had allowed it. Their defensiveness is expressed as distrust for family, each other, the poltergeist, and the group experience. When the group members begin to express negatively toned affects to one another, it is our opinion that with lower functioning patients their perceptions should be acknowledged generally without specific accusation, but that the negative venom must be suctioned away from the group members and be contained by the therapists. In this case, the therapists declare themselves as ultimately responsible for the group's safety and management of the group process.

Such a problem could take many different directions depending upon the capacities of the group. The fears of criticism, either direct (e.g., Dan's blaming members for Ally's leaving) or indirect (e.g., being shut out of entering the solution into group dialogue), for participation need to be outweighed by the belief and hope that this group and its process will allow for an improvement in these skills and an overall augmentation in social functioning. Therapists attempt to reframe these concerns by formulating them as dilemma and balance between enthusiastically contributing and listening.

STATUS OF THE RESEARCH

Much empirical work has examined problem-solving abilities, the relationship to psychopathology, and the impact treatment has on these (Malouff et al., 2007). Several reliable and valid measures of problem-solving attitudes and skills have been developed (see Chang et al., 2004, for a more thorough review). When used in conjunction with symptom evaluation, researchers and clinicians are able to specifically evaluate problem-solving skills in relation to psychiatric symptoms before and after the treatment. The Means-Ends Problem-Solving Test, most frequently used in inpatient settings, presents predetermined scenarios to measure ability to conceptualize the steps required to achieve a goal, the capacity to anticipate obstacles involved in goal achievement, and the appreciation that this task takes time for successful implementation (Gilbride & Hebert, 1980; Marx, Williams, & Claridge, 1992; Platt & Spivack, 1975; Schotte & Clum, 1982; Spivack, Shure, & Platt, 1985). Many early outcome studies utilized this assessment tool.

Another tool, the Social Problem-Solving Inventory—Revised, is a 52-item Likert-type inventory which assesses the five dimensions in the D'Zurilla social problem-solving model, including positive problem orientation, negative problem orientation, rational problem-solving skills, the impulsivity/carelessness style, and the avoidance style. A score on each of these dimensions is available to ascertain specific deficits in pre- and post-treatment assessment (D'Zurilla, Nezu, & Maydeu-Olivares, 2004). A 25-item short form is available, but no subscales scores can be obtained.

Compared with nonclinical populations, psychiatric populations are deficient in particular problem-solving abilities. Problem-solving training improves problem-solving abilities, often ameliorates symptomatology and thus has the potential to increase adaptive functioning and reduce the effects of stress. There is now a good deal of evidence that supports the efficacy of the problem-solving model in residential, inpatient, and partial programs, but most studies use an individual rather than group delivery format. Proponents of the model tout the versatility in delivering it in the individual and group format, although acknowledge that a group format may require an increased number of sessions (Nezu et al., 2012). We summarize evidence of its effectiveness in hospital and residential settings using a group format.

Acute Care Psychiatric Setting Studies

As detailed in our 1993 book (Brabender & Fallon, 1993), initial research on this model was based upon a closed-ended, eight-session group with mixed-gender, mixed-diagnostic populations in acute settings. In comparison with a supportive group treatment or no group treatment, patients from problem-solving groups had shorter hospital stays and improved their problem-solving skills (E. Coché & Douglas, 1977; D. Jones, 1981). Depressive symptoms, psychotic thinking, and impulsivity improved. Patients felt greater self-esteem and feelings of competence. Patients were less critical of themselves, less worried and frightened, and less dependent on other people, and they felt better able to handle the exigencies of everyday living than were patients in either more supportive groups or no-treatment groups. Although hospitalization alone improved capacity to generate relevant means (i.e., the sequence of steps to achieve an endpoint), participation in problem-solving groups additionally enhanced abilities to produce an even greater number of alternative solutions. Some evidence suggested that those who participated in the problem-solving group were more interested in and able to form and maintain interpersonal relationships. Those patients with more severe psychopathology made greater gains in problem-solving skills (E. Coché & Flick, 1975).

In comparison with other types of group models, there is some limited evidence that certain patients seem to profit more from problem-solving training. For example, men seem to gain more from problem-solving training, whereas women do better in interpersonal groups (E. Coché, Cooper, & Petermann, 1984). When separated by diagnostic category, schizophrenics showed greater gains with social interaction training, whereas depressed patients made greater progress with problem-solving training (Cohen, 1982).

A critical variable in these acute care inpatient studies is the number of sessions—with eight being the norm. When fewer sessions are provided, some problem-solving skills may improve, such as ability to generate relevant alternatives, and patients may have a more positive attitude about their ability to solve problems, but patients' perceptions of their problems and evidence that learned skills translate into more functional and adaptive behavior may not be present (Grey, 2007; D. Jones, 1981; Radcliffe & Bird, 2016).

Diagnostic and Symptom Groups

Patients With Schizophrenia

Although the problem-solving model aids patients with acute schizophrenic episodes, its efficacy with chronic and severe psychopathology has been more difficult to demonstrate (McLatchie, 1981). In longer term facilities, a more expanded version of problem solving has improved abilities to generate alternatives to a greater degree than control or other active treatments (Edelstein et al., 1980; Siegel & Spivack, 1976). This can take the form of increased number of sessions (11–24 sessions) for 80 to 90 minutes (e.g., Barbieri et al., 2006).

In a study with chronic PHP patients (twice a week for 15 sessions), patients were required to master each step before tackling the next (e.g., problem definition, generation of alternatives) instead of completing all the steps with a single problem (Hansen, St. Lawrence, & Christoff, 1985). Each step included instruction, rationale, modeling, behavioral rehearsal, feedback, and verbal reinforcement. This method effectively improved problem-solving abilities for these patients on trained situations and did generalize to novel situations. Improvement was largely maintained even at 4-month follow-up, although there was decreased retention of individual component steps.

Another approach is to structure the content of the session. Liberman et al. (2001) used videocassettes that demonstrated each problem-solving step. Fifteen specific scenarios then were presented by videotape. For example: "A disability recipient has not received her monthly check. She informs a clerk that her rent is past due and asks her to look into it. The clerk suggests that the check has probably been delayed in the mail and turns her attention to the next person in line" (p. 32). After some discussion of the steps and alternatives, videocassettes demonstrate poor and good examples of managing each interpersonal problem. Falloon, Barbieri, Boggian, and Lamonaca (2007) used a similar structured approach over 24 sessions, moving from simple, practical, everyday problems to more complex and emotionally charged interpersonal crises. Both studies yielded positive results in terms of improved problem solving and reduction in hospitalization. Including families in problem-solving training for the patient also improves outcomes (Calvo et al., 2014).

Patients With Depression

Meta-analyses reveal that problem-solving treatment for depression is as effective as other treatments and more effective than treatment as usual (Bell & D'Zurilla, 2009b; Cuijpers et al., 2007; Kirkham, Choi, & Seitz, 2016). Although this treatment is very promising, setting (inpatient, outpatient), format (group, individual), and psychiatric severity were not further delineated or compared. Most of the studies contributing to analyses had individual administration of problem-solving treatment, and most were community settings. When directly compared, the group format demonstrated larger effect sizes than the individual format; however, samples of patients with severe depression yielded small effect sizes (Cuijpers et al., 2007).

Patients With Personality Disorders

Patients with personality disorders have difficulties in problem solving, although specific deficits depend on the diagnostic cluster of symptoms. In particular, Cluster B patients score high on the impulsive/carelessness style, whereas Cluster C patients have a negative problem orientation (McMurran, Nezu, & Nezu, 2008). Stop & Think is a relatively new problem-solving program with emphasis on techniques to slow down the process of decision making (McMurran, Maguth Nezu, & Nezu, 2010; Nezu et al., 2012). Problem recognition includes learning that negative emotions are signals that a problem is present and a rational problem-solving approach is required.[7] A pilot program in a group format with criminal detainees revealed improvement in problem-solving skills (McMurran, Fyffe, McCarthy, Duggan, & Latham, 2001; McMurran et al., 2016). Male offenders also report that the training is helpful (McMurran & Wilmington, 2007). A larger study with community-based personality disorder patients utilizing a combination of nine group and three individual sessions showed significantly better social functioning at 6-month follow-up (Huband, McMurran, Evans, & Duggan, 2007).

Patients With Suicidality

Adults and children who have attempted suicide or have suicidal ideation also have been found to have defective problem-solving skills and inflexibility in their thinking (Patsiokas & Clum, 1985; Schotte & Clum, 1982). Meta-analyses have revealed that problem-solving treatment after deliberate self-harm improves depression, hopelessness, and social problems compared with treatment as usual (Townsend et al., 2001), but some of this effect may have been due to ongoing follow-up (Inagaki et al., 2015). Neither analysis differentiated IHP or RTC from outpatient, or group from individual formats. Adult IHP participants who attempt suicide do benefit even 3 months posttreatment from individual problem-solving treatment (Lerner, 1990; Salkovskis, Atha, & Storer, 1990). Likewise, children's problem-solving skills dramatically improve with individual problem-solving training (Cohen-Sandler, 1982). An IHP pilot program with group-based treatment for self-poisoning females (eight sessions of 2.5 hours each) was effective in reducing levels of depression, hopelessness, and suicidal ideation, and improved problem-solving skills (Bannan, 2010). Joiner, Voelz, and Rudd (2001) studied suicidal young adults with comorbid anxiety and depressive disorders in an intensive (10 days, 9 hours per day) structured group problem-solving therapy

---

[7]Six key questions are used to guide the process: Am I feeling bad? What's my problem? What do I want? What are my options? What is my plan? How am I doing?

in a PHP. Patients who received this treatment had symptom reduction and improved problem-solving skills compared with those that received treatment as usual.

Substance-Abuse Patients

Patients with drug and alcohol problems are deficient in problem-solving skills compared with normal individuals (Platt & Spivack, 1975). In our 1993 book we detailed four studies (three with inpatient/rehab alcoholics, one with incarcerated heroin addicts) who participated in homogeneous groups with 6 to 10 problem-solving sessions (Brabender & Fallon, 1993). All reported significant improvement in problem-solving skills at discharge and up to 1-year follow-up (Chaney, O'Leary, & Marlatt, 1978; S. L. Jones, Kanfer, & Lanyon, 1982; Platt et al., 1973). Since then only one additional study with mixed psychiatric and mixed substance abuse patients has been published. Although patients were able to learn problem-solving steps, they could not apply them to common social problems and were not more confident of their problem-solving skills at discharge (Carey, Carey, & Meisler, 1990). One major difference from previous studies was that the groups were not homogeneous, as encouraged by Platt and Spivack (1975). Unlike the previous studies, patients included polysubstance abuse as well as abuse of alcohol and cannabis. Psychiatric diagnosis also ranged from psychotic to mood disorder.

Patients Who Are Incarcerated

Individuals who are incarcerated have many problem-solving deficits (Antonowicz, 2005). Many offenders fail to think about the consequences of an action before they act and then fail to reflect back on their behavior after they act. Platt's earlier success with heroin addicts suggests that acquiring problem-solving skills will improve recidivism (Platt, Scura, & Hannon, 1973). The Reasoning and Rehabilitation program is an interpersonal problem-solving treatment specifically tailored to this population. In a Canadian sample of more than 4,000 offenders who completed this program, recidivism was reduced by 19% for violent offenders, 29% for drug offenders, and 39% for sex offenders (Robinson, 1995). Similarly, incarcerated juveniles in the state of Georgia had a rearrest rate of 39% after treatment compared with 75% of the control group (Antonowicz, 2005).

Problem Solving Across the Developmental and Intellectual Spectrum

Problem-solving skills develop early and continue a more nuanced development across the life span.

Problem Solving With Patients With Intellectual Disabilities

Because problem-solving training involves considerable cognitive processing, one reasonable question might be the extent to which an individual with less-than-average intelligence could benefit from this type of treatment. In a vocational training setting, individuals with mild to moderate intellectual disabilities do learn problem-solving skills and demonstrate greater problem-solving capacity and leadership capacity when given at least 14 to 15 group sessions compared with those who have not had the treatment (Benson, Rice, & Miranti, 1986; Castles & Glass, 1986). Those with mild disabilities improved more, although transfer of the skill to other social situations was limited (Castles & Glass, 1986).

Only one study has examined the effects of problem-solving training and assertiveness training on mildly cognitively impaired adults who also have both substance abuse and psychiatric diagnoses. When the five sessions of assertiveness training followed five sessions of problem-solving training, problem-solving skills improved, but there was no improvement when the format was reversed (Nezu et al., 1991). Both treatment conditions had increased levels of social functioning at posttreatment.

Problem Solving With Geriatric Patients

Many of the outcome studies have included a wide age range of adult patients up to 70 years of age, but small numbers did not allow a separate analysis (Brabender & Fallon, 1993). Toseland and Rose (1978) compared a role-playing (interpersonal skills training) group with a problem-solving group and a social work group in a nursing home population. They found that the role-playing and problem-solving groups showed significant gains compared with the social work group. This finding is consistent with the study demonstrating effectiveness with groups of older adults in outpatient problem-solving groups (Arean et al., 1993). In contrast, Mellinger (1989) found that five sessions were not sufficient to achieve improved problem-solving skills. The efficacy of problem-solving training with older adults is supported by a meta-analysis of problem-solving training with older adults who have major depressive disorders. Although not analyzed by setting or format, problem-solving training was effective in reducing depressions and decreasing disability (Kirkham et al., 2016).

Problem Solving With Children

Much of the original work on problem-solving training was designed to teach primary grade-school children a problem-solving style that could help them cope more successfully with their day-to-day problems (Spivack & Shure, 1974). This worked well with nonclinical populations in a large-group (e.g., classroom) format. Similarly, when antisocial inpatient children were given problem-solving training, relationship therapy, or treatment contact for 20 sessions, problem-solving training led to a decrease in externalizing and aggressive behavior at home and school immediately after discharge and 1 year later in comparison with the other treatment conditions (Kazdin, Esveldt-Dawson, French, & Unis, 1987).[8]

Emotionally disturbed preadolescent boys in an RTC were given group problem-solving training, interpersonal skill training, a combination of these two, or discussion only (Small & Schinke, 1983). Results indicated that boys in the combined problem-solving and interpersonal skill training conditions had better conceptual abilities and social behavior than did boys in the problem-solving training or discussion-only conditions. Similar positive results were obtained when children receiving 12 sessions of problem-solving training or another social-cognitive training approach (e.g., social perspective taking) were compared with those receiving a behavioral contingency approach without cognitive training (Urbain & Kendall, 1980). Results indicated that all three approaches led to increases in performance on the social-cognitive measures (e.g., problem-solving and perspective taking) but not on teacher ratings of socially impulsive behavior.

Problem Solving With Adolescents

The benefits of either direct didactic problem-solving training, a role-playing approach (videotaped role playing with corrective feedback), a combined didactic problem-solving and videotaped corrective feedback approach, or the making of a documentary film (attention-control group) for seven sessions (10.5 hours) were evaluated with a group of male adolescent offenders (Chudy, 1981). Results revealed that all three training groups were equally effective in improving the adolescent offenders' interpersonal problem-solving skills and decreasing their use of aggressive solutions. Follow-up indicated that training groups had a 10% recidivism rate compared with a 33% rate for the attention-control group.

Young incarcerated males with an identified suicidal risk received either five group sessions of problem solving or treatment as usual. Even with only brief exposure to problem solving, psychological distress decreased and offenders experienced enhanced perception of problem-solving abilities compared with those who received treatment as usual (Biggam & Power, 2002). This improvement was still evident at a 3-month follow-up. However, improvement in solution implementation and verification did not occur. Perhaps a greater number of sessions would have augmented these skills.

---

[8]Sessions 12 and 20 had an individual format.

In summary, problem-solving training has a more substantial base of empirical support for its efficacy within acute care settings and longer term RTCs than most models. Moreover, the benefits accrued from training have been shown to be maintained for at least some follow-up period. When the treatment has not been effective, it is unclear whether a specific modification in the procedure, such as an increased number of training sessions or more emphasis on the role-playing aspect, would have aided its efficacy (Youssef-Shalala, Ayres, Schubert, & Sweller, 2014).

CONTEXTUAL DEMANDS OF THE MODEL

Clinical Mission

The problem-solving model is grounded in the belief that psychiatric populations are deficient in problem-solving abilities. The use of this model is compatible with the mission of any setting that permits this skill to be taught and practiced. This model can coexist with almost any theoretical orientation. Its value may be most salient in a setting that endorses the interpersonal or biopsychosocial view of psychopathology; here, the acceptance of the notion that problem-solving deficits can lead to a reoccurrence of symptoms is natural. Treatment and support staff do not need to actively embrace this model, although its efficacy is likely to be enhanced in a setting wherein members are encouraged to complete homework or review material or suggestions made by the group. It can coexist with a strictly biological model of psychopathology. Problem-solving deficits do not need to be viewed as an essential component in the etiology of or recovery from symptoms; rather, the training could be viewed as an additional life enhancer (e.g., with an attitude such as "antidepressants will eliminate your symptoms of depression, but life would be easier if you had better problem-solving skills"). Settings holding a strong psychoanalytic orientation might regard the problem-solving approach as a Band-Aid solution. In its more behavioral form, its presence as part of the treatment may encourage affective suppression and may destroy the nurturing of a deeper understanding of one's difficulties, given that patients often prefer the easier, quicker solution. By suppressing areas of conflict, it may render a more intensive exploration in outpatient psychotherapy difficult.

Context of the Group

Groups using the problem-solving approach can coexist with any number of other activities and therapies. The versatility in the range of human problems that can be explored in the group is one of the strengths of this model. The group can focus on problems that members introduce, or it can focus on a particular problem such as discharge planning. Such a group is not constrained by where the patients reside. Although material from shared residential living can be brought to the group for exploration, the approach does not necessarily use that context as a source for material. If temporal requirements are met, this model can be used with IHP, PHP, and RTC patients.

This training can be used in conjunction with other types of psychosocial treatments. For example, it can be used either as a prelude to participating in another, more traditional inpatient group or concomitantly with another model of group therapy that may or may not have overlapping membership. Because it can also be used in combination with other techniques, it provides additional clinical armamentarium for therapists to aid patients (e.g., Benson et al., 1986; Pekala, Siegel, & Farrar, 1985). For example, Pekala et al. (1985) combined the problem-solving approach with a somewhat less-structured approach of the interpersonal model. In addition to teaching problem-solving skills and improving abilities to deal with interpersonal interactions, the combination helped members realize how they may have been contributing to their problems (insight), to recognize the universality of their feelings, and to enhance ego functioning vis-à-vis current problems. When problem-solving training is combined with other techniques, a number of outcome studies have suggested an increase in effectiveness (e.g., Kanfer & Busemeyer, 1982).

Temporal Variables

Stability of membership and the length of time required to complete the training are the factors that most limit the applicability of the problem-solving model. Research and clinical reports suggest that for a group in which the content is not prespecified, a minimum of six sessions is required and eight or more sessions are recommended. Within an acute care setting, given that the average length of hospitalization is less than 10 days, this is certainly a challenge. As severity of psychopathology increases, more sessions may be required. Most clinical and empirical reports support the use of a closed-ended group in an acute care setting for good reason. In groups wherein the content is dependent on what problems members choose to present, stability of membership is needed to free the group from addressing every member's concern. A closed-ended group allows for the possibility that a problem tabled one day can be scrutinized the next day. Even when the content is preordained, it takes more than a few sessions to understand and incorporate the problem-solving steps into members' everyday response repertoires to problems.

When the content is limited to a specific topic, or when the group works on hypothetical (but usually relevant) problems, the number of sessions may be reduced. However, without allowing members to apply the model directly to their particular problems, members' success in generalizing their learning to their own lives may be limited. Groups can be scheduled every day as long as the total number of sessions is achieved. Although closed-ended groups are not required, some stability of membership is highly recommended to obviate the need to review the problem-solving method in every session attended by a new member. Such a review of the process in its abstract form may not benefit and may even be tedious to those members who have already attended several sessions. As suggested in the clinical example, if admissions to the group are frequent, members should be involved in the explanation of the method. It is recommended that entrance to the group occur only once every four to five sessions. If the suggested length and stability requirements are met, short-term psychiatric facilities would not be able to support such a group given the frequency of turnover of patients. Thus, its utility may be largely limited to inpatient programs that are frequently admitting larger numbers of chronic individuals or residential and partial programs that are at least of 2 to 3 weeks duration.

Size of the Group

Clinical reports suggest that groups should have no fewer than three members and no more than 12 (e.g., Pekala et al., 1985). Most of the research that reports on groups in acute care setting have used groups with between four and 10 members (Brabender & Fallon, 1993). Studies with chronic patients tend to have groups with fewer members (around five; Edelstein et al., 1980; McLatchie, 1981). Patients were more active and gained more from the experience when they were placed in the smaller groups (E. Coché & Flick, 1975). In prison settings, a meta-analysis suggests that smaller groups are more effective (Antonowicz, 2005).

Composition of the Group

The problem-solving model offers tremendous latitude in terms of appropriate group composition. The approach can be used with all age groups—children (over 5 years old), adolescents, adults (18–70 years old), and geriatric patients. With the exception of the combination of both young and older adults, groups ideally should be composed of a single-age category because the problem-solving training in part is dependent on cognitive processing abilities. Moreover, the training for children who have a limited ability to think abstractly is different from that for adults who under normal circumstances are capable of formal operations. Similarly, individuals with intellectual disabilities can benefit from this training but should be placed in a group separate from those of average intelligence given that the procedure does require some modification. One group that has been systematically excluded from this model has been those individuals with severe memory impairment or other more severe organic brain impairments, including those receiving ECT.

Diagnostically, a tremendous range of patients benefits from problem-solving training. The modification of techniques required for the transition of use from one group to another is well articulated in the manuals available. This approach also has been used successfully with populations that are often considered difficult to treat, such as patients with acute psychosis and chronic schizophrenia, patients with impulsivity disorders, patients with suicidal ideation and depression, drug and alcohol addictions, patients with intellectual deficiency, and juvenile and adult offenders. In the previous section, we presented substantial empirical evidence for the model's efficacy in an inpatient group setting for both acute and long-term care, including its superiority over no treatment and it equivalency or superiority over other types of groups (e.g., social skills, supportive, nonstructured) for improving problem-solving skills.

Groups can be diagnostically homogeneous or heterogeneous. Effective groups have been conducted with mixed-gender, mixed-diagnostic composition, and mixed-adult age ranges. Some evidence suggests that patients may benefit from groups that are homogeneous with respect to chronicity and how longstanding and unremitting their symptoms are, although this is seldom an issue because facilities are often segregated along these lines (e.g., acute, chronic, and intermediate care). In addition, some research that we have discussed suggests that depressed patients may respond better to this model than to a social skills model, whereas chronic schizophrenics may respond better to a social skills model (Cohen, 1982). If individuals with different diagnoses have difficulties at different stages of problem solving, using diagnostically homogeneous groups might be advantageous (Marx et al., 1992). For example, violent offenders often have an impulsive problem-solving style, whereas those who are depressed may have an avoidant style. Segregating these groups would help the therapist to hone in on that stage of processing in which a particular diagnostic group is most deficient.

For some patient populations (e.g., those with borderline personality disorders and depression patients), the problem-solving model may ignore and suppress angry thoughts and aggressive behaviors. This approach may foster a defensive primitive idealization, particularly when the therapy is approached from a more behavioral orientation. With such an emphasis, the priority is not recognizing and understanding the member's aggression but rather encouraging an analysis of the problem in concrete and measurable terms. In a highly structured problem-solving program (appropriate for those with intellectual disabilities), it may be impossible for patients to learn to accept and manage what for them may be a central problem—the containment of their aggressive impulses (Swenson, 1989). As always, the treatment must be tailored to the diagnosis.

Therapist Variables

Leaders can work alone or in cotherapy pairs. The most ideal therapist is someone who has group dynamics training along with some background in cognitive behavior therapy. However, compared with other models, this model permits the use of relatively untrained personnel who may have limited theoretical knowledge about psychopathology or group dynamics. Young college graduates, graduate students, social workers, psychiatric aides, or even nonpsychology personnel (Rosenblum, 1983) can function as cotherapists; they can learn the model usually by reading literature in cognitive behavior modification and working as coleaders in a group with an experienced leader.

SUMMARY

The problem-solving model is a method of enhancing members' adjustments by increasing abilities and positive attitudes to address interpersonal problems. Its techniques are based on the assumptions that (a) psychiatric patients are deficient in problem-solving skills; (b) this deficiency in part is responsible for their psychological symptoms; and (c) problem-solving training will improve their abilities to function effectively in everyday life, increase self-esteem, and potentially attenuate their psychiatric symptoms. Leaders actively assess specific problem-solving skills, encourage hopeful and positive attitudes toward problem-solving, and impart a specific set of steps and techniques for members to learn and practice in the group setting. Members are assessed, given a general orientation and then are taught specific steps to follow after which they immediately begin to apply the techniques to either hypothetical problems or ones from their own lives. The steps include: aiding patients in recognizing one's problem orientation and style; presenting and clarifying the problem; generating alternatives; evaluating the alternatives; assessing steps of implementation role playing; and reporting back to the group at a later time their successes or failures with the particular solutions. Strong evidence exists that psychiatric patients are deficient in problem-solving skills. Moreover, a relationship between the severity of the psychopathology and deficiencies in interpersonal social skills and problem-solving has been fairly well-established. The evidence that a wide range of ages, diagnostic categories, and levels of intellectual functioning can benefit from this training is considerable.

The model can be used in a variety of settings and is minimally constrained by the clinical mission and theoretical orientation of the setting. Compared with other models in this book, much less training of the therapist is required, and the therapist is only minimally required to have a working knowledge of the cognitive behavior theoretical framework. The most limiting requirement of this model is the time that is necessary to have members recognize their problem-solving attitudes and styles, develop a positive orientation, and learn and practice the problem-solving technique. Overall, the model works best if the groups are closed-ended and last for at least six to eight sessions. Perhaps one of the most remarkable aspects of this model is that given its robust empirical base, it has received so little attention in the general group psychotherapy literature.

REFERENCES

Antonowicz, D. H. (2005). The Reasoning and Rehabilitation Program: Outcome evaluations with offenders. In M. McMurran & J. McGuire (Eds.), *Social problem-solving and offending* (pp. 163–181). Chichester, England: Wiley. http://dx.doi.org/10.1002/9780470713488.ch9

Arean, P. A., Perri, M. G., Nezu, A. M., Schein, R. L., Christopher, F., & Joseph, T. X. (1993). Comparative effectiveness of social problem-solving therapy and reminiscence therapy as treatments for depression in older adults. *Journal of Consulting and Clinical Psychology, 61*, 1003–1010. http://dx.doi.org/10.1037/0022-006X.61.6.1003

Bannan, N. (2010). Group-based problem-solving therapy in self-poisoning females: A pilot study. *Counselling & Psychotherapy Research, 10*, 201–213. http://dx.doi.org/10.1080/14733140903337292

Barbieri, L., Boggian, I., Falloon, I., Lamonaca, D., & the Centro Diurno 5 (CD5) collaborators. (2006). Innovations: Rehab rounds: Problem-solving skills for cognitive rehabilitation among persons with chronic psychotic disorders in Italy. *Psychiatric Services, 57*, 172–174. http://dx.doi.org/10.1176/appi.ps.57.2.172

Bedell, J. R., & Michael, D. D. (1988). Teaching problem-solving skills to chronic psychiatric patients. In D. Upper & S. M. Ross (Eds.), *Handbook of behavioral group therapy* (pp. 83–118). New York, NY: Plenum Press.

Bell, A. C., & D'Zurilla, T. (2009a). The influence of social problem solving ability on the relationship between daily stress and adjustment. *Cognitive Therapy Research, 33*, 439–448. http://dx.doi.org/10.1007/s10608-009-9256-8

Bell, A. C., & D'Zurilla, T. J. (2009b). Problem-solving therapy for depression: A meta-analysis. *Clinical Psychology Review, 29*, 348–353. http://dx.doi.org/10.1016/j.cpr.2009.02.003

Bellack, A. S., Morrison, R. L., Wixted, J. T., & Mueser, K. T. (1990). An analysis of social competence in schizophrenia. *The British Journal of Psychiatry, 156,* 809–818. http://dx.doi.org/10.1192/bjp.156.6.809

Bellack, A. S., Sayers, M., Mueser, K. T., & Bennett, M. (1994). Evaluation of social problem solving in schizophrenia. *Journal of Abnormal Psychology, 103,* 371–378. http://dx.doi.org/10.1037/0021-843X.103.2.371

Benson, B. A., Rice, C. J., & Miranti, S. V. (1986). Effects of anger management training with mentally retarded adults in group treatment. *Journal of Consulting and Clinical Psychology, 54,* 728–729. http://dx.doi.org/10.1037/0022-006X.54.5.728

Biggam, F. H., & Power, K. G. (2002). A controlled, problem-solving, group-based intervention with vulnerable incarcerated young offenders. *International Journal of Offender Therapy and Comparative Criminology, 46,* 678–698. http://dx.doi.org/10.1177/0306624X02238162

Brabender, V. (2002). *Introduction to group therapy.* New York, NY: Wiley.

Brabender, V., & Fallon, A. (1993). *Models of inpatient group psychotherapy.* Washington, DC: American Psychological Association. http://dx.doi.org/10.1037/10121-000

Calvo, A., Moreno, M., Ruiz-Sancho, A., Rapado-Castro, M., Moreno, C., Sánchez-Gutiérrez, T., . . . Mayoral, M. (2014). Intervention for adolescents with early-onset psychosis and their families: A randomized controlled trial. *Journal of the American Academy of Child & Adolescent Psychiatry, 53,* 688–696. http://dx.doi.org/10.1016/j.jaac.2014.04.004

Carey, M. P., Carey, K. B., & Meisler, A. W. (1990). Training mentally ill chemical abusers in social problem-solving. *Behavior Therapy, 21,* 511–519. http://dx.doi.org/10.1016/S0005-7894(05)80362-4

Castles, E. E., & Glass, C. R. (1986). Training in social and interpersonal problem-solving skills for mildly and moderately mentally retarded adults. *American Journal of Mental Deficiency, 91,* 35–42.

Chaney, E. F., O'Leary, M. R., & Marlatt, G. A. (1978). Skill training with alcoholics. *Journal of Consulting and Clinical Psychology, 46,* 1092–1104. http://dx.doi.org/10.1037/0022-006X.46.5.1092

Chang, E. C., D'Zurilla, T. J., & Sanna, L. J. (Eds.). (2004). *Social problem solving: Theory, research, and training.* Washington, DC: American Psychological Association. http://dx.doi.org/10.1037/10805-000

Chudy, J. F. (1981). *The effectiveness of integrated vs. independent training in interpersonal problem-solving and role-taking with juvenile delinquents* (Doctoral dissertation, University of Southern Mississippi). Available from ProQuest Dissertations and Theses Database.

Coché, E. (1987). Problem-solving training: A cognitive group therapy modality. In A. Freeman & V. Greenwood (Eds.), *Cognitive therapy: Applications in psychiatric and medical settings* (pp. 83–102). New York, NY: Human Sciences Press.

Coché, E., Cooper, J. B., & Petermann, K. J. (1984). Differential outcomes of cognitive and interactional group therapies. *Small Group Behavior, 15,* 497–509. http://dx.doi.org/10.1177/104649648401500404

Coché, E., & Douglas, A. A. (1977). Therapeutic effects of problem-solving training and play-reading groups. *Journal of Clinical Psychology, 33,* 820–827. http://dx.doi.org/10.1002/1097-4679(197707)33:3<820::AID-JCLP2270330345>3.0.CO;2-2

Coché, E., & Flick, A. (1975). Problem-solving training groups for hospitalized psychiatric patients. *The Journal of Psychology: Interdisciplinary and Applied, 91,* 19–29. http://dx.doi.org/10.1080/00223980.1975.9915793

Coché, J., & Coché, E. (1986). Group psychotherapy: The severely disturbed patient in hospital. *Carrier Foundation Letter, 113,* 1–6.

Cohen, S. R. (1982). A comparison of the effects of interpersonal problem solving training groups and social interaction training groups on hospitalized psychiatric patients. *Dissertation Abstracts International, 42,* 2981B.

Cohen-Sandler, R. (1982). *Interpersonal problem-solving skills of suicidal and nonsuicidal children: Assessment and treatment* (Doctoral dissertation, American University). Available from ProQuest Dissertations and Theses Database.

Cuijpers, P., van Straten, A., & Warmerdam, L. (2007). Problem solving therapies for depression: A meta-analysis. *European Psychiatry, 22,* 9–15. http://dx.doi.org/10.1016/j.eurpsy.2006.11.001

Dammann, G., Riemenschneider, A., Walter, M., Sollberger, D., Küchenhoff, J., Gündel, H., . . . Gremaud-Heitz, D. J. (2016). Impact of interpersonal problems in borderline personality disorder inpatients on treatment outcome and psychopathology. *Psychopathology, 49,* 172–180. http://dx.doi.org/10.1159/000446661

Davila, J., Hammen, C., Burge, D., Paley, B., & Daley, S. E. (1995). Poor interpersonal problem solving as a mechanism of stress generation in depression among adolescent women. *Journal of Abnormal Psychology, 104,* 592–600. http://dx.doi.org/10.1037/0021-843X.104.4.592

Douglas, M. S., & Mueser, K. T. (1990). Teaching conflict resolution to the chronically mentally ill: Social skills training groups for briefly hospitalized patients. *Behavior Modification, 14,* 519–547. http://dx.doi.org/10.1177/01454455900144007

D'Zurilla, T. J., & Goldfried, M. R. (1971). Problem solving and behavior modification. *Journal of Abnormal Psychology, 78,* 107–126. http://dx.doi.org/10.1037/h0031360

D'Zurilla, T. J., & Nezu, A. M. (2007). *Problem-solving therapy: A positive approach to clinical intervention* (3rd ed.). New York, NY: Springer.

D'Zurilla, T. J., & Nezu, A. M. (2010). Problem-solving therapy. In K. Dobson (Ed.), *Handbook of cognitive-behavioral therapies* (3rd ed.; pp. 197–225). New York, NY: Guilford Press.

D'Zurilla, T. J., Nezu, A. M., & Maydeu-Olivares, A. (2004). Social problem-solving: Theory and assessment. In E. C. Chang, T. J. D'Zurilla, & L. J. Sanna (Eds.), *Social problem solving: Theory, research, and training* (pp. 11–27). Washington, DC: American Psychological Association. http://dx.doi.org/10.1037/10805-001

Edelstein, B. A., Couture, E., Cray, M., Dickens, P., & Lusebrink, N. (1980). Group training of problem-solving with psychiatric patients. In D. Upper & S. M. Ross (Eds.), *Behavioral group therapy: An annual review* (pp. 85–102). Champaign, IL: Research Press.

Falloon, I. R. H., Barbieri, L., Boggian, I., & Lamonaca, D. (2007). Problem-solving training for schizophrenia: Rationale and review. *Journal of Mental Health, 16,* 553–568. http://dx.doi.org/10.1080/09638230701494910

Gilbride, T. V., & Hebert, J. (1980). Pathological characteristics of good and poor interpersonal problem-solvers among psychiatric outpatients. *Journal of Clinical Psychology, 36,* 121–127. http://dx.doi.org/10.1002/1097-4679(198001)36:1<121::AID-JCLP2270360110>3.0.CO;2-5

Goldfried, M. R., & Davison, G. (1976). *Clinical behavior therapy.* New York, NY: Holt, Rinehart & Winston.

Gotlib, I. H., & Asarnow, R. F. (1979). Interpersonal and impersonal problem-solving skills in mildly and clinically depressed university students. *Journal of Consulting and Clinical Psychology, 47,* 86–95. http://dx.doi.org/10.1037/0022-006X.47.1.86

Grey, S. J. (2007). A structured problem-solving group for psychiatric inpatients. *Groupwork: An Interdisciplinary Journal for Working with Groups, 17*(1), 20–33. http://dx.doi.org/10.1921/0951824X.17.1.20

Grover, K., Green, K., Pettit, J., Monteith, L., Garza, M., & Venta, A. (2009). Problem solving moderates the effects of life event stress and chronic stress on suicidal behaviors in adolescence. *Journal of Clinical Psychology, 65,* 1281–1290. https://dx.doi.org/10.1002/jclp.20632

Hansen, D. J., St. Lawrence, J. S., & Christoff, K. A. (1985). Effects of interpersonal problem-solving training with chronic aftercare patients on problem-solving component skills and effectiveness of solutions. *Journal of Consulting and Clinical Psychology, 53,* 167–174. http://dx.doi.org/10.1037/0022-006X.53.2.167

Huband, N., McMurran, M., Evans, C., & Duggan, C. (2007). Social problem-solving plus psychoeducation for adults with personality disorder: Pragmatic randomised controlled trial. *The British Journal of Psychiatry, 190,* 307–313. http://dx.doi.org/10.1192/bjp.bp.106.023341

Hussian, R. A. (1987). Problem-solving training and institutionalized elderly patients. In A. Freeman & V. Greenwood (Eds.), *Cognitive therapy: Applications in psychiatric and medical settings* (pp. 199–212). New York, NY: Human Sciences Press.

Hussian, R. A., & Lawrence, P. S. (1981). Social reinforcement of activity and problem-solving training in the treatment of depressed institutionalized elderly patients. *Cognitive Therapy and Research, 5,* 57–69. http://dx.doi.org/10.1007/BF01172326

Im-Bolter, N., Cohen, N. J., & Farnia, F. (2013). I thought we were good: Social cognition, figurative language, and adolescent psychopathology. *The Journal of Child Psychology and Psychiatry, 54,* 724–732. http://dx.doi.org/10.1111/jcpp.12067

Inagaki, M., Kawashima, Y., Kawanishi, C., Yonemoto, N., Sugimoto, T., Furuno, T., . . . Yamada, M. (2015). Interventions to prevent repeat suicidal behavior in patients admitted to an emergency department for a suicide attempt: A meta-analysis. *Journal of Affective Disorders, 175,* 66–78. http://dx.doi.org/10.1016/j.jad.2014.12.048

Joiner, T. E., Voelz, Z. R., & Rudd, M. D. (2001). For suicidal young adults with comorbid depressive and anxiety disorders, problem-solving treatment may be better than treatment as usual. *Professional Psychology: Research and Practice, 32,* 278–282. http://dx.doi.org/10.1037/0735-7028.32.3.278

Jones, D. E. (1981). Interpersonal cognitive problem-solving training: A skills approach with hospitalized psychiatric patients. *Dissertation Abstract International, 42,* 2060B.

Jones, S. L., Kanfer, R., & Lanyon, R. I. (1982). Skill training with alcoholics: A clinical extension. *Addictive Behaviors, 7,* 285–290. http://dx.doi.org/10.1016/0306-4603(82)90057-0

Kanfer, F. H., & Busemeyer, J. R. (1982). The use of problem solving and decision making in behavior therapy. *Clinical Psychology Review, 2,* 239–266. http://dx.doi.org/10.1016/0272-7358(82)90014-9

Kazdin, A. E., Esveldt-Dawson, K., French, N. H., & Unis, A. S. (1987). Problem-solving skills training and relationship therapy in the treatment of antisocial child behavior. *Journal of Consulting and Clinical Psychology, 55,* 76–85.

Kirkham, J. G., Choi, N., & Seitz, D. P. (2016). Meta-analysis of problem solving therapy for the treatment of major depressive disorder in older adults: Problem-solving therapy for depression. *International Journal of Geriatric Psychiatry, 31,* 526–535. http://dx.doi.org/10.1002/gps.4358

Leff, S. S., Crick, N. R., Angelucci, J., Haye, K., Jawad, A. F., Grossman, M., & Power, T. J. (2006). Social cognition in context: Validating a cartoon-based attributional measure for urban girls. *Child Development, 77,* 1351–1358. http://dx.doi.org/10.1111/j.1467-8624.2006.00939.x

Leff, S. S., Gullan, R. L., Paskewich, B. S., Abdul-Kabir, S., Jawad, A. F., Grossman, M., . . . Power, T. J. (2009). An initial evaluation of a culturally adapted social problem-solving and relational aggression prevention program for urban African-American relationally aggressive girls. *Journal of Prevention & Intervention in the Community, 37,* 260–274. http://dx.doi.org/10.1080/10852350903196274

Lerner, M. S. (1990). Treatment of suicide ideators: A problem-solving approach. *Dissertation Abstracts International, 51,* 435.

Levenson, M., & Neuringer, C. (1971). Problem-solving behavior in suicidal adolescents. *Journal of Consulting and Clinical Psychology, 37,* 433–436. http://dx.doi.org/10.1037/h0031985

Leykin, Y., Roberts, C. S., & DeRubeis, R. J. (2011). Decision-making and depressive symptomatology. *Cognitive Therapy and Research, 35,* 333–341. http://dx.doi.org/10.1007/s10608-010-9308-0

Liberman, R. P., Eckman, T. A., & Marder, S. R. (2001). Rehab rounds: Training in social problem solving among persons with schizophrenia. *Psychiatric Services, 52,* 31–33. http://dx.doi.org/10.1176/appi.ps.52.1.31

Linehan, M. (1987). Dialectical behavior therapy for borderline personality disorder: Theory and method. *Bulletin of the Menninger Clinic, 51*, 261–267.

Linehan, M., & Wagner, A. (1990). Dialectical behavior therapy: A feminist-behavioral treatment of borderline personality disorder. *Behavior Therapist, 13*, 9–14.

Loumidis, K. S., & Hill, A. (1997). Training social problem-solving skill to reduce maladaptive behaviours in intellectual disability groups: The influence of individual difference factors. *Journal of Applied Research in Intellectual Disabilities, 10*, 217–237. http://dx.doi.org/10.1111/j.1468-3148.1997.tb00018.x

Malouff, J. M., Thorsteinsson, E. B., & Schutte, N. S. (2007). The efficacy of problem solving therapy in reducing mental and physical health problems: A meta-analysis. *Clinical Psychology Review, 27*, 46–57. http://dx.doi.org/10.1016/j.cpr.2005.12.005

Marx, E. M., Williams, J. M., & Claridge, G. C. (1992). Depression and social problem solving. *Journal of Abnormal Psychology, 101*, 78–86. http://dx.doi.org/10.1037/0021-843X.101.1.78

McGuire, J. (2005). Social problem solving: Basic concepts, research, and applications. In M. McMurran & J. McGuire (Eds.), *Social problem solving and offending: Evidence, evaluation and evolution* (pp. 3–29). Chichester, England: Wiley.

McLatchie, L. R. (1981). *Interpersonal problem-solving group therapy: An evaluation of a potential method of social skills training for the chronic psychiatric patient* (Doctoral dissertation, The Pennsylvania State University). Available from ProQuest Dissertations and Theses Database.

McMurran, M., Crawford, M., Reilly, J., Delport, J., McCrone, P., Whitham, D., . . . Day, F. (2016). Psychoeducation in problem-solving (PEPS) therapy for adults with personality disorder: A pragmatic randomised controlled trial to determine the clinical effectiveness and cost-effectiveness of a manualised intervention to improve social functioning. *Health Technology Assessment, 20.* http://dx.doi.org/10.3310/hta20520

McMurran, M., Fyffe, S., McCarthy, L., Duggan, C., & Latham, A. (2001). "Stop & Think!": Social problem-solving therapy with personality-disordered offenders. *Criminal Behaviour and Mental Health, 11*, 273–285. http://dx.doi.org/10.1002/cbm.401

McMurran, M., Nezu, C., & Nezu, A. M. (2010). Problem-solving therapy for people with personality disorders. In C. Morgan & D. Bhugra (Eds.), *Principles of social psychiatry* (pp. 449–459). Chichester, England: John Wiley & Sons. http://dx.doi.org/10.1002/9780470684214.ch34

McMurran, M., Nezu, A., & Nezu, C. (2008). Problem solving therapy for people with personality disorders. *Mental Health Review, 13*, 35–39.

McMurran, M., & Wilmington, R. (2007). A Delphi survey of the views of adult male patients with personality disorders on psychoeducation and social problem-solving therapy. *Criminal Behaviour and Mental Health, 17*, 293–299. http://dx.doi.org/10.1002/cbm.663

Meichenbaum, D., & Goodman, J. (1971). Training impulsive children to talk to themselves: A means of developing self-control. *Journal of Abnormal Psychology, 77,* 115–126.

Mellinger, D. J. (1989). *Problem-solving orientation in nursing home residents: An intervention featuring the recognition of choice and perceived control* (Doctoral dissertation, Antioch New England Graduate School). Available from ProQuest Dissertations and Theses Database.

Nezu, A. (1980). Component analyses of three stages of the social problem solving training model. *Dissertation Abstracts International, 40,* 929B.

Nezu, A. M. (1986). Efficacy of a social problem-solving therapy approach for unipolar depression. *Journal of Consulting and Clinical Psychology, 54,* 196–202. http://dx.doi.org/10.1037/0022-006X.54.2.196

Nezu, A. M., Nezu, C. M., & D'Zurilla, T., (2012). *Problem-solving therapy: A treatment manual.* New York, NY: Springer.

Nezu, A. M., & Perri, M. G. (1989). Social problem-solving therapy for unipolar depression: An initial dismantling investigation. *Journal of Consulting and Clinical Psychology, 57,* 408–413. http://dx.doi.org/10.1037/0022-006X.57.3.408

Nezu, A. M., Wilkins, V. M., & Nezu, C. M. (2004). Social problem-solving, stress, and negative affect. In E. C. Chang, T. J. D'Zurilla, & L. J. Sanna (Eds.), *Social problem-solving* (pp. 49–65). Washington, DC: American Psychological Association.

Nezu, C. M., Nezu, A. M., & Arean, P. (1991). Assertiveness and problem-solving training for mildly mentally retarded persons with dual diagnoses. *Research in Developmental Disabilities, 12,* 371–386. http://dx.doi.org/10.1016/0891-4222(91)90033-O

Osborn, A. F. (1963). *Applied imagination: Principles and procedures of creative problem-solving* (3rd ed.). New York, NY: Scribner's.

Patsiokas, A. T., & Clum, G. A. (1985). Effects of psychotherapeutic strategies in the treatment of suicide attempters. *Psychotherapy: Theory, Research, Practice, Training, 22,* 281–290. http://dx.doi.org/10.1037/h0085507

Pekala, R. J., Siegel, J. M., & Farrar, D. M. (1985). The problem-solving support group: Structured group therapy with psychiatric inpatients. *International Journal of Group Psychotherapy, 35,* 391–409. http://dx.doi.org/10.1080/00207284.1985.11491424

Platt, J. J., Scura, W. C., & Hannon, J. R. (1973). Problem-solving thinking of youthful incarcerated heroin addicts. *Journal of Community Psychology, 1,* 278–281. http://dx.doi.org/10.1002/1520-6629(197307)1:3<278::AID-JCOP2290010307>3.0.CO;2-I

Platt, J. J., Siegel, J. M., & Spivack, G. (1975). Do psychiatric patients and normals see the same solutions as effective in solving interpersonal problems? *Journal of Consulting and Clinical Psychology, 43,* 279. http://dx.doi.org/10.1037/h0076518

Platt, J. J., & Spivack, G. (1972a). Problem-solving thinking of psychiatric patients. *Journal of Consulting and Clinical Psychology, 39,* 148–151. http://dx.doi.org/10.1037/h0033211

Platt, J. J., & Spivack, G. (1972b). Social competence and effective problem-solving thinking in psychiatric patients. *Journal of Clinical Psychology, 28,* 3–5. http://dx.doi.org/10.1002/1097-4679(197201)28:1<3::AID-JCLP2270280102>3.0.CO;2-R

Platt, J. J., & Spivack, G. (1974). Means of solving real-life problems: I. Psychiatric patients vs. controls and cross-cultural comparisons of normal females. *Journal of Community Psychology, 2,* 45–48. http://dx.doi.org/10.1002/1520-6629(197401)2:1<45::AID-JCOP2290020117>3.0.CO;2-X

Platt, J. J., & Spivack, G. (1975). *Means-ends problem-solving procedure (MEPS): A measure of interpersonal cognitive problem-solving skill.* Philadelphia, PA: Department of Mental Health Science, Hahneman Medical College & Hospital.

Platt, J. J., Spivack, G., Altman, N., Altman, D., & Peizer, S. B. (1974). Adolescent problem-solving thinking. *Journal of Consulting and Clinical Psychology, 42,* 787–793. http://dx.doi.org/10.1037/h0037564

Pollack, L. E. (1991). Problem-solving group therapy: Two inpatient models based on level of functioning. *Issues in Mental Health Nursing, 12,* 65–80. http://dx.doi.org/10.3109/01612849109058210

Radcliffe, J., & Bird, L. (2016). Talking therapy groups on acute psychiatric wards: Patients' experience of two structured group formats. *BJPsych Bulletin, 40,* 187–191. http://dx.doi.org/10.1192/pb.bp.114.047274

Raeff, C., & Benson, J. B. (2003). *Social and cognitive development in the context of individual, social, and cultural processes.* London: Routledge.

Richard, B. A., & Dodge, K. A. (1982). Social maladjustment and problem solving in school-aged children. *Journal of Consulting and Clinical Psychology, 50,* 226–233. http://dx.doi.org/10.1037/0022-006X.50.2.226

Robinson, D. (1995). *The impact of cognitive skills training on post-release recidivism among Canadian federal offenders* (Research Report No. R-41). Ottawa, Canada: The Correctional Service of Canada. Retrieved from http://www.csc-scc.gc.ca/research/092/r41e_e.pdf

Rosenblum, B. (1983). ROSEBUD: An interpersonal problem-solving enhancement program for kindergarteners. A primary prevention mental health program. *Dissertation Abstracts International, 23,* 2565A.

Rubin, K. H., & Rose-Krasnor, L. (1992). Interpersonal problem solving and social competence in children. In V. B. Van Hasselt & M. Hersen (Eds.), *Handbook of social development: Perspectives in developmental psychology* (pp. 283–323). Boston, MA: Springer. http://dx.doi.org/10.1007/978-1-4899-0694-6_12

Salkovskis, P. M., Atha, C., & Storer, D. (1990). Cognitive-behavioural problem solving in the treatment of patients who repeatedly attempt suicide: A controlled trial. *The British Journal of Psychiatry, 157,* 871–876. http://dx.doi.org/10.1192/bjp.157.6.871

Schotte, D. E., & Clum, G. A. (1982). Suicide ideation in a college population: A test of a model. *Journal of Consulting and Clinical Psychology, 50*, 690–696. http://dx.doi.org/10.1037/0022-006X.50.5.690

Shure, M. B. (1997). Interpersonal cognitive problem solving: Primary prevention of early high-risk behaviors in the preschool and primary years. In G. W. Albee & T. P. Gullotta (Eds.), *Primary prevention works* (pp. 167–188). Thousand Oaks, CA: Sage. http://dx.doi.org/10.4135/9781452243801.n8

Shure, M. B., & Spivack, G. (1972). Means–ends thinking, adjustment, and social class among elementary-school-aged children. *Journal of Consulting and Clinical Psychology, 38*, 348–353. http://dx.doi.org/10.1037/h0032919

Shure, M. B., & Spivack, G. (1982). Interpersonal problem-solving in young children: A cognitive approach to prevention. *American Journal of Community Psychology, 10*, 341–356. http://dx.doi.org/10.1007/BF00896500

Shure, M. B., Spivack, G., & Jaeger, M. (1971). Problem-solving thinking and adjustment among disadvantaged preschool children. *Child Development, 42*, 1791–1803. http://dx.doi.org/10.2307/1127585

Siegel, J. M., Platt, J. J., & Peizer, S. B. (1976). Emotional and social real-life problem-solving thinking in adolescent and adult psychiatric patients. *Journal of Clinical Psychology, 32*, 230–232. http://dx.doi.org/10.1002/1097-4679(197604)32:2<230::AID-JCLP2270320205>3.0.CO;2-2

Siegel, J. M., & Spivack, G. (1976). Problem solving therapy: The description of a new program for chronic psychiatric patients. *Psychotherapy: Theory, Research and Practice, 13*, 368–373.

Small, R. W., & Schinke, S. P. (1983). Teaching competence in residential group care: Cognitive problem solving and interpersonal skills training with emotionally disturbed preadolescents. *Journal of Social Service Research, 7*, 1–16. http://dx.doi.org/10.1300/J079v07n01_01

Spivack, G. (1984). *Interpersonal cognitive problem-solving, mental health and prevention: An annotated bibliography.* Unpublished manuscript.

Spivack, G., & Levine, M. (1963). *Self-regulation in acting-out and normal adolescents* (Report No. M-4531). Washington, DC: National Institutes of Health.

Spivack, G., Platt, J. J., & Shure, M. B. (1976). *The problem-solving approach to adjustment.* San Francisco, CA: Jossey-Bass.

Spivack, G., & Shure, M. B. (1974). *Social adjustment of young children.* San Francisco, CA: Jossey-Bass.

Spivack, G., Shure, M. B., & Platt, J. J. (1985). *Means-ends problem-solving (MEPS): Stimuli and scoring procedures supplement.* Philadelphia, PA: Department of Mental Health Sciences, Hahneman Medical College.

Swenson, C. (1989). Kernberg and Linehan: Two approaches to the borderline patient. *Journal of Personality Disorders, 3*, 26–35. http://dx.doi.org/10.1521/pedi.1989.3.1.26

Tannenbaum, M. (1991). *Social-cognitive therapy for children* (Unpublished doctoral dissertation). Institute for Graduate Clinical Psychology of Widener University, Chester, PA.

Tarrier, N., Beckett, R., Harwood, S., Baker, A., Yusupoff, L., & Ugarteburu, I. (1993). A trial of two cognitive-behavioural methods of treating drug-resistant residual psychotic symptoms in schizophrenic patients: I. Outcome. *The British Journal of Psychiatry, 162*, 524–532. http://dx.doi.org/10.1192/bjp.162.4.524

Thoma, P., Friedmann, C., & Suchan, B. (2013). Empathy and social problem solving in alcohol dependence, mood disorders and selected personality disorders. *Neuroscience and Biobehavioral Reviews, 37*, 448–470. http://dx.doi.org/10.1016/j.neubiorev.2013.01.024

Toseland, R., & Rose, S. D. (1978). A social skills training program for older adults: Evaluation of three group approaches. *Social Work Research Abstracts, 14*, 873–874.

Townsend, E., Hawton, K., Altman, D. G., Arensman, E., Gunnell, D., Hazell, P., . . . Van Heeringen, K. (2001). The efficacy of problem-solving treatments after deliberate self-harm: Meta-analysis of randomized controlled trials with respect to depression, hopelessness and improvement in problems. *Psychological Medicine, 31*, 979–988. http://dx.doi.org/10.1017/S0033291701004238

Urbain, E. S., & Kendall, P. C. (1980). Review of social-cognitive problem-solving interventions with children. *Psychological Bulletin, 88*, 109–143. http://dx.doi.org/10.1037/0033-2909.88.1.109

Wessler, R., & Hankin-Wessler, S. (1989). Cognitive group therapy. In A. Freeman, K. M. Simon, L. E. Beutler, & H. Arkowitz (Eds.), *Comprehensive handbook of cognitive therapy* (pp. 196–223). New York, NY: Plenum Press. http://dx.doi.org/10.1007/978-1-4757-9779-4_28

Wilhelm, K., Siegel, J. E., Finch, A. W., Hadzi-Pavlovic, D., Mitchell, P. B., Parker, G., & Schofield, P. R. (2007). The long and the short of it: Associations between 5-HTT genotypes and coping with stress. *Psychosomatic Medicine, 69*, 614–620. http://dx.doi.org/10.1097/PSY.0b013e31814cec64

Youssef-Shalala, A., Ayres, P., Schubert, C., & Sweller, J. (2014). Using a general problem-solving strategy to promote transfer. *Journal of Experimental Psychology: Applied, 20*, 215–231. http://dx.doi.org/10.1037/xap0000021

8

THE BEHAVIORAL MODEL: SOCIAL SKILLS TRAINING

Behavioral therapy is an approach that has evolved considerably over its history. Since its development, many factions have formed based on philosophical, theoretical, and technical differences with one another. Use of the group format by behavioral therapists led to further splintering, resulting in the generation of many variations in the technical application of the model. This diversity has left the behavioral therapists struggling to find identity and to articulate characteristic features that are common to their many variations. Nonetheless, the behavioral family of group models offers a plenitude of techniques that aim to change a particular set of behaviors. This model, in all its myriad forms, is unique in its emphatic commitment to empirical methods as the crucible for successful treatment. In this chapter, we highlight a particular version of the behavioral model, social skills training, which is applicable to a wide range of inpatient hospital program (IHP), partial hospital program (PHP), and residential treatment center (RTC) patients,

http://dx.doi.org/10.1037/0000113-009
Group Psychotherapy in Inpatient, Partial Hospital, and Residential Care Settings, by V. Brabender and A. Fallon

but particularly to those who have more severe and chronic psychopathology such as schizophrenia. The basic premise of social skills training is that adjustment to life in the community is predicated on an individual's psychosocial functioning, which social skills training can enhance (Kurtz & Mueser, 2008; Mueser & Bellack, 2007).

THEORETICAL UNDERPINNINGS

Relation of Behaviorism to Learning Theory and Behavioral Therapy

Behavioral models of group psychotherapy come out of a rich theoretical tradition.

Levels of Analysis

Behaviorism, learning theory, and behavior therapy are not synonymous terms; rather, they represent three separate levels of analysis. First, behaviorism is most generally a philosophy of science, which carries with it a philosophy of the mind, specific assumptions about human nature, and a set of values and goals concerning the pursuit and evaluation of scientific activity, including objectivity and empiricism (Zuriff, 1985). Second, learning theory draws upon philosophical assumptions about human nature to develop principles describing how organisms learn, modify, and extinguish behaviors. Classical conditioning and operant conditioning are examples of theories that attempt to explain and predict observable phenomena. Third, behavior therapy is associated with a methodology and set of techniques that are aimed at changing certain behaviors in identifiable and predictable ways. In summary, behavioral therapists' clinical practice is informed by theoretical proclivities. The philosophical lens by which they view human behavior, in turn, determines their conceptual leanings. Although this notion applies to all of the therapy models described in this book, it is particularly central to the behavioral family of models, given that variation in behavioral approaches is rooted in the different philosophical shadings within behaviorism.

Types of Behaviorism

Watson (1924) defined *behaviorism*, which originally began as a movement in opposition to introspection, as the study of muscle movements and glandular secretions. Mental events such as thoughts or feelings were not seen as the purview of psychology because no public agreement as to their occurrence could be achieved (Watson, 1924). This philosophy became known as *metaphysical behaviorism* and is reflected in the early writings of Wolpe (1958) and his use of desensitization in a group setting, and in the current practice of social skills training, which emphasizes observable behaviors. Skinner (1974) also rejected the idea that cognitions and emotions were necessary to the prediction and control of behavior; however, his reasoning was based on the notion that those contingencies that give rise to feelings or cognitions are isomorphic to those that produce the concomitant behaviors. Thus, for Skinner, the focus in theory and clinical practice should be on observable behaviors rather than on an individual's emotions or cognitions. Skinner's philosophy, known as *radical behaviorism*, also deviated from the metaphysical philosophy in that behavior was seen as an interaction between the organism and its environment. In a contemporary radical behaviorism, context continues to assume a central focus. Unlike Skinner's radical behaviorism, some contemporary radical behaviorists, known as *contextual behaviorists*, see cognitions as having a legitimate status in determining behavior (Hayes, 2016). They argue that the cognitive/social history of an individual influences overt behavior in a manner that cannot be predicted simply by knowing the history of reinforcement with the stimulus event. (For example, a man's response to a woman might be influenced not only by his direct experiences with previous women but also by what verbal rules he has learned in the social context without direct experience.) Thus, metaphysical, radical, and contextual behaviorists agree on the acceptable method of study (the empirical method) but vary on the unit of study (e.g., public versus private behavior; overt mechanistic units of behavior versus behavior and its context; observable behavior versus cognition or verbalization).

Watson (1924) is also known for a method he developed for studying behavior, which has come to be known as *methodological behaviorism*. This form of behaviorism is commonly regarded as the *sine qua non* of behavioral therapy. It claims that science can study only public (observable) events; private events such as thoughts and feelings are unsuitable targets of inquiry. Over time, however, contemporary methodological behaviorists have attempted to address cognition and emotion by conceding that the scientifically analyzable world must be used to make inferences about what is scientifically unanalyzable. Although thoughts cannot be seen directly, their influence on other types of human behavior can be observed and measured. For example, cognitive mastery of a task improves the efficacy of behavioral rehearsal and modeling techniques (Mahoney & Kazdin, 1979). Although they might not necessarily label themselves methodological behaviorists, most group behavioral therapists, including those practicing in IHPs, PHPs, and RTCs, are influenced by this philosophical tradition. Therapists might vary on the particular behavioral unit they believe worthy of study, but they all agree on the acceptable method of study, namely, the empirical method.

Common Features of Behavioral Approaches

Contemporary behavioral therapy is based on a broad set of theoretical and methodological assumptions and principles rather than either a unitary theoretical framework or a fixed set of techniques. It is a therapy in which theory and practice are complementary and scientific rigor and clinical acumen are interwoven. The central features common to most types of behavioral therapy include an emphasis on (a) an empirical orientation, (b) a behavioral focus, (c) an action orientation, (d) environmental factors, (e) an ahistorical focus, and (f) an ideographic approach (Wixted, Bellack, & Hersen, 1990).

Empirical Orientation

The nexus of all behavioral approaches is an empirical orientation, which entails the application of findings and principles derived from experimental and social psychological research to the design of the treatment. Basic research in psychology serves as a source of hypotheses about the efficacy of various techniques. The criterion for acceptability of a particular intervention is that it has been found to be effective on the basis of empirical validation rather than clinical intuition or general impression.

Behavioral therapy involves the systematic application of experimentally confirmed techniques within a setting that uses an empirical framework. Such an approach encourages the generation of hypotheses related to the nature of the problem behavior, the use of techniques most suitable to ameliorate the problem behavior, and the collection of data relevant to evaluating the utility of these interventions for treating the patient's identified problems. Although all psychotherapy models adopt a set of hypotheses regarding a theory of the nature of abnormal behavior, it is the use of these hypotheses in an experimental paradigm that distinguishes the behavioral model from many other approaches. In this model, problems are clearly delineated and operationally defined. Interventions are concretized and systematically applied, and thus can be reproduced (Flowers, 1979). In the behavioral approaches, the evaluation of the efficacy of the intervention is specified in objective and measurable terms, with an emphasis on overt change as the main criterion (although some meditational variables [e.g., attributions] are considered acceptable).

Focus on Behavior

Related to the model's empirical foundation and consistent with the philosophy of behaviorism is the focus on behavior rather than underlying causes or traits. Whereas traits are only inferred, behaviors are directly observed. Whereas traits are general, behaviors capture the individuality of the person (Spiegler, 2016). Many psychotherapy models assume that human response (including behavior, cognition, and affect) can be changed through a process of unlearning or relearning. The particular form that this learning process takes depends on the type of therapy model selected. It is a commonly held belief that behavioral therapists use only learning theory that contains a concomitant empirical methodology as a conceptual basis for intervention and change (Flowers, 1979). Although this view is not incorrect, other theoretical frameworks affect contemporary behavioral applications (Hollander & Kazaoka, 1988).

At one time, therapists thought that most manifestations of maladaptive behavior were either the failure of the individual to learn adaptive coping skills or the sometimes accidental acquisition of unacceptable and often self-defeating behaviors. Nowadays, however, most behavioral therapists accept biological contributions to abnormal behavior. Still, how symptoms are acquired is less relevant to treatment than the symptoms themselves because the empirical method cannot easily be applied to a retrospective analysis, one cannot be entirely sure of causality, and even knowing the cause of maladaptive behaviors does not necessarily lead to effective treatment.

Maladaptive behaviors can be categorized as (a) behavioral excesses, (b) behavioral deficits, or (c) behavior under inappropriate stimulus control (Hollander & Kazaoka, 1988). Behavioral excesses are those behaviors that in isolation are not unacceptable but become so when used to an extreme degree. These behaviors can interrupt the individual's routine (e.g., frequent checking of the stove interfering with leaving the house) and engender discomfort in others (as in the case of an individual who frequently exhibits aggressive behavior). Individuals exhibit behavioral deficits when they are unable to perform a behavior that would be appropriate in a situation (e.g., acts of self-assertion). Behaviors under inappropriate stimulus control are not deemed abnormal in isolation. They are maladaptive when they work to the person's detriment in specific circumstances. For instance, a person's attempt to acquire emotional support is not abnormal; the individual seeking sexual interaction via sexting with strangers places him or herself in peril. Behavior therapy aims to increase an individual's flexibility by enabling him or her to select responses from a broad repertoire that are adaptive within a particular environment context (Antony & Roemer, 2011).

Action Orientation

Behaviorists believe that behavioral changes occur by actively practicing newly targeted behaviors or by being exposed to critical cues (Antony & Roemer, 2011). Behavioral change is accomplished by rehearsing appropriate behaviors in the session followed by in vivo practice (i.e., homework). A consequence of the emphasis on activity is a need for the therapist to be directive within the treatment (Antony & Roemer, 2011) such that the therapist structures the patient's activities or behaviors.

Environmental Factors: Antecedents and Consequences

The behavioral approach emphasizes the study of the environmental factors and behavior–environment interaction, which are seen as playing an essential function in shaping and maintaining behavior. A systematic assessment of the behavior in its context is then made to assess whether a behavior is adaptive. This process involves a study of the interactions among antecedents, behaviors, and consequences. The antecedents determine under what circumstances certain target responses occur; they are identified by systematic study of the factors that exist each time the objectionable behaviors occur. The evaluation of consequences is also important in clinical assessment because such consequences strengthen, weaken, or maintain previously acquired behaviors.

Ahistorical Focus

The focus is on the individual's current focus and contemporary factors rather than historical ones. The critical factors involved in producing dysfunctional behaviors are not assumed to be the same factors that maintain behavior. A child with autism, for example, might be taught to speak using operant methods (Kodak & Grow, 2011), but behavioral therapists would not claim that autism is caused by operant factors. This ahistorical focus and the belief that an individual's problems are subject to the same processes that influence normal behavior help attenuate the potential for problems to be viewed as manifestations of intrapsychic disease.

An Ideographic Approach

Traditionally, the emphasis in this model is on the prominent features of each individual case rather than nosological labels (Eifert, 1996). This individually centered approach applies to both assessment and treatment. From the perspective of assessment, behavioral therapists are concerned more with how an individual acts in a situation than with his or her diagnosis. Such labels are often of little value, behaviorists hold, in correcting or remediating specific skill deficiencies, or even in identifying what the relevant behaviors are. For instance, if an individual is described as depressed, one does not know if that means that the individual is socially isolated, does not make eye contact, does not groom, and so on.

From a treatment standpoint, the multitude of behavioral techniques liberate the therapist from using a single method for all problems (Bandura,

1979, p. 89) with every problem. For example, whereas with a chronic hospitalized schizophrenic individual, the therapist might set up a token economy to increase the patient's social contact on the unit, a less-regressed psychotic person might receive social skills training to foster more appropriate social interaction. Despite the advantages of this ideographic approach, some behavioral therapists hold that the availability of manualized approaches for many processes creates the potential for integration of the ideographic with more nomothetic (group-based) approaches (Eifert, 1996).

BEHAVIORAL THERAPY IN A GROUP SETTING

The extent to which behavioral therapists focus on the unique properties of the group varies considerably from a lack of interest at the one end of the continuum to a significant investment in them at the other. Those practitioners with the least interest in group process apply the same behavioral principles and technical interventions used in an individual format. The trend of applying behavioral interventions to groups can be seen in the extension of behavioral techniques such as assertion training or social skills training to IHP, PHP, and RTC groups. This application often is motivated by the pragmatic effort to conserve resources (economic or personnel). These groups often do not use member–member interactions to promote change, are generally more didactic, have a structured format, and have patients with homogeneous target problems and similar treatment goals. Goals for these kinds of groups often center on issues of self-management and solving practical problems that emerge in social contexts. For example, Kern, Glynn, Horan, and Marder (2009) described the use of groups as a venue for schizophrenic individuals to practice skills, such as those associated with attention and memory, acquired in cognitive enhancement therapy (Hogarty et al., 2004). Initially, the patient might perform individual computer-based work, and then he or she might transition to using the cognitive skills in a group setting.

In contrast, those practitioners showing a keen interest in group factors view the group format as offering a unique context for the modification of behaviors that might not otherwise occur or at the very least would be difficult to change in an individual therapy context. Associated with this perspective is the importance of the group setting (i.e., group structure and group process) as a vehicle of change. At the same time, this view pays homage to the essence of behavioral methodology. Group process is empirically defined as the changes over time in observable and measurable elements of the environment (including member-to-member interaction) that affect members' behaviors.

Learning Mechanisms and Group Psychotherapy

Clinicians pragmatically approach the behavioral group from an empirical and applied perspective (Hollander & Kazaoka, 1988). Behavioral group therapists regard principles of learning as the core of its intervention strategies in this treatment (Antony & Roemer, 2011). The operant conditioning approach is based on the notion that the frequency or intensity of a response will increase if it is followed by a reinforcing event and will decrease if it is followed by no reinforcement or punishment (Domjan, 2015).

The classical conditioning approach, a more useful intervention when attempting to change maladaptive emotional reactions such as fear or anger, is based on the theoretical assumption that a negative emotional response is acquired when an originally neutral stimulus becomes associated with an unpleasant experience. When an originally neutral object is presented, it elicits the emotional response as if the original unpleasant experience were going to take place. Systematic desensitization is a technique that uses this notion of classical conditioning in its treatment of fear or anxiety. In his theory of reciprocal inhibition, Wolpe (1958) put forth the idea that if the feared stimulus (e.g., a crowd of people) is paired with the fear's opposite, that is, relaxation, the strength of the original conditioning process will gradually lessen and the emotional response extinguish.

Mechanisms of Change

Behavioral group therapists range in their views of the mechanisms responsible for change depending on whether they emphasize the nonmediational and mechanistic bases of behavior or higher order constructs such as expectancies. In either case, the primary causal factors are the individual's transactions with the environment rather than personality traits. Behavioral group therapists predicate their interventions on traditional learning theory and social learning theory's postulates. What social learning theory adds to traditional learning theory is the notion that learning can occur indirectly through vicarious or observation experiences as well as through direct behavioral experiences and that individual behavior (and change) is a result of ongoing reciprocal interactions between the environment and the individual's behavioral and cognitive processes. This "reciprocal determinism" (Bandura, 1978, p. 384)—the notion that individuals act on their environment, which in turn influences the individual in an interactive loop—crucially affects the interventions of the behavioral group therapist. Learning and change occur when new behaviors are acquired or when existing responses are modified. The change process is enhanced by the patient's engagement in a self-observation process (by way of self-monitoring). The importance of the group context is that members provide one another with both examples of new appropriate behaviors (vicarious learning) and valued feedback and reinforcements.

Although many behavioral group therapists believe that cognitive change is important in therapeutic change, most view cognitive techniques alone as less efficacious in facilitating change. Furthermore, cognition is considered to be either isomorphic to behavioral change (Skinner, 1974) or simply one part of the behavior–cognition–environment loop in which none of these components is primary (Arkowitz & Hannah, 1989). Similarly, affective arousal is viewed as a phenomenon to be changed rather than as a mediator of behavioral change as it is in the more psychoanalytically based models (see Chapter 4, this volume). In fact, a basic assumption of the behavioral models is that the subjective experience of an emotion follows the acquisition of a targeted behavioral manifestation of the emotion (Mueser, Wallace, & Liberman, 1995). Although some believe that change in behavior must be accompanied by affective arousal (e.g., Arkowitz & Hannah, 1989), most proponents of the behavioral model regard teaching the demonstrable and measurable behaviors of affective expression as a more efficient means of fostering emotional change. In fact, evidence suggests that behavioral manifestations of one's ability to manage interpersonal exchange is highly correlated with aspects of intrapsychic functioning such as motivation, curiosity, and sense of humor (Bellack, Morrison, Wixted, & Mueser, 1990). Such findings support the emphasis on providing the patient with new behavioral experiences to modify behavior with the expectation that positive inner life changes (e.g., higher self-esteem) will follow.

Goals of Treatment

Behavioral group therapy is most noted for the treatment of problems that involve troubled interactions with others. Even so, proponents of this model believe that most target symptoms amenable to individual behavioral therapy are equally suitable for treatment in the group setting (Hollander & Kazaoka, 1988). In fact, the group environment is regarded as more desirable because even problems seeming to have little to do with social interaction (e.g., snake phobia) often have a social aspect to their maintenance that is likely to remain unnoticed in an individual therapy setting.

A central feature of this model is its emphasis on the therapist and patient's agreeing on observable and measurable goals (Hollander & Kazaoka, 1988). The goals are specific to the individual in that they involve the acquisition or modification of a person's target behaviors. They can also focus on the individual in that the behaviors or experiences of concern occur whether the member is alone or with others. Examples include a foot fetish, panic attack, or suicidal attack. In such instances, the group facilitates progress toward individual goals by providing enhanced reinforcement options. Because the group setting is highly controlled, members can practice newly acquired or modified behaviors spontaneously without the negative consequences of failure and with continuous feedback from members and the therapist.

Alternatively, identified goals can be interactional, as in the case of an individual who is socially avoidant or inappropriately aggressive. For social goals, the group setting has a number of advantages. The format allows the assessment of members' behaviors by sampling and monitoring behaviors inside the group. Problem behaviors are enacted in the group setting so that the therapist and members have firsthand experience of observing the problem behaviors. The group provides abundant opportunities for members to learn and practice new target social behaviors in a safe environment in which they can obtain feedback and reinforcement from the therapist and other members. The therapist's control over the therapeutic environment allows members to try new behaviors or modify existing ones in a setting in which the penalty for mistakes is attenuated. In addition, the presence of multiple individuals makes possible learning more flexible response patterns that enable members to cope better with people in their environment because each group member offers an idiosyncratic style of response as do people outside the group with whom patients will need to interact (Hollander & Kazaoka, 1988).

TECHNICAL CONSIDERATIONS

Although many types of behavioral groups exist, one format that has especial relevance to IHPs, PHPs, and RTCs is the social skills training model, a treatment format that has been practice for over 50 years (Mueser & Bellack, 2007). This type of group involves augmenting or modifying an individual's behavioral repertoire, particularly in the domain of interpersonal exchange but also in that of practical life skills. Social skills can be defined as those behaviors occurring in the interpersonal transactions that enable an individual to fulfill social emotional needs and to achieve independent living in the community (Bellack, Mueser, Gingerich, & Agresta, 2004).

Role of the Leader

Social skills training requires therapists with particular skills, personal qualities, and knowledge bases as well as a particular leadership style.

Leader Qualities and Responsibilities

The function of therapeutic relationships within a social skills model is to facilitate behavioral change. As a credible and authoritative source of information and education, the therapist is able to motivate members and provide a comfortable environment in which skills can be learned. The social skills model requires therapists who are expressive, active, and lively. Optimism on the part of the therapist is extremely important. As Bellack et al. (2004) wrote, "The leaders need to convey the expectation that the group will help people to achieve personal goals and that they will enjoy attending" (p. 121). An enthusiastic therapist is particularly important for more chronic patients who lack spontaneity and affect. Liberman, DeRisi, and Mueser (1989) likened the therapist to a theater director or an athletic coach. Therapists are encouraged to gesture broadly and speak with greater volume than usual, even if it seems overdone. In fact, Liberman et al. suggested that the therapist remain standing throughout most of the session, moving freely about the room, unless otherwise required by the practice situation. The therapist creates an ambience that is somewhere "between an elementary school classroom and a revival meeting" (p. 75), with plenty of good humor and positive reinforcement, including cheering and applause. Sessions should never be boring; a "boring" session is likely to be the result of too much talking and not enough action. The therapist downplays speculation on motives and emphasizes action and behavior.

The therapist closely monitors group events. For example, during a role play, the therapist moves about the room to observe and direct the member and terminates the role play when (a) it is successfully completed, (b) the main theme gets lost in details and irrelevancies, (c) too much material is presented in a single role play so that the member is overwhelmed, or (d) the member begins to founder for other reasons. This type of intervention is particularly important because members' practicing of ineffective responses might make later change even more difficult.

The social skills therapist carefully manages the treatment environment, striving to provide a highly reinforcing and comfortable setting for members to learn new behaviors by having an upbeat attitude and offering abundant positive reinforcement. If possible, the therapist ignores inappropriate social behavior; members are not confronted with their deficits. Rather, the therapist solicits, acknowledges, and socially reinforces members' constructive behaviors. Those techniques that lessen members' anxiety are employed. For example, therapists provide snacks, use tokens and other rewards, allow sessions to exceed their specified length, and so on.

In social skills training, the therapist's task is to teach members the complex social skills required to communicate their needs and feelings to others in a socially acceptable and productive way. The social skills therapist is a teacher who creates a structured plan for the session and spends the session enacting the plan. In advance of the session, the therapists decide what role plays should occur, with two or three role plays per member being typical (Bellack et al., 2004).

Leadership Structure

Although it is possible to conduct the sessions with a single therapist, a cotherapy team is preferred because it enables therapists to share the planning and distribution of the many duties required for the implementation of an extensive set of techniques. When a cotherapy team is used, at least one of the therapists should be experienced in the social skills model. The second leader can be a cotherapist who has some basic knowledge of group treatment.

The cotherapists should establish in advance of the sessions how the responsibilities are shared. One possible delineation is that one therapist be actively involved with presenting the content of the day's lesson while the other serves as a role-play partner, with a period in which the roles are switched (Monti & Kolko, 1985). Another division is in the cotherapists' attentions to members at different levels of functioning (Bellack et al., 2004). Variability in member functioning creates challenges as, for example, when lower functioning members engage in behaviors that disrupt the work of other members. To remedy this problem, one leader might teach and organize the role plays while the other focuses on the lower functioning clients, calibrating the role plays so that they are able to be completed by these individuals.

Relationship With Other Staff

When social skills training occurs in a larger training program, the therapist should cultivate a positive relationship with the staff, helping them to understand the approach. Staff members perform three functions. First, they can support group attendance (Bellack et al., 2004). Second, they assist in the execution of the homework. Specifically, they encourage members to do their homework and "sign off" on the homework assignment cards. They might even prompt the actual use of the newly acquired skill in vivo. They participate in role plays as part of the homework assignments for members when they are beginning their training or when their skills are not sufficient to allow them to successfully complete their assignments with other patients. Generally, the more severe the social skill deficits and chronic the patient population, the more active a role the staff must have in bolstering the importance of the group, in reinforcing group attendance and in participating in the homework practice. Third, program staff usually control privileges and token incentives, which can motivate members to practice and use their newly developing and acquired skills.

Steps in a Social Skill Training Group

Group participation unfolds in a series of steps, the first of which occurs before the member even enters the group.

Assessment of Social Skill Deficits and Choice of Goals

Before group participation, the therapist identifies which particular skills are in need of cultivation. To assist the therapist, a number of tools have been developed such as the Social Functioning Interview (Remington & Tyrer, 1979), the Social Adaptive Functioning Evaluation (Harvey, Davidson, Mueser, Parrella, White, & Powchik, 1997), and the Social Skills Checklist (Bellack et al., 2004). Role-play assessments are also employed, which involve the presentation of a simulated interpersonal situation to which the prospective member is asked to respond. The particular role play is dependent on the nature of the IHP, PHP, or RTC, as well as the patient's level of functioning. Social skills evaluation should be macroscopic enough to indicate whether the behavior occurred and was appropriate but microscopic enough to capture such paralinguistic phenomena as eye contact, body posture, facial expressions, and verbal phenomena such as latency of response, loudness regulation, and language appropriateness.

All of this information is used in order to formulate the patient's goals. According to Morrison and Bellack (1987), four questions are especially important in this effort: (a) Does the person show difficulties in at least one interpersonal behavior? (b) When is this problem most likely to be manifest? (c) What accounts for the problem—a primary absence or weakness of a social skill or another problem that creates the social skills issue? and (d) What, specifically, is the social deficit? In some cases, the therapist will have direct evidence of interpersonal difficulties from observation of the person elsewhere in the program. This information can be integrated with that derived from self-report instruments and the clinical interview.

Format of the Sessions

The format varies somewhat, depending on whether the group has an open or closed membership and on whether a specific skill is being taught in a series. The level of skill deficit is also relevant.

Introductions. Whereas in a close-ended group the therapists encourage all members to introduce themselves, in an open-ended group introductions might be confined to the new members. A brief description of the goals and methods of the group is presented, ideally, by seasoned members. At a minimum, why practice and rehearsal of verbal and nonverbal behaviors, both in the session and for homework, should be explained. As with all steps, any contributions made by members should be amply rewarded with praise. The therapist fills in any essential information not mentioned by members. Members' participation in the orientation increases their sense of responsibility for the group as well as creates for new members realistic but positive expectations of what the group can do. In an ongoing group in which some member continuity exists from session to session, the next step is to check homework assignments and formulate goals.

Homework Review and Goal Development. Checking homework assignments and formulating goals can be done either as two separate steps or as a single go-around that incorporates both elements. If the homework report is a separate step, groups with more chronic patients should not only report on their assignment but also role play the target skills because such members are often not accurate observers of their own performance. Elucidating details are sought from the reporting member. For example, if a member says, "My homework got all messed up," the therapist should find out in what way it happened, at what point, and what else was occurring. The success or failure of the homework assignment will influence the goals and situations chosen to address within that particular session. For example, suppose a member were given the assignment of inviting another patient to take a walk. Were that member to report that she approached and greeted the person but was unable to ask that person to take a walk, that specific scene would be role played so that the person could be assisted in taking the step avoided outside the session. Regardless of outcome, members are praised for completing homework. At the discretion of the therapist, sometimes members who fail to complete their homework might be asked to perform the assignment in the session.

Teaching a New Skill. Not all sessions necessarily involve teaching a new skill, because learning a new skill typically involves multiple sessions. However, when new skills are being taught, the therapist must calibrate the level of the skill. For example, a group of chronic schizophrenic persons in a long-term PHP might need to learn how to begin a conversation by first, working on eye contact, interpersonal distance, or different types of greetings. The therapist might assist a group of higher functioning depressives by helping them generate a variety of topics with which to initiate conversations.

When teaching a new skill, the therapist must offer a rationale so that group members can recognize its usefulness. As members come to appreciate its importance, their motivation levels to pursue ensuing steps increase. Ideally, the cultivation of this understanding occurs via discussion rather than a lecture. Members can be assisted in recognizing for themselves why the possession of the skill might improve their lives (Bellack et al., 2004). For example, the following exchange might occur:

Therapist: Can anybody tell me why it might be not such a great thing if a person can't say "goodbye" after having started a conversation?

Blake: You could be standing there all day.

Shauna: If you just walk away, the other person might think you're crazy.

This framing of the skill is so crucial that before the therapist moves on, he or she should take pains to ensure that the members grasp the rationale.

After the rationale is presented, clear, concrete, and brief instructions are presented for performing the response. Each step of the skill is presented and discussed. To the extent that members realize why the step is necessary, they will be likely to complete it fully and effectively. When sending skills are taught, therapists can cultivate specific verbal and nonverbal behaviors (e.g., "When you begin a conversation, make eye contact, stand at an appropriate distance, and give a greeting"). The therapist would take each element and have members consider its importance ("Why should you make eye contact?"). When receiving skills are taught, the therapist might pose questions that get the individual to think about what the other is thinking, feeling, and intending (e.g., "Exactly what did George say?" "What do you think George was thinking when he asked you to make up your mind?" "What was he feeling?"). Processing skills include having the patient state short- and long-term goals, generate possible alternative strategies, and predict long- and short-term consequences of each of the strategies. The therapist should pose questions to the patient to elicit such responses: "In the short run, what did you want to accomplish?" "If you gave your boss a piece of your mind, what do you think would happen immediately?" "How do you think speaking up would affect your overall relationship?"

Instructions are not sufficient. The skill needs to be modeled by the therapist or by another who is competent in the skill. As Bellack et al. (2004) noted, "Demonstrating the skill helps translate the abstract steps of the skill into a concrete reality" (p. 52). Here, the presence of a cotherapy team presents an advantage in that cotherapists can serve as partners in the role play, thereby allowing for the enactment of a well-planned production. Following their role play, cotherapists help the group members to recognize the various elements that were incorporated into the role play.

Behavioral Rehearsal. In this step, also called the *dry run*, each member role plays, receives feedback, attempts the role play again, and receives more feedback. The therapist aids each member is setting up the role play. To the extent that members are able, they should participate in delineating and designing the role-play scene. The therapist should begin with a seasoned and enthusiastic member of the group, although a pattern should not emerge wherein the more able members participate prior to the less able members (Bellack et al., 2004). Role play times vary, but they should not be longer than 5 minutes for higher functioning patients and 2 minutes for chronically ill patients (K. T. Mueser, personal communication, July 21, 1992). The therapist must elicit the who, what, when, where, how, and how often of the scene when attempting to select a recent situation or one that is likely to occur in the near future (Flowers & Schwartz, 1985). It is important that efforts be made to have group members who resemble the individual with whom the patient has difficulty be active in the role play. However, replaying a role play a number of times with different people aids in fostering interpersonal flexibility and a broader behavioral repertoire. Any props that help to make the scenario realistic should be employed.

A series of situations should be devised, each slightly more difficult for the member to handle than the previous one. It is essential that the member experience success early on in the process so that he or she is encouraged to continue working on the skill. Occasionally, members refuse to participate in a role play. Generally, members should neither be confronted nor unduly pressured to engage in the role play. Initially, such individuals might be encouraged to participate in a way that they might experience as less threatening. For example, they might be asked to give feedback or take on a nondemanding role in a role play. The therapist's goal should be for members to move toward the level of participation that would enable their acquisition of social skills.

Constructive Feedback and Additional Modeling. The therapist uses every available opportunity to provide realistic praise to the member. Positive feedback is also encouraged from other members. If members have more serious deficits in social skills, it might be necessary for the therapist to request feedback about more specific elements of the member's performance. For example, rather than asking, "What was positive about the way he handled that situation?" the therapist might pose a more focused query: "How has his voice tone improved since last time?" The number of comments that a member can successfully incorporate is also related to his or her level of functioning. More chronically impaired patients usually can absorb only one or two suggestions. If the member receives more comments than he or she is likely to assimilate, the leader directs the member to a subset of them. The therapist handles off-topic, hostile, or negative statements made by members whose feedback was invited by ignoring them, when possible.

After a group member has received feedback from others on the role play, members can benefit from witnessing a model exhibit the skill in which the feedback is very explicitly and conspicuously incorporated. Following the modeling, the therapist asks the member to state what he or she noticed; this step better ensures that the member has understood and observed the demonstrated. The modeling process can be augmented through videotaping of role playing. One advantage of this tool is that it can be stopped at various points to allow the therapist to comment about elements of it.

Behavioral Rehearsal With Coaching. The member then practices the same scene again so that the therapist can assess skill acquisition and the member can strengthen the skill further. This step is important, given the evidence that improvement in social skills is more closely linked to the number of role plays in which a member participates than the number of sessions that a member attends (Douglas & Mueser, 1990). If the member does not improve sufficiently, more active coaching with hand signals might be necessary, an intervention involving positive "online" feedback during the role play from the therapist (e.g., "Just the right distance"). After the therapist has terminated the role play, specific positive feedback is again solicited from the other group members as well as the member performing the behavior (e.g., "What were you able to do this time that enabled you to accomplish your goal?"). For programs that treat depressed or higher functioning patients, this step is especially important, whereas it is used much less frequently with more severely impaired patients.

Assignment of Homework. Assignments outside of group sessions help increase the possibility of transfer of learning and overcome the problem of generalization, that is, performing the behavior only in the sessions and not in the member's everyday life (Kopelowicz, Liberman, & Zarate, 2006). For assignments to have the best chance of success, it is important for the cotherapist to provide each member with an assignment card that gives clear, simple, detailed instructions. The card is given to the member who carries it about as a reminder to complete the task before the next group convenes. Assignments are gradually adjusted to increasing levels of difficulty as the member develops skills and confidence. They should directly follow from the training. For example, if the member has practiced making a request of another patient, such as to turn down his or her radio, the homework assignment should focus on making the same or similar request of someone else on the unit. To increase the likelihood of success, the specific assignment should be based on a proficiency that has been achieved in the session. The homework should specify the circumstances under which the new skill should be attempted—when, where, and with whom.

With more chronic patients, involvement of the nursing staff can be critical in the designing, monitoring, and carrying out of assignments, given that chronic patients respond more adversely to failure and are less likely to carry out an assignment if not encouraged by staff (Bellack et al., 2004).

For all populations, it is not necessary to provide different assignments each time, because repeated assignments can increase the member's sense of effectiveness.

The basic features of the social skills training model appear in Table 8.1.

CLINICAL ILLUSTRATION OF THE SOCIAL SKILLS TRAINING MODEL

The group took place in a chronic-care RTC. The group met daily for 35 to 40 minutes. As each member developed goals and specific skills on which to work, the therapist noted this information on a poster. Another poster containing the nonverbal and paralinguistic skills (e.g., eye contact, body posture, distance and physical contact) was a permanent wall fixture.

Group Members

Although the group had six members, we focus on only three of them.

Tony—a 45-year-old man diagnosed with chronic schizophrenia who had been hospitalized a dozen times since he was 22 years old. The long-term task was to increase the quantity and quality of Tony's social interactions by increasing the quality of his social skills. When Tony first entered the

TABLE 8.1
Social Skills Training Model

Elements of the model	Characteristics of the model
View of psychological problems	Psychological problems are rooted in the absence or lack of coordination of core social skills, often due to faulty instrumental or classical conditioning.
Goals of model	To foster the acquisition and coordination of social skills
Methods of action	An educational, skill-training approach
Intervention techniques	Therapist modeling, positive reinforcement for desired behaviors, practice opportunities inside and outside the group, processing of home-work assignments
Adaptation of the model to a brief time frame	Delimitation of number of skills to be taught
Use of group process	Members are encouraged to develop an esprit de corps, which helps them take risks in attempting new behaviors. The group is used as a laboratory to help members develop social skills.

program, he began an individual social skills program with one of the group therapists because of staff concern that the group would be overwhelming. Once he had learned to approach people, make a greeting, and pose basic requests, he joined the group. Although initially he wanted only to watch the other members engage in the training, he moved onto offering feedback, then serving as a confederate, and finally being the target actor in the role play itself. The group leaders discovered that he had an interest in Parcheesi, a game that patients often played in the program. Tony worked in the group on learning how to initiate conversations by greeting another person and then inviting another person to join him in a game.

WillieMae—a 56-year-old woman with a 30-year history of hearing voices. She had had a long-standing delusion that a homing radio had been implanted in her head, a conviction spawned by a course of electroconvulsive shock therapy, 25 years ago. Her frequent mumbling and inexplicable laughing led others to avoid her. Therapists assessed WillieMae as having good eye contact, a nice smile, and an ability to respond to others' greetings in passing. The therapists observed that although she was able to start an appropriate response to others' questions and requests, WillieMae would then have bursts of laughter and begin to refer to some aspect of her delusions. The therapists concluded relevant goals would include improving her ability to initiate conversation and to respond to others without wandering off into delusional material. Another goal was to decrease her inappropriate laughter and replacing it with an alternative skill, namely, active listening.

Gina—a 32-year-old woman who had been making deep cuts in her arms and legs since age 12. She also experienced transient psychotic episodes. The staff suspected that she had occasional dissociative experiences. Her two interpersonal goals included strengthening her ability to be appropriately assertive and expressing her needs and feelings with clarity. The second goal—essential to an ability to hold a job—concerned her frequent misperception that others were transgressing against her. The therapists sought to enhance her skill in correctly perceiving others.

The Session

> *Therapist:* Today, we have a new member, so let's begin with some introductions.
>
> [*Members introduce themselves and indicate how long they have been in the group.*]
>
> *Therapist:* Let's begin with talking about the goals of the social skills group. [*Silence*] WillieMae, what can you tell John about our group?

WillieMae [*laughs*]: I did my homework [*holding out an assignment card, which has her assignment on it; she laughs again loudly*].

Therapist: Good, WillieMae, and we will get to that in a moment. But you told John about an important part of our group. Every day, we leave with a homework assignment. We have an assigned job that we do before the next time we meet. The more you can practice with other people, the better you will become at the skill, and it will be easier, too. First, we try out new skills in here. We get some help from the other group members; then, we do homework. When you practice out there, it's more like real life.

WillieMae: Safe [*laughs*].

Therapist: Yes, WillieMae, good thought! It is safer here. What else can we tell John about the way our group works? [*Silence*]

Gina: Why don't you just tell him? It's such a waste of time to have these people try to struggle through this. It will take all of our time! And if that's all we're going to do, I'm out of here. It's just too boring.

Therapist: I'm glad you are excited to get started, Gina. [*Notice the bypassing of hostility.*] Before we do, we should tell John that what you illustrated by your request is exactly the kind of thing we are working on in here. You have been working on making requests of people in a way that they can hear you and respond to you. And that one was a pretty good request. Maybe the group can look at that a little later when we do your role plays. But first we need to explain to John what you did that was so clear and how that relates to our goals. Maybe you can explain to him what you were able to do so much better than when you started.

Gina: Well, I get emotional real easy. When I get mad, I used to let people have it. So, I've been working on how to get what I want, you know, ask for what I want without having everyone get mad at me. So I guess you're here so that you can work on something that will make it easier for you to get along with other people.

Therapist: Yes, good, Gina, really good explanation! Tony, do you have anything you want to add, like what you've been working on?

Tony: I want to play Parcheesi.

Therapist: Yes, very good, Tony. Tony has been learning how to introduce himself to others and to make requests of people. What in particular have you been practicing?

Tony: Looking at people right and saying the right words.

Therapist: Yes, indeed! We try to improve the way we talk to people, both what we say and how we say it [*points to poster of paralinguistic skills on the wall*]. Tony is working very hard to make good eye contact. Did you notice that he looked up while he was speaking? Very good! We work on our facial expressions, where we should stand, and the quality of our voice. We learn to say what we think and feel, and to make requests rather than hoping someone will know what we want. And we also learn [*looking at the relevant members*] how to better hear what others say to us because often we don't hear it quite right. One of the things we do in here is role play. Who can tell John what a role play is? Tony?

Tony: Pretend.

Therapist: That's right, Tony. A role play is a pretend interaction. It gives us a chance to practice what we've learned and for others to help by giving us feedback about the way that we come across to them.

[*This introduction is long compared with those of many other models. It serves multiple purposes in that it (a) continues to teach methods of social skills training to old members, (b) aids in the development of healthy group norms such as taking an active role in the group, (c) enhances members' abilities to communicate by modeling positive feedback, and (d) fosters accurate expectations of the group in new group members.*]

Therapist: Terrific introduction! Let's go on to your homework assignments. Let's begin with you, WillieMae, since you told John how important homework is. You have been working very hard, learning how to let others know what you are thinking and feeling and what it is you want from them. [*Therapist reads assignment from index card that WillieMae has given him.*] Your homework assignment was to call your caseworker to see if she would take you to the public assistance office so you could get your housing situation straightened out. I saw that the aide signed the card that you completed. Maybe you can show us how it went.

WillieMae [*laughs*]: Yeah, and she knew already what I was going to say. Dr. Smith must have wired her [*laughs, referring to her belief of the implanted radio tracker in her head*].

Therapist: That is great that you were able to carry out the assignment [*ignoring the opportunity to get into delusional material and finding something in the performance to reward*]. Here is a phone you can use in showing us. Were you standing or sitting?

WillieMae:	Standing up. [laughs]
Therapist:	Good. We'll put the phone here. Did the aide say anything? [WillieMae nods.] How about if Dr. X [the cotherapist] plays the aide, and you show us where and how he was standing? [WillieMae does so and starts laughing.] Now, was anyone else in line to use the phone? [WillieMae nods.] Did they say anything to you?
WillieMae:	No, he was listening. Dr. Smith couldn't hear with the phone interfering with the transmitter . . .
Therapist [interrupts]:	Okay, Tony, how about if you stand in line behind WillieMae and not say anything? Your caseworker is Ms. Yarrow. Gina, how about if you be Ms. Yarrow and stand over here with the other phone line? Now, what did Ms. Yarrow say exactly?
	[A great deal of effort is spent to make the role play realistic to foster generalization. The effort to involve as many people as possible in the role play serves to make it believable and to keep the members active in the session, even when they are not themselves working on their skill.]
WillieMae:	I did talk to my doctor about it, and then I knew that Dr. Smith told her to say that.
Gina [exasperated]:	Dr. Smith left years ago. Why do you keep focusing on him? He's not even here.
Therapist:	Well, Gina, that's an interesting question, but right now, let's focus on exactly what was said [moves away from whys and speculation in favor of observing the behavior]. WillieMae, did Ms. Yarrow say anything else? [WillieMae shrugs.] Okay, Gina, maybe when we get to that part, you can say whatever you think that Ms. Yarrow may have said under the circumstances. Whenever you're ready, WillieMae, you can begin. [She starts to laugh and continues for about 20 seconds.] Okay, WillieMae, what was your goal in this assignment? What are you going to try and do?
WillieMae:	Well, it's to talk to Ms. Yarrow to see if she can take me out of the hospital to take care of my housing problem [laughs a bit more quietly].
Therapist:	Yes, very good. Start whenever you are ready.
WillieMae:	Ms. Yarrow, this is WillieMae. I want to go out on a pass [tries to suppress a laugh] 'cause I got a letter in the mail [laughs].

Gina: WillieMae, I was thinking about you. Well, I need to see the letter. I could take you, but did you speak to your doctor about getting a pass?

WillieMae: So you know, I will lose my apartment. Does he want me to lose my apartment? [*She laughs but quickly places her hand over her mouth.*]

Gina [*looks uncertain; the cotherapist whispers what Gina can say*]: No, WillieMae! No one wants you to lose your apartment, but I can't take you anywhere until your doctor gives you permission to travel with me. Why don't you call me back after you speak with your doctor, or would you like me to call him?

Therapist: Okay, why don't we stop right here. WillieMae, is that what Ms. Yarrow said? [*WillieMae nods.*] What was very good about WillieMae's performance, Gina?

Gina: Well, her voice was loud and clear and she had a good start. I mean, she said who she was.

Therapist: Good, Gina! What else do you think she did well, Tony? Did she state the purpose of the call? [*Tony nods.*] Yes, she did. Thank you, Tony. What would have made what she did even better?

Gina: I think Ms. Yarrow didn't know that WillieMae already spoke with her doctor. She could have said that she did.

Therapist: What would that have done?

Gina: Well, maybe WillieMae thought that Ms. Yarrow already knew something and was against her, but I think she was just making sure that WillieMae had permission.

Therapist: Do you see what Gina means, WillieMae? [*She nods.*] Maybe we can work on adding that piece of information to help you clarify what Ms. Yarrow knew. The role play was a good one. We'll see if we can make it even better. [*WillieMae starts laughing.*] WillieMae, how would you let Ms. Yarrow know that you had spoken with your doctor? What would you say?

WillieMae: I would say, "Ms. Yarrow, I already asked my doctor."

Therapist: Good, that is a clear way to say it. Let's try it again in a role play. [*WillieMae rehearses again with the same actors. This time she makes the above statement but adds at the end that she thinks Ms. Yarrow is in collusion with Dr. Smith.*] Okay, let's stop right there. Tony, was she able to clarify that she had already spoken with her doctor? [*Tony nods.*] Yes, she did. You did that well, WillieMae. After we finish the homework assignments, we will come back to this role play and see if we can help you be able to really listen to what Ms. Yarrow has to say.

Comment on the Session

After the introduction of the new member, the checking of homework occurs. In this example, checking homework is combined with two behavioral rehearsals and setting of the day's tasks and goals. In higher functioning groups, this initial homework checking might be merely a verbal check. However, because these members might be better able to demonstrate than narrate, a role play was used.

The reader undoubtedly has noticed that the therapist does not establish as a focus WillieMae's laughing. The presumption is that doing so would create a negative cast to the treatment and raise WillieMae's anxiety to an unproductive level. Learning to suppress a response is generally more difficult than mastering a response. Possibly, her willingness to attend the group would be undermined were the laughter to be a treatment target. Instead, the therapist focuses on the cultivation of positive behaviors, such as clear verbal expression, that ultimately might lead to the diminishment of the disruptive laughing behavior. This positive emphasis can be challenging in that it requires the therapist to contain members' negative reactions to a given member's behavior but also to his or her own.

The vignette illustrates the fact that staff members outside of the group play a role in members' group work. As noted previously in this chapter, not only do staff help members to complete homework assignments but they also find new opportunities for members to practice skills. For example, staff might ask WillieMae about her preferences and attend to whether she responds with the kinds of clear communications that she practiced in the group. This function is crucial because practice increases the likelihood of skill acquisition.

A final note concerns diversity. With individuals with severe and persistent mental illness, it is not uncommon for them to face challenges with negotiating various social systems such as Medicare and Medicaid. Often, the social skills members are seeking to develop can assist them in interacting with these systems. The therapist's familiarity with these systems will enable him or her to be more specific during role play. In this example, WillieMae is working on communication skills that she will need in order to have continued access to housing. To the extent that the therapist appreciates the specificities of this challenge, she will able to incorporate elements into the role play that will make it believable to WillieMae and others.

STATUS OF THE RESEARCH

In recent years, meta-analyses have been published on social skills training models. Many of the studies included in the meta-analyses involve a combination of group therapy studies, individual therapy studies, or programs with both components. Pilling et al. (2002) obtained unfavorable results for a meta-analysis of nine studies involving participants with schizophrenia or schizoaffective disorder. In their study, social skills training failed to foster an improvement in psychosocial and global functioning, relapse rate, and treatment compliance. The possible benefits of social skills training might have been hidden by Pilling et al.'s combination of different types of outcome measures (Mueser & Penn, 2004). Pfammatter, Junghan, and Brenner (2006) examined 19 studies and found strong effect sizes for basic skill acquisition and moderate effects for assertiveness and social functioning. All of these positive effects were sustained on a long-term basis. Kurtz and Mueser (2008) describe a meta-analysis of 22 studies in which social skills training protocols were implemented with schizophrenic individuals. Thirty-seven percent of these studies were conducted with inpatients. They found that the effect sizes for content-mastery examinations (paper and pencil, interviews, or role plays) were very large, whereas those for social and independent living and psychosocial functioning were in the moderate range. Relapse rate yielded a small effect size.

Social skills training approaches are also commonly used with children and adolescents who are in the formative years of acquiring and refining social skills. A meta-analysis by Weisz, Weiss, Han, Granger, and Morton (1995) focused on 23 studies conducted with these populations. Their analysis yielded a weighted effect size of .28 and an unweighted effect size of .37, suggesting a mildly to moderately positive effect of treatment. Although a number of other meta-analyses (e.g., Forness & Kavale, 1996) have been conducted with children and adolescents, they are primarily focused on school settings and hence, of questionable relevance to patients in clinical settings.

Increasingly, social skills training is blended with other types of intervention. For example, in their review article, Kopelowicz et al. (2006) described the blending of cognitive remediation with social skills training. The notion here is that underlying deficits in social skills are particular cognitive problems, the lessening of which enable the patient to be more amenable to social skills interventions. Some empirical support for this notion exists (e.g., see Silverstein et al., 2005). Kopelowicz et al. also pointed to the increasing practice of social skills training being embedded in a much larger program of carefully constituted components. They note that an exemplar of such groundbreaking work is the optimal treatment program designed by Falloon and colleagues (Falloon, 1999). In addition to social skills training, the package includes such components as assertiveness training, medication and compliance training, and family psychoeducation. Staff members are trained intensively trained in delivering interventions. The treatment package was evaluated in a randomized clinical trial with 100 schizophrenic individuals who had been symptomatic for no longer than 10 years. In comparison with the treatment as usual group, the treatment groups showed a higher level of psychosocial functioning, particularly after 6 months of treatment. An ongoing cross-cultural data collection effort on the Optimal Treatment Program continues to show exceedingly favorable results (Falloon et al., 2004).

In summary, the research shows quite clearly that social skills can be learned. As Kurtz and Mueser (2008) usefully noted, the more proximal the measure is to the training, the larger the size of effect tends to be. The biggest challenge continues to be in ensuring that those skills mastered in sessions are transferred to the individual's day-to-day life (Mueser & Bellack, 2007). One means to accomplish this goal is to integrate social skills training with other therapeutic elements such as cognitive retraining.

CONTEXTUAL DEMANDS OF THE SOCIAL SKILLS TRAINING MODEL

Clinical Mission and Context of the Group

This model, a version of behavioral group therapy, proposes to improve social competence, which is viewed as the individual's repertoire of social skills. As such, the model is compatible with any clinical setting that considers these skills to be important and permits them to be taught or modified. As Kopelowicz et al. (2006) noted, social skills training is appropriate for all three types of settings featured in this book. This model is, in principle, compatible with a biological or pharmacological approach; in fact, one available module teaches medication management. This model is likely to have more difficulty thriving in a purely psychoanalytic setting in which underlying motivation and the affects and impulses that sustain behavior are considered the *sine qua non* of treatment. Social skills training explicitly does not attend to unconscious underpinnings of behavior.

Although often not specifically addressed in the literature, the attitude of the unit staff toward the treatment is important, particularly in long-term settings with chronic patients; the model is optimally applied when staff are enthusiastic participants, willing to reinforce, prompt, and rehearse the target skills with the patient outside the group setting.

The quality and efficacy of the group is unaffected by whether the group is constituted of members from one unit or members from multiple units. The therapists can be part of the unit staff or can be outside consultants so long as unit staff are apprised of members' homework assignments and are attuned to the goals of social skills training.

Temporal Variables

This model can be structured to be successful in a closed-ended or open-ended format. In some ways, a closed-ended group is more efficient because each skill can be taught to all the members together. If the group is open-ended, two options are available: Either single skills can be taught continuously, such as how to start a conversation, or in a longer term setting, each individual can be uniquely assessed, and goals can be designed to teach the specific social skills in which that individual might be deficient. Specific skills can be introduced and taught when patients are ready to acquire those particular target behaviors. In this design, members can broaden their skill set through vicarious learning. This same process will help to reinforce skills previously mastered.

An advantage of this model is the degree to which the therapist can tailor the structure and specific skills taught to the number of sessions in which the average member participates. For example, Goldstein, Sprafkin, and Gershaw (1976) developed a program to teach 36 skills, whereas Douglas and Mueser (1990) reported teaching only two skills. In general, the greater the number of sessions that the patient can attend, the more likely he or she is to acquire, generalize, and maintain a particular skill. Moreover, longer participation enables the patient to acquire multiple skills, which is important given that most inpatients with social skills deficits are deficient in more than a single skill. In addition, with social skills training, the intersession interval is important because smaller intervals facilitate skill acquisition. This is particularly true for the more severely mentally ill. In a meta-analysis of 27 studies examining social skills training for schizophrenics (only some of which were in a group format), Benton and Schroeder (1990) found that 41% of the studies used 10 hours of training or less but that some used more than 100 hours; the amount of training appeared to have no relation to outcome. There is no study or technique paper that suggests a single session is beneficial (Benton & Schroeder, 1990). Training in most studies continued until acquisition of the skill had occurred. Bellack et al. (2004) pointed out that with more severely disturbed patients, a greater number of sessions is necessary. However, they also aver that the therapist must be sensitive to whether members continue to be interested in working on a given skill; when members' attention flags, little progress can be made.

Size of the Group

This model has considerable flexibility in terms of numbers of patients attending the group, particularly with higher functioning patients. The recommended number of group members is between four and 16. For more chronic patients, a smaller group, sometimes with as few as two members and two therapists but no more than four or five members, is recommended.

Composition of the Group

Social skills training has been found to be effective with persons with affective disorders, chronic and acute schizophrenia, arson, alcoholism, anxiety disorders, impulsive disorders, and aggressive behavior in acute care settings, day hospitals, and the longer-term state hospital programs. The optimal arrangement for groups appears to be that in which the level of functioning is relatively homogeneous and the social skills deficits are largely shared. Successful treatments have been developed with heterogeneous populations, although care must be taken to teach a skill on which all members can improve. Perhaps one of the most difficult arrangements is that wherein chronic schizophrenics with acute exacerbations are in the same group with patients who primarily have personality disorders; in these cases, the higher functioning personality disordered patients often become uninterested in the group, the demonstration of which raises the anxiety levels of the schizophrenic members.

Most of the programs have been used with adults ranging from ages 18 to 65. However, since our last edition, significant development has occurred in the application of the model to child and adolescent populations (e.g., Spence, 2003) and elderly populations (e.g., Granholm, Holden, Link, McQuaid, & Jeste, 2013). The emphasis, though, has been on outpatient applications. Almost all the work that has been reported has used homogeneous age groupings. It is not clear whether this is by design or because of population availability and unit groupings. No outstanding evidence for gender differences seems to be available, with the exception of training of compromise and negotiation and expression of negative feelings: males appeared to be better able to acquire the skills than were females (Douglas & Mueser, 1990; Mueser, Levine, Bellack, & Douglas, 1990).

Therapist Variables

Therapists come from a broad spectrum of disciplines: psychology, psychiatry, social work, occupational therapy, nursing, vocational counseling, and other human-service occupations. Neophyte group therapists who have a methodological behaviorist orientation would be at ease with this model. However, it is not necessary for a therapist to be a behaviorist to be able to successfully and enthusiastically use this model. It is essential that the therapist view the alteration of social behaviors as beneficial either in its own right or because it produces a secondary benefit such as increase in self-esteem. Additionally, the therapist must be comfortable with the high level of activity required of a therapist in this model. A flare for the dramatic is also helpful but not essential. Finally, the therapist needs a minimum amount of social skill and comfort with other people.

In terms of technical expertise, this model is one of the few that does not require an extensive training background or prior exposure to the model through a mentor. Use of this model has been taught with positive results in a 12-hour course to interested people who have at least a high school education; the outcome for patients who were taught by a "professional" versus a "nonprofessional" did not differ (Thompson, Gallagher, Nies, & Epstein, 1983). For those with a background in the mental health field, training manuals are available that spell out in great detail and assessable language the procedures that the therapist follows.

Cotherapy is important for this model. The cotherapy team is a very active one; therapists physically move about more than most. Cotherapy is often very important in the role play, particularly with chronic patients. While the therapist is busily directing the format and flow of the session, the cotherapist assists in watching the other members, writing homework assignments, keeping track of goals, and participating in role plays.

SUMMARY

In our 1993 book, we described behavior therapy as a newcomer to the group psychotherapy scene. This statement is no longer accurate; the model is now well-established in many IHP, PHP, and RTC environments. At the nexus of the model is an empirical foundation that focuses primarily on measurable behavior and current environmental antecedents and consequences in an action-oriented therapeutic setting. The central goal of therapy is to change behavior.

Because the range of technical considerations and research to date for all the variants of this model are so vast, we chose social skills training as a representative variant of the behavioral model to explore in more detail. Social skills training focuses on the acquisition or modification of interpersonal behavior. Technically, this model is extraordinarily well developed, with a multitude of manuals available for the neophyte therapist. The therapist is very active in structuring the session, which provides instruction, discussion, and modeling of the particular skill to be learned. Participants then role play, receive and give feedback, and complete homework.

The research on the efficacious use of group social skills in IHPs, PHPs and to a lesser extent RTCs is extensive. This model accommodates a wide range of diagnoses and uniquely offers a procedure to train schizophrenic persons. This model has been extended to the treatment of children, adolescents, and geriatric patients. The model can be geared to various lengths of stay but does require multiple sessions. The most notable challenge of this approach is assisting group members to generalize their newly acquired skills to the natural environment. This problem is twofold. Are patients capable of discriminating the particular cues that call for the use of the skill? Are there conditions under which certain skills are not retained? These questions continue to be the objects of empirical inquiry.

REFERENCES

Antony, M. M., & Roemer, L. (2011). *Behavior therapy*. Washington, DC: American Psychological Association.

Arkowitz, H., & Hannah, M. T. (1989). Cognitive, behavioral, and psychodynamic therapies: Converging or diverging pathways to change? In A. Freeman, K. M. Simon, L. E. Beutler, & H. Arkowtiz (Eds.), *Comprehensive handbook of cognitive therapy* (pp. 143–167). New York, NY: Plenum Press. http://dx.doi.org/10.1007/978-1-4757-9779-4_8

Bandura, A. (1978). The self system in reciprocal determinism. *American Psychologist, 33,* 344–358. http://dx.doi.org/10.1037/0003-066X.33.4.344

Bandura, A. (1979). *Principles of behavioral modification*. New York, NY: Holt, Rinehart & Winston.

Bellack, A. S., Morrison, R. L., Wixted, J. T., & Mueser, K. T. (1990). An analysis of social competence in schizophrenia. *The British Journal of Psychiatry, 156,* 809–818. http://dx.doi.org/10.1192/bjp.156.6.809

Bellack, A. S., Mueser, K. T., Gingerich, S., & Agresta, J. (2004). *Social skills training for schizophrenia: A step-by-step guide*. New York, NY: Guilford Press.

Benton, M. K., & Schroeder, H. E. (1990). Social skills training with schizophrenics: A meta-analytic evaluation. *Journal of Consulting and Clinical Psychology, 58,* 741–747. http://dx.doi.org/10.1037/0022-006X.58.6.741

Domjan, M. (2015). *The principles of learning and behavior* (7th ed.). Stamford, CT: Cengage.

Douglas, M. S., & Mueser, K. T. (1990). Teaching conflict resolution skills to the chronically mentally ill: Social skills training groups for briefly hospitalized patients. *Behavior Modification, 14,* 519–547. http://dx.doi.org/10.1177/0145445590014400

Eifert, G. H. (1996). More theory-driven and less diagnosis-based behavior therapy. *Journal of Behavior Therapy and Experimental Psychiatry, 27*, 75–86. http://dx.doi.org/10.1016/0005-7916(96)00008-0

Falloon, I. R. (1999). Optimal treatment for psychosis in an international multisite demonstration project. Optimal Treatment Project Collaborators. *Psychiatric Services, 50*, 615–618. http://dx.doi.org/10.1176/ps.50.5.615

Falloon, I. R., Montero, I., Sungur, M., Mastroeni, A., Malm, U., Economou, M., . . . Gedye, R., & the OTP Collaborative Group. (2004). Implementation of evidence-based treatment for schizophrenic disorders: Two-year outcome of an international field trial of optimal treatment. *World Psychiatry, 3*(2), 104–109.

Flowers, J. V. (1979). Behavioral analysis of group therapy and a model for behavioral group therapy. In D. Upper & S. M. Ross (Eds.), *Behavioral group therapy 1979: An annual review* (pp. 5–37). Champaign, IL: Research Press.

Flowers, J. V., & Schwartz, B. (1985). Behavioral group therapy with heterogeneous clients. In D. Upper & S. M. Ross (Eds.), *Handbook of behavioral group therapy* (pp. 145–170). New York, NY: Plenum Press. http://dx.doi.org/10.1007/978-1-4684-4958-7_6

Forness, S. R., & Kavale, K. A. (1996). Treating social skill deficits in children with learning disabilities: A meta-analysis of the research. *Learning Disability Quarterly, 19*, 2–13. http://dx.doi.org/10.2307/1511048

Goldstein, A. P., Sprafkin, R. P., & Gershaw, N. J. (1976). *Skill training for community living: Applying structured learning therapy.* New York, NY: Pergamon Press.

Granholm, E., Holden, J., Link, P. C., McQuaid, J. R., & Jeste, D. V. (2013). Randomized controlled trial of cognitive behavioral social skills training for older consumers with schizophrenia: Defeatist performance attitudes and functional outcome. *The American Journal of Geriatric Psychiatry, 21*, 251–262. http://dx.doi.org/10.1016/j.jagp.2012.10.014

Harvey, P. D., Davidson, M., Mueser, K. T., Parrella, M., White, L., & Powchik, P. (1997). Social-adaptive functioning evaluation (SAFE): A rating scale for geriatric psychiatric patients. *Schizophrenia Bulletin, 23*, 131–145. http://dx.doi.org/10.1093/schbul/23.1.131

Hayes, S. C. (2016). Why contextual behavior science exists: An introduction to Part 1. In R. D. Zettles, S. C. Hayes, D. Barnes-Holmes, & A. Biglan (Eds.), *The Wiley handbook of contextual behavioral science* (pp. 9–16). West Sussex, England: Wiley.

Hogarty, G. E., Flesher, S., Ulrich, R., Carter, M., Greenwald, D., Pogue-Geile, M., . . . Zoretich, R. (2004). Cognitive enhancement therapy for schizophrenia: Effects of a 2-year randomized trial on cognition and behavior. *Archives of General Psychiatry, 61*, 866–876. http://dx.doi.org/10.1001/archpsyc.61.9.866

Hollander, M., & Kazaoka, K. (1988). Behavior therapy groups. In S. Long (Ed.), *Six group therapies* (pp. 257–326). New York, NY: Plenum Press. http://dx.doi.org/10.1007/978-1-4899-2100-0_6

Kern, R. S., Glynn, S. M., Horan, W. P., & Marder, S. R. (2009). Psychosocial treatments to promote functional recovery in schizophrenia. *Schizophrenia Bulletin*, *35*, 347–361. http://dx.doi.org/10.1093/schbul/sbn177

Kodak, T., & Grow, L. L. (2011). Behavioral treatment of autism. In W. W. Fisher, C. C. Piazza, & H. S. Roane (Eds.), *Handbook of applied behavior analysis* (pp. 402–416). New York, NY: Guilford Press.

Kopelowicz, A., Liberman, R. P., & Zarate, R. (2006). Recent advances in social skills training for schizophrenia. *Schizophrenia Bulletin*, *32*(Suppl. 1), S12–S23. http://dx.doi.org/10.1093/schbul/sbl023

Kurtz, M. M., & Mueser, K. T. (2008). A meta-analysis of controlled research on social skills training for schizophrenia. *Journal of Consulting and Clinical Psychology*, *76*, 491–504. http://dx.doi.org/10.1037/0022-006X.76.3.491

Liberman, R. P., DeRisi, W. J., & Mueser, K. T. (1989). *Social skills training for psychiatric patients*. New York, NY: Pergamon Press.

Mahoney, M. J., & Kazdin, A. E. (1979). Cognitive behavior modification: Misconceptions and premature evaluation. *Psychological Bulletin*, *86*, 1044–1049. http://dx.doi.org/10.1037/0033-2909.86.5.1044

Monti, P. M., & Kolko, D. J. (1985). A review and programmatic model of group social skills training for psychiatric patients. In D. Upper & S. M. Ross (Eds.), *Handbook of behavioral group therapy* (pp. 25–61). New York, NY: Plenum Press. http://dx.doi.org/10.1007/978-1-4684-4958-7_2

Morrison, R. L., & Bellack, A. S. (1987). Social functioning of schizophrenic patients: Clinical and research issues. *Schizophrenia Bulletin*, *13*, 715–725. http://dx.doi.org/10.1093/schbul/13.4.715

Mueser, K. T., & Bellack, A. S. (2007). Social skills training: Alive and well? *Journal of Mental Health*, *16*, 549–552. http://dx.doi.org/10.1080/09638230701494951

Mueser, K. T., Levine, S., Bellack, A. S., & Douglas, M. S. (1990). Social skills training for acute psychiatric inpatients. *Hospital & Community Psychiatry*, *41*, 1249–1251. Retrieved from http://dx.doi.org/10.1176/ps.41.11.1249

Mueser, K. T., & Penn, D. L. (2004). Meta-analysis examining the effects of social skills training on schizophrenia. *Psychological Medicine*, *34*, 1365–1367. http://dx.doi.org/10.1017/S0033291704213848

Mueser, K. T., Wallace, C. J., & Liberman, R. P. (1995). New developments in social skills training. *Behaviour Change*, *12*(01), 31–40. http://dx.doi.org/10.1017/S0813483900004368

Pfammatter, M., Junghan, U. M., & Brenner, H. D. (2006). Efficacy of psychological therapy in schizophrenia: Conclusions from meta-analyses. *Schizophrenia Bulletin*, *32*(Suppl. 1), S64–S80. http://dx.doi.org/10.1093/schbul/sbl030

Pilling, S., Bebbington, P., Kuipers, E., Garety, P., Geddes, J., Martindale, B., . . . Morgan, C. (2002). Psychological treatments in schizophrenia: II. Meta-analyses of randomized controlled trials of social skills training and cognitive remediation. *Psychological Medicine*, *32*, 783–791. http://dx.doi.org/10.1017/S0033291702005640

Remington, M., & Tyrer, P. J. (1979). The social functioning schedule: A brief semi-structured interview. *Social Psychiatry, 14,* 151–157. http://dx.doi.org/10.1007/BF00582182

Silverstein, S. M., Hatashita-Wong, M., Solak, B. A., Uhlhaas, P., Landa, Y., Wilkniss, S. M., . . . Smith, T. E. (2005). Effectiveness of a two-phase cognitive rehabilitation intervention for severely impaired schizophrenia patients. *Psychological Medicine, 35,* 829–837. http://dx.doi.org/10.1017/S0033291704003356

Skinner, B. F. (1974). *About behaviorism.* New York, NY: Vintage.

Spence, S. H. (2003). Social skills training with children and young people: Theory, evidence and practice. *Child and Adolescent Mental Health, 8,* 84–96. http://dx.doi.org/10.1111/1475-3588.00051

Spiegler, M. D. (2016). *Contemporary behavior therapy.* Boston, MA: Cengage Learning.

Thompson, L. W., Gallagher, D., Nies, G., & Epstein, D. (1983). Evaluation of the effectiveness of professionals and nonprofessionals as instructors of "coping with depression" classes for elders. *The Gerontologist, 23,* 390–396. http://dx.doi.org/10.1093/geront/23.4.390

Watson, J. B. (1924). *Behaviorism.* New York, NY: Norton.

Weisz, J. R., Weiss, B., Han, S. S., Granger, D. A., & Morton, T. (1995). Effects of psychotherapy with children and adolescents revisited: A meta-analysis of treatment outcome studies. *Psychological Bulletin, 117,* 450–468. http://dx.doi.org/10.1037/0033-2909.117.3.450

Wixted, J. T., Bellack, A. S., & Hersen, M. (1990). Behavior therapy. In A. S. Bellack & M. Hersen (Eds.), *Handbook of comparative treatments for adult disorders* (pp. 17–33). New York, NY: Wiley.

Wolpe, J. (1958). *Psychotherapy by reciprocal inhibition.* Stanford, CA: Stanford University Press.

Zuriff, G. E. (1985). *Behaviorism: A conceptual reconstruction.* New York, NY: Columbia University Press.

9

THE SIX MODELS:
A COMPARATIVE ANALYSIS

This final chapter provides a comparative exploration of the six broad approaches discussed in this book. This analysis is followed by an examination of the relations of the models to different features of inpatient hospital programs (IHPs), partial hospital programs (PHPs), and residential treatment centers (RTCs). We consider what environmental characteristics strengthen or diminish the effectiveness of each model. As in Chapter 2, we define the treatment environment in terms of broad institutional variables, immediate contextual variables, and factors pertaining to the therapeutic frame, the patient population, and the therapist as an individual. We close this chapter by providing examples of several treatment environments and by walking the reader through the process of model selection.

http://dx.doi.org/10.1037/0000113-010
Group Psychotherapy in Inpatient, Partial Hospital, and Residential Care Settings, by V. Brabender and A. Fallon
Copyright © 2019 by the American Psychological Association. All rights reserved.

COMMONALITIES AMONG MODELS

Commonalities among models are important because they are likely to reveal the essential characteristics of any effective approach conducted in an IHP, PHP, and RTC setting. That is, if most or all model builders in these contexts have seen fit to include some particular feature, it might be that that feature has broad utility. The models in this text share five features listed in Exhibit 9.1. One such feature is a high level of specificity in treatment goals, characterization of change processes, and methods of intervention. At first, this point might appear to be circular given that we selected these models partly for their specificity. However, it is noteworthy that even 35 years ago, detailed approaches for these settings did not exist. It seems that greater specificity in goals, methods, and the like, occurred because clinicians came to recognize that their clinical circumstances demanded it.

Despite this shared specificity, the models differ on which of their aspects are best developed. For example, relative to other models, the object relations/systems (OR/S), mentalization, and acceptance and commitment therapy–group (ACT-G) models provide particularly refined expositions of the assumptions made about psychopathology in relation to the group's change processes. The interactional agenda and interpersonal psychotherapy–group (IPT-G) versions of the interpersonal model, as well as the problem-solving and social skills training model, involve an especially programmatic description of the methods used in the group. ACT-G

EXHIBIT 9.1
Commonalities and Differences Between Inpatient Hospital Program, Partial Hospital Program, and Residential Treatment Center Models of Group Psychotherapy

Commonalities
- Highly specific treatment goals, change processes, and interventions
- Provision of an explicit cognitive framework for organizing the affect that emerges in sessions
- Leadership qualities of warmth, responsiveness, active pursuit of goals, and moderate transparency
- Maintenance of consistent and clear boundaries
- Focus on the here and now

Differences
- A deficit- versus conflict-based view of psychopathology
- Target area of change: intrapsychic, experiential, behavioral, or administrative
- Relationship of group to the treatment unit in which it is embedded
- Leadership emphasis on technique versus relationships, leader focus on the group as a whole, subgroups, dyads, or individuals, and the leader's adoption of a directive versus reactive stance

distinguishes itself by the robust set of tools it offers the therapist to assess a member's progress. These respects in which models favorably distinguish themselves enable them to serve as examples of how other models might be developed further.

The second shared feature pertains to how the models handle the relation between affect and cognition in the group. Relative to earlier approaches, current approaches appear to offer members a much more substantial cognitive framework for organizing and understanding their affective lives. This provision derives from a common recognition of the disorganizing effects of unconstrained affective expression. The models vary in how they provide this cognitive framework. For example, consider the following excerpt from a session:

> Max, a patient with an anxiety disorder (among other problems), storms into the session. He announces he is going off his medication because a staff member admitted to him that the day prior, he was given another patient's medication. Other members immediately categorized this event as being a "one-in-a-million" occurrence and suggested that he was worrying about it needlessly. Max responded by pulling his chair back several inches, staring out the window, and nervously fidgeting with a paper cup.

All models have some mechanisms for helping Max and the group organize the affect he brought to the group and that he stimulated in other members (despite their appearance of unresponsiveness). The therapist implementing the problem-solving model would help the group identify the alternatives available to Max (and, by implication, to others) besides taking the medication compliantly or rejecting it altogether. Max's awareness of the diversity of options and his power to choose among them would be expected to serve as an antidote to his and others' anxiety. The OR/S model would immediately accept the reasonableness of Max's fright about this rather egregious error. The acknowledgment of the reality of the event would itself bridle Max's anxiety because the definition of the event limits its scope and, hence, its effect. Moreover, in this model, through clarifications, the therapist would help members accept identification with Max's fright. In assisting members in tolerating their identification with Max's discomfort, the therapist would interrupt a sequence of escalating projective identifications. In a mentalization approach, the therapist might encourage Max to elaborate on any fears he has about the ramifications of that mistake. The therapist would assist Max and others in recognizing that the presence of a fear does not establish the reality of the feared consequence (thereby helping Max to challenge psychic equivalence). In a cognitive behavioral model, the cognitive distortion of overgeneralization, which might have interfered with Max's ability to recognize alternate solutions, would be identified. In an ACT-G group, Max might consider whether going off of his medications is a form of experiential avoidance and whether this action has worked for him in the past. He might also consider whether this way of addressing his fears is consonant with his goals and values. Although the mechanisms of the models differ, their intended shared effect is to help members achieve affect regulation.

A third common feature is the posture of the leader: No model in this text advocates that the leader assume a posture of passivity and inscrutability. Rather, the recommended attributes of the leader in IHP, PHP, and RTC groups are warmth, responsiveness, and a moderate level of transparency. In all models, the leader is extremely active in pursuing goals and establishing and supporting norms that are compatible with the group's goals. Still, differences exist. In some models, such as the interactional focus group and social skills training models, the therapist is unstinting in offering individual members praise for desired behaviors. In others, such as the interactional agenda and mentalizing approaches, the therapist fosters others giving individual members positive and negative feedback. In still others, such as the OR/S and classic psychodynamic approaches, the groups strive to promote a secure and nurturing group climate, which supports individual members' reconstitution and development.

A fourth shared attribute is an insistence on the maintenance of consistent and clear internal and external boundaries. Again, the models differ on how boundary stability is to be achieved. For example, one respect in which the interactional agenda version of the interpersonal model creates a stable boundary is through the therapist's meticulous attendance to the starting time of the group session, as is seen, for example, in the therapist's refusal to allow late members entrance into the group. In the cognitive behavioral model, the boundary is created by the stipulation that no member can be accepted into the group unless he or she can remain in the group for several sessions. Despite this variability in methods of boundary setting, models are in accord in seeing the stability of boundaries as a prerequisite of a group's accomplishing its goals.

A fifth characteristic is a strong emphasis on the domain of experience tapped for the group's focus—namely, the here and now as opposed to the there and then. The *here* refers to the geographic immediacy of the social context of the group. The *here* in those groups taking place in larger treatment environments extends to the treatment environment itself. It is distinguished from *there*, which pertains to experiences that a given member might have outside the group to which other members are likely not privy. For example, an event that occurred at a member's home would be considered *there* rather than *here*. The *now* is a temporal concept that refers to the patient's recent (but not necessarily present) experience in the setting. For example, *now* might include an altercation between two group members in the lounge of the RTC in the evening before a session. By way of contrast, an event in a member's childhood would belong to *then*. IPT provides an exception to these definitions of the here and now. In IPT, here and now constitutes those events occurring within the person's contemporary life, whether they happen in the group or not. The problem-solving model similarly frames here-and-now events.

All the models in this text have some here-and-now aspect, an inclusion based on the presumption that the here and now provides more accurate data and more potential for engaging members in the group (Ferencik, 1991) than less immediate foci. Each of the models highlights a slightly different aspect of the here and now. ACT and mentalization groups encourage patients to focus on disturbing inner experiences activated by events in the group. The problem-solving model delves into members' here-and-now interpersonal information processing. It also gives priority to the examination of interpersonal problems that emerge among group members. The interpersonal model considers the present social interactions among members. The behavioral model analyzes the microscopic features of members' social behaviors. As we have written previously (Brabender & Fallon, 1993) and continues to be true, an example of a model placing little emphasis on the here and now is the cognitive behavioral model. However, even this model contains here-and-now elements. For example, members' reports on their homework experiences on the unit tap the extended here and now. More significant, the discussion of all events, inside or outside the group, enables the recognition of each member's automatic thoughts and cognitive schemes, which are assumed to be in continuous operation. Although many of these models permit members to make excursions into the there and then, they are used either to provide a transition to the here and now or to enable the group to discern what present elements are most worthy of the group's consideration.

In summary, any adequate approach to psychotherapy groups conducted in IHP, PHP, or RTCs must involve the following: (a) well-articulated goals and methods, (b) mechanisms for the containment of affect, (c) a leader who is highly active and emotionally available, (d) consistent internal and external boundaries that serve as a framework for the group, and (e) a focus on the here and now.

DIFFERENCES AMONG MODELS

Differences among models are important because they highlight critical areas of controversy, many of which can be addressed empirically. The identification of differences also leads to the delineation of important contextual and population variables that must be considered in selecting a model for a given setting. We consider differences among models in four areas: (a) their philosophical underpinnings, (b) their goals, (c) their perspectives on the group-treatment program relationship, and (d) the role of the leader.

Philosophical Underpinnings

The most basic area of difference among the models is the set of assumptions they make about psychopathology. One heuristic distinction for capturing philosophical differences among the models is whether a model sees psychopathology as deficit or conflict based (Jang, 2005; Karasu, 1994). *Deficit models* regard psychopathology as a result of a developmental arrest or loss that deprives the person of the necessary structures, processes, or repertoires of behaviors essential for maintaining a stable sense of well-being. In contrast, *conflict models* seek modification in already-present structures and processes. They assume that psychological problems are rooted in the individual's difficulty in managing the presence of conflicting cognitions, affects, and impulses.

Among the models in this book, those most clearly falling into the conflict framework are the classic psychodynamic model, the OR/S model, and the unstructured version of the interpersonal model. The OR/S model (Kibel, 2003) explicitly defines itself as a conflict model and addresses such tensions as those between a person's negative affects and the mechanisms he or she uses to defend against those affects. Although less explicit, the unstructured version of the interpersonal model seems to have a conflict foundation given that its application frequently entails members' gaining awareness of how their warded-off affects and impulses control maladaptive social behaviors.

The clearest examples of a deficit model are those models that entail members' acquisitions of a skill in the group. The problem-solving model, which regards members' psychopathologies as fundamental to their lack of effective decision-making processes, is a deficit model par excellence. Other models that appear to be most accurately classified as having a deficit rather than conflict orientation are the social skills version of the behavioral model, the mentalization model, the focus group, interactional and IPT versions of the interpersonal model, and Meichenbaum's (2007) stress inoculation and self-instruction training versions of the cognitive behavioral model. As Kibel (1987a) pointed out, although these models do not always explicitly declare their assumptions about psychopathology, they hold that individuals in need of extensive care lack a particular psychological commodity essential to the achievement of a sense of well-being: a lack of knowledge of others' reactions to their behaviors.

Although the deficit–conflict distinction is useful in that it enables an understanding of other differences among models, it does not provide a perfect framework for comparison because the notions of conflict and deficit do not represent endpoints of a univariate continuum. It is possible for models to have both conflict and deficit elements. Even the OR/S model, which is a prime example of a conflict model, has deficit components—namely, members' lack of tolerance for their negative affects and their inability (at the time of admission) to engage in splitting, or the partitioning of representations according to their positive or negative valence.

Despite these deficit components, the Kibel (1987a, 1987b) model emphasizes the conflict over the deficit aspect. With other models, the emphasis is less obvious, particularly those models that have been influenced by widely diverging theoretical orientations. Beck's (1976, 1991) version of the cognitive model, with its complex theoretical foundations, is an example. Reflecting its psychoanalytic roots, the model seeks to alter preexisting structures—specifically, the cognitive schemes responsible for the individual's disturbing affects. Like the conflict models, the model assumes (without embracing the notion of defense, however) that these schemes are not entirely within conscious awareness and that part of the therapeutic task is to make them so. In consonance with both the behavioral roots of the model and a deficit perspective, the model emphasizes the acquisition of adaptive skills such as the ability to correct distorted thoughts. Although we see the deficit aspect as being more conspicuous in this model, we recognize that others might reasonably disagree.

Particularly for those models that are easily classified using the deficit–conflict distinction, this philosophical difference concerning defining psychopathology sets the stage for other differences on how psychopathology is best treated. An important difference is the therapist's response to the emergence of affect in the group. It was suggested earlier that although all models help members organize affect, especially hostility, models vary in the extent to which negative feelings are allowed entrance in the sessions. Some models (e.g., interactional agenda) actively discourage aggression in the group in anything but the most muted form. Others (e.g., mentalizing groups) welcome the emergence of strong negative feeling but provide some scaffolding for it so it stays in a mild to moderate range. Still others create such a high level of cognitive structuring of experience (e.g., cognitive behavioral, problem solving) such that, although hostility is not explicitly discouraged, it is given little room to surface.

Another feature of models that is related to the conflict–deficit distinction is whether the model accepts members' communications on a manifest level or whether it seeks to unlock latent or hidden meanings in the members' communications. Whereas the deficit models might focus on either the latent or manifest aspects, the conflict models invariably require the therapist to search for latent content. According to conflict-based models, the individual's intolerance of some (or any) polarity in experience necessitates defensive activity. Defended-against contents emerge symbolically rather than directly. The therapist who is interested in helping the member be more tolerant of opposing cognitions, feelings, or impulses can assist the member in identifying (and eventually accepting) unwanted psychological elements by listening to the member's communications as metaphors, symbols, or derivatives. For example, within the OR/S model, the therapist listens to material with an ear to how it might reflect reactions to events on the unit. Although attendance to the covert level of communication is certainly compatible with the unstructured version of the interpersonal model, it seems to be less of an emphasis in the interactional and focus group versions.

Deficit models do not preclude the therapist's search for latent meanings because the notion of individuals protecting themselves from psychological discomfort is wholly compatible with at least some of these models. For example, an individual could speak in metaphorical terms about the deficit itself when the full and direct acknowledgment of its existence would be intolerable. Alternately, the model might hold that members discover parts of themselves once particular experiences no longer serve as a camouflage for those parts. For example, in ACT-G (Westrup & Wright, 2017), individuals often discover the values that had been obscured by their efforts to control their private experiences. The effort to control is not a defense against values per se but nonetheless can mask values. However, the deficit perspective does not require attendance to latent meaning: Some deficit models (e.g., behavioral) take members' comments largely at face value.

Goals of the Group

Related to, but separate from, the philosophical underpinnings of a model are the goals of the groups. Models vary in what they establish as the primary target of change. What Erickson noted in 1984 holds true today: A taxonomy of goals has yet to be established for group psychotherapy. However, one distinction that can be made among different approaches is whether the type of change they seek is intrapsychic, experiential, behavioral, or administrative. These goals are not mutually exclusive.

Models that target intrapsychic or dynamic change seek to alter the balance of psychological forces within the psyche, forces that might or might not be conscious. All conflict-based models fall into this category. All the psychodynamic models presented in Chapter 4 entail some reorganization of an individual's representations of self and other. They also seek to effect a shift in those psychic processes that create emotional experiences. For example, the mentalization model nurtures the individual's capacity to engage in self-reflection. The OR/S model seeks to help the individual use more mature defenses, specifically those premorbid defenses that permit life in the community. The unstructured version of the interpersonal model also can, at least by design, produce intrapsychic change on the notion that as individual interpersonal experiences change, their scheme of self and others also changes. Moreover, interpersonal approaches at times work toward the goal of helping individuals obtain access to preconscious affects and impulses that control their maladaptive social behaviors.

In the second category are those models that assume that the member's phenomenology or conscious experience can be altered through group participation. Models that seek experiential change can be divided into those that emphasize affective versus cognitive aspects of experience. In the former category are the interpersonal, OR/S, and ACT-G models. For example, the interpersonal model attempts to increase the member's openness to interactions with others. The OR/S model aims to lessen a member's hostility toward self and others. ACT-G entails members' engaging in valued living, which involves a willingness to have negative private events in the context of pursuing one's values. Models that target a more cognitive type of experiential change are the problem-solving and cognitive behavioral models. The experiential changes sought by the problem-solving model are the following: recognition of the problem-solving style, greater clarity in defining the problem at hand, enhanced awareness of the diversity of solutions to a problem, and strengthened confidence in choosing among them. It is presumed that these changes are accompanied by a fortified sense of control and competence in facing life's tasks. The cognitive behavioral model, including dialectical behavior therapy (DBT) applications of it, seeks a change in both the cognitions that induce painful affect and the painful affects themselves.

Many of the models in this text claim to produce behavioral change. The type of change and level of specificity is highly variable from model to model, and some models expect to produce either general or specific changes. On a general level, the interpersonal, OR/S, and mentalization models all expect that members' group participation will awaken in them a desire for relationships. Members should exhibit a greater frequency of engagement behaviors as a result of group involvement. Other models are designed to enable the achievement of more specific goals. The unstructured version of the interpersonal model attempts to lessen those interpersonal behaviors that lead to alienation between a member and others in his or her life. The monopolizer should monopolize less; the interrupter should interrupt less. Application of the cognitive behavioral model should diminish the frequency and intensity of whatever behaviors were associated with the individual's negative cognitions and affects. For example, depressed individuals who benefit from this approach might show less avoidance of interpersonal contacts and a greater frequency of positive statements. At the endpoint of the continuum of specificity is the behavioral model, which demands concrete, measurable changes in a member's communication behaviors before the model can be deemed successfully applied. For example, a particular group member might be expected to show better voice modulation or fewer interrupting behaviors as a function of group involvement.

All the aforementioned types of goals concern changes in the individual. As Erickson (1984) pointed out, certain models seek more systemic changes as a consequence of successful application. He referred to goals that pertain either to the broader context in which the group takes place or to the individuals' behaviors in that context as *administrative goals*. Certain of the models featured in this text explicitly posit administrative goals. The OR/S model sees the group as a place in which tensions on the unit can be diminished. The interactional agenda and focus group versions of the interpersonal model and the OR/S model hold that successful group participation leads to patients' increased receptivity to other modalities.

THE MODELS' PERSPECTIVES OF THE GROUP WITHIN THE SYSTEM

Models vary in how they conceptualize the relation between the group and the treatment context in which the group is embedded. Although most models seem to recognize that the group exists within a hierarchy of systems, a point of difference is whether any given model views the group as capable of becoming a system in its own right. On one end of the continuum is the perception of the group as so completely open to the influence of the unit that it is unable to achieve its own integrity as a system; it remains forever a subsystem. Within that perspective, because the group is unable to have a life of its own (i.e., its own dynamic process and its own structural features), the group therapist must necessarily focus on group–unit relations. This view leads inexorably to the notion that no event in the group can be adequately understood simply in relation to the group itself. Group events are elucidated by referral to life on the unit. Representing this position is the OR/S model. The system of meaning proposed by this model is one wherein the group events are seen as reflecting unit dynamics. The key interventions associated with this model are designed to help members recognize the connection between group and unit events.

On the other end of the continuum is the position that the psychotherapy group, even within a larger program or unit, can potentially achieve the status of a bona fide system with sufficiently limited boundary permeability to permit the group to develop its own dynamic concerns, goals, norms, and so on. An example of this view of the group–program relation is the problem-solving model, which teaches members a method of thinking that is assumed to have value independent of the particular problems with which members are struggling, including problems emerging on the unit. The behavioral and cognitive behavioral models are additional examples of models that treat the group as autonomous from the unit.

Those models that might be positioned more centrally on this continuum of group–unit separateness are ones that see the group as having a high level of boundary permeability but not so much that the group is unable to pursue its goals independently of the unit. These models tend to view the external environment as a resource to the group and vice versa. For example, the interactional agenda model looks to members' interactions with one another as a source of material for the establishment of agendas. It also sees the group as a place in which unit-level problems can be productively addressed, thereby leading to a diminishment of tension on the unit. IPT regards the key interpersonal difficulties members are having outside the program as of primary interest. Group or program social difficulties are of exploratory interest only if they reflect these external problems. Similarly, the mentalization model sees life in the program as providing events that members can then endeavor to mentalize within the group.

An implication of the group's conceptualized relationship to the program or unit in which it is embedded is in the extent to which the therapist can make decisions independently of what is occurring in the broader context. A group conceptualized as a subsystem of a system requires the therapist's careful attendance to system dynamics and events in the treatment context. Those groups that are viewed as autonomous accord the therapist much more independence in working with members. However, in no circumstance should the therapist be indifferent to the broader context. All group therapists working in a larger treatment context do well to develop strong alliances with the other staff members who work with group members. A cultivated understanding on the part of staff members of a model's goals and the processes through which the goals are met nurture such alliances.

Role of the Leader

Although the models agree on particular features that are ascribed to the effective leader, important differences exist among them in their characterization of the leader's role.

Emphasis on Techniques Versus the Patient–Therapist Relationship

Some models see the relationship between the therapist and group member as a focus of the group's work and an instrument in members' progress. For example, psychodynamic models, in general, assume that the therapist is likely to evoke the reactions that members have toward authority figures. These models further posit that the exploration of these reactions can serve important therapeutic goals, such as the lessening of members' dependency on authority. Other models that are more technique oriented see the patient–therapist relationship as having a more collateral effect on the treatment. A positive therapist–patient relationship is useful in that it supports group members' receptiveness to the techniques that the therapist presents. However, it is the techniques and not the relationship from which members directly benefit. Probably the best example of a technique-oriented model is the social skills version of the behavioral model. In this approach, the therapist is primarily a technician. The quality of the relationship is important but only in that it affects members' openness to the therapist's techniques.

The problem-solving model places a more moderate level of emphasis on the relationship. Because the therapist in this model takes a fairly directive role, the members must have sufficiently positive regard for the leader to follow. Beyond this factor, however, the model has a proviso that problems that arise within the sessions have priority over those that emerge outside the group. Hence, if a member were to experience him- or herself as having a problem with the leader (or any group member, for that matter), that problem would be given priority in relation to problems external to the group. The mentalizing model takes a somewhat similar position as the problem-solving model in that preference is given to the exploration of relationships in the group.

Level of Conceptualization

Another dimensional difference is whether the model conceptualizes the group primarily at the group-as-a-whole (and subgroup), interpersonal, and individual level. We discuss each level in turn.

Some models assume that dynamics exist pertaining to the group as a social system apart from the issues that surface for any individual member. They further hold that the therapist's attendance to these group-as-a-whole phenomena has therapeutic utility. An example of a model in this category is the OR/S model. It might be noted that the group-as-a-whole perspective does not mandate the exclusive or even predominant use of group-as-a-whole interpretations. Models involving this level of conceptualization also require the use of interventions at the individual, interpersonal, and subgroup levels. However, those interventions deemed to be most powerful in advancing the goals of the group are ones formulated at the subgroup and group-as-a-whole levels. Other levels of intervention might be seen as developing members' receptivity to an eventual group-as-a-whole interpretation.

Another set of models featured in this text involves the therapist's conceptualization of occurrences in the group on an interpersonal or dyadic level. Specific member–member or leader–member interactions are the primary units of analysis. Examples of models that emphasize the interpersonal level of conceptualization are all versions of the interpersonal model. Once again, although this level of analysis represents the emphasis of these models, it is by no means the exclusive focus. For example, the interpersonal model stresses the importance of building cohesiveness within the group, which implies the presence of an aspect of the group that exists apart from the feelings any two members have toward one another. Also, these models specifically underscore the importance of the therapist's intervening on the individual level to deal with particularly withdrawn or anxious members or to respond to emergencies that might develop with any given member, as when a member attempts to leave the group.

For the third category of models, the conceptualization of problems at the individual level is key to members' progress. Examples of approaches within this category are the cognitive behavioral, problem-solving, DBT, schema-focused therapy, and the behavioral models. These models involve not only conceptualization but also intervention at the individual level. Although some proponents of these models talk about the necessity of developing a certain emotional atmosphere in the group that is propitious for individual work, group-level factors are less of a focus in the cognitive behavioral model than they are in the other two models. Also, interventions having somewhat of an interpersonal cast are occasionally used within this model, as when members participating in a cognitive behavioral group test out dysfunctional beliefs using feedback from other group members. However, unlike their use in the interpersonal models, these interventions are designed to benefit only one person rather than both members of the dyad.

Directive Versus Reactive

Another set of variables that distinguishes each model is the extent to which the therapist assumes a directive versus a reactive posture in relation to the content and the process of the session.

Direction on Content. Models vary in the freedom they accord members in determining the content of the session. Here, *content* refers to what the group talks about (in contrast to how it talks about it). For example, if in a segment of a session, members talk about their relationships with their psychiatrists, that topic is the content of the segment. In some models, the therapist intervenes in such a way as to guarantee the emergence of specifically defined material and support the submergence of other topics. Such models require a highly directive posture on the part of the therapist in determining the topics the group will address. Contrasting with this posture is one in which the therapist is reactive to whatever is spontaneously produced in the group. Although the therapist might guide the group to some broad realm of exploration, such as the here and now, the group is nonetheless given considerable latitude in the particular concerns it addresses. Models that require a reactive posture in relation to content frequently emphasize the importance of the therapist's accurate discernment of the concerns (explicit or implicit) occupying the group's attention. That is, reactive models highlight the therapist's diagnostic activity vis-à-vis group, subgroup, interpersonal, or individual dynamics.

An example of a model that is directive vis-à-vis the session's content is a behaviorally oriented assertiveness-training group. To enhance members' engagement in appropriate assertive behaviors, the therapist might ask them to recount situations in which they had either failed or succeeded in exhibiting assertive behaviors. The therapist categorizes other material as "irrelevant" or used as a segue to discussing assertiveness-related situations. The interpersonal agenda model is also directive, albeit to a lesser extent. Once the agenda is established, that becomes the focus of the member's work. Any other emerging issues are likely related back to the agenda. In some instances, the therapist might point to new material as forming the basis for an agenda in an ensuing session.

Direction on Process. Process is distinct from content in that *process* refers to how a group pursues its work. In the former example in which members were talking about their psychiatrists, the process of the group might refer to a format that evolved in the group wherein each member made a comment and waited for the therapist to respond. Some models specify in a highly detailed and programmatic way how problems are to be addressed. Usually, these models require that sessions be highly formatted. Other models provide only general guidelines that can be observed in various ways both by the group members and by the therapist.

Two examples of models that require a high level of therapist direction regarding the group process are the cognitive behavioral and problem-solving models. Within each, the sessions have a highly articulated format, and the patient–therapist and member–member interactions are clearly proscribed by the model. In contrast, such models as the unstructured interpersonal and OR/S models provide the therapist with a set of goals and a range of interventions that might be helpful in pursuing group goals. However, what interventions should be deployed at any moment of the group's life is largely left to the judgment of the therapist.

A model's stance on the deficit–conflict issue has a bearing on the therapist's levels of reactivity and directiveness on both content and process dimensions. Conflict models assume that what creates a problem for patients is not what is missing but what is present. They posit that if members are provided with the conditions to speak openly about their experience, the therapist will have the necessary material for the work of the group. The therapist then reacts to the surfacing of such material with interventions designed to foster its organization. Hence, conflict therapists are inclined to assume a primarily reactive posture concerning both process and content.

However, some directive elements might be present such as when the thera-pist fosters a process of members giving feedback to one another. The deficit models emphasize what is missing or insufficiently present in the patient. The therapist must create the necessary experiences within the group so that some structure, process, or repertoire of behaviors can either be acquired or strengthened. Hence, deficit models tend to place the therapist in a position of being directive. To the extent that the model sees the deficit as being one of process, the therapist is likely to be directive with respect to how the group functions. A relevant example is the problem-solving model, which sees patients as lacking effective means to solve problems. Members are directed to focus on specific problems using a highly prescribed process. Although members might be free to identify the particular problems targeted, once a problem is selected, members focus on it for a protracted interval within the session using a highly specific and invariable sequence of steps.

VARIATION IN SETTINGS

In this text, we have undertaken the task of describing models that might be used in one or more of three types of settings: IHPs, PHPs, and RTCs. We now examine each setting with a consideration of the models most suited to application within that treatment context.

Inpatient Hospital Programs

Almost always, inpatient treatment in the United States is brief. Individuals receive inpatient treatment only as long as they are regarded as an immediate threat to themselves or others. Consequently, appropriate treatment models are those that can be applied over an exceedingly brief duration. Some individuals might remain in the group for only a single ses-sion. The challenge for the group therapist is to find a model that can have utility within that extremely limited time frame. Many models in this text are ideally suited to time frames longer than most inpatient stays. However, with adaptation, these models can be serviceable. Two examples are ACT-G and mentalization models. These models are used to best effect when the therapist has a sufficient number of sessions to present concepts sequentially, allowing members to practice the application of each element and obtain feedback on the practice before moving on. However, a subset of elements of both of these models can be introduced in a psychoeducational way, thereby providing a foundation for later work on an outpatient basis. For example, in an IHP group, the therapist might focus on goals and values over two ses-sions. In doing so, the therapist would cultivate the members' appreciation of how allowing goals and values to guide action enables the member to achieve a meaningful life, even amidst psychological suffering. For ACT-G, investigators have observed benefit over as few as two sessions (e.g., Tyrberg, Carlbring, & Lundgren, 2017). For models that can be adapted in this way, the learning is intensified if unit staff members are familiar with the goals' models and processes and can engage patients therapeutically with the model's concepts outside the session.

Some models have been developed in recognition that a member might be in the group for only a single session. Our prime examples of group formats designed for a brief time frame are the OR/S models (or Kibel groups) and the interactional agenda and focus group models. These models distinguish themselves for positing goals that can be achieved in even a single session. For example, the interactional agenda model establishes as a goal enabling members to have a positive group experience by seeing themselves fulfill an agenda within the confines of a session. The OR/S model helps members to reacquire the defense of splitting by members' having their negative emotional experiences validated within the session. Unfortunately, although the interactional agenda model has been studied on a limited basis (e.g., see Pollack, Harvin, & Cramer, 2001), the OR/S model has received no empirical scrutiny, to the best of our knowledge. We recommend that other models establish limited goals that can be accomplished in one or two sessions so that a broader array of models will be available in our current inpatient environments. Often, the abbreviated delivery of a model entails the extraction of one or two concepts that can be delivered in a psychoeducational format. Both ACT and mentalization approaches make use of this flexibility and, as the research suggests, to good effect.

As we discussed in Chapter 1, much of the contemporary research on inpatient groups is taking place in Europe. In many European countries, individuals remain for a longer duration of treatment than in the United States. Psychodynamic approaches, in particular, have been subject to empirical scrutiny, but much of the emphasis of the research is on the linkage between process and outcome. An example is Kirchmann et al.'s (2009) study examining attachment characteristics, group climate, and outcomes in the context of psychodynamic group psychotherapy. The researchers found definite links between member characteristics, process characteristics of the group, and outcome. They identified a link, for instance, between attachment security and outcome. Such research not only teaches us whether a given model is effective but also how we can catalyze its application.

Partial Hospital Programs

The reader might recall that in Chapter 1, we distinguished three forms of PHPs: day hospital, day treatment, and day care programs (Piper,

Rosie, Joyce, & Azim, 1996). These forms distinguish themselves from one another on the basis of the acuteness versus chronicity of the population, with day care involving the treatment of individuals at the lowest level of ego functioning. Group therapy is a key modality across all these types of PHPs (Neuhaus, Christopher, Jacob, Guillaumot, & Burns, 2007). Most of the models described in this text are suitable for clients in day hospital and day treatment programs. A few, such as the social skills training model, the problem-solving model, and the focus group interpersonal model, would be appropriate for a day care population.

A subset of the models featured in this text has been studied in PHP contexts. Most of the studies are limited by lack of random assignment, small sample size, insufficient examination of model adherence, and other methodological problems. Nonetheless, these studies are mentioned because the findings are promising:

- Application of the mentalization model in a PHP with persons with borderline personality disorder showed diminished frequency of suicide attempts and acts of self-harm, diminished depression and anxiety, improved interpersonal functioning, and reduced social services use (Bateman & Fonagy, 2001, 2006). These positive changes were sustained over an 8-year period following treatment (Bateman & Fonagy, 2008). Moreover, such treatment was more cost-effective than the treatment-as-usual (TAU) condition (Bateman & Fonagy, 2003).

- A 2-week cognitive behavioral program emphasizing group therapy was offered to PHP patients with heterogeneous symptoms (Neuhaus et al., 2007). A comparison of self-report measures administered before, 1 week after and 2 weeks after treatment shows a diminishment in symptoms. For example, Beck Depression Inventory (Beck & Steer, 1987) scores moved from the severe to the moderate range. A significant limitation of the study is the lack of a control group. Reisch, Thommen, Tschacher, and Hirsbrunner (2001) obtained similar findings. In both of these studies, the group is not investigated separately from the treatment program in which it is embedded. The treatment is designed to be a program-wide, consistent experience. Wilberg, Karterud, Urnes, Pedersen, and Friis (1998) found medium to high effect sizes on the Global Assessment of Functioning (American Psychiatric Association, 1994), Global Severity Index of the Symptom Checklist–90–Revised (Derogatis & Unger, 2010), and Inventory of Interpersonal Problems (Alden, Wiggins, & Pincus, 1990) with the implementation of a program emphasizing cognitive behavior therapy (CBT) groups with poorly functioning patients with personality disorders. Again, the absence of a control group limits our ability to infer causality. Borderline patients participated in a 3-week program in DBT consisting of both individual and group treatment (McQuillan et al., 2005). Participants showed a decline in scores on depression and hopelessness scales. Women diagnosed with borderline personality disorder participated in a 5-day DBT day hospital program combining individual and group psychotherapies (Yen, Johnson, Costello, & Simpson, 2009). A 3-month follow-up demonstrated significant declines in hopelessness, depression, dissociation, anger expression, and general psychopathology.

The fact that multiple models might be useful in a PHP setting is positive given that a variety of factors, such as staff theoretical orientation, might recommend one over another in a specific context.

Residential Treatment Centers

RTCs have become increasingly popular because they provide many of the treatment advantages of inpatient hospitalization at a much lower cost. Group psychotherapy of many varieties is a staple of these programs. As in the case of PHPs, the study of particular models of group psychotherapy in RTCs is at an early stage. Nonetheless, investigators have made some preliminary findings, many of which were discussed at greater length in earlier chapters:

- A trend was found for patients with eating disorders to exhibit less eating pathology with TAU plus ACT than TAU alone (Juarascio et al., 2013).
- Individuals with social phobia were assigned to either cognitive or interpersonal group therapy with four sessions a week over 10 weeks. Although patients received some individual therapy, 88% of the work occurred in groups. Patients in both groups showed diminished fear, avoidance, distress, and thought interference after treatment and at a 1-year follow-up, yet the two groups did not differ from each other in the extent of change. Notably, the attrition rate was 8% and 20% for the interpersonal and cognitive treatments, respectively (Borge et al., 2008).
- Individuals receiving four sessions of interactional agenda group psychotherapy showed less difficulty with symptoms and

negative behaviors (e.g., addictive behaviors) 3 months after being discharged from the hospital relative to their admission levels in comparison with a self-management group (Pollack et al., 2001).

- Steil, Dyer, Priebe, Kleindienst, and Bohus (2011) investigated a program of DBT (including both individual and group elements) in a pilot study of individuals with posttraumatic stress disorder (PTSD) from child sexual abuse. Patient acceptance was high, reflected by the fact that no patient dropped out of treatment. Patients showed a significant decline in symptoms of PTSD and continued to improve 6 weeks after the conclusion of treatment.

CASE EXAMPLES

The premise of this book is that in selecting a model, the therapist should take into account an array of contextual features of the setting. In this section, we illustrate the process through a case example from each of the settings we featured in this text. Although these cases are fictive, they represent common situations in these settings.

Case 1: Inpatient Hospital Program

Description

A group psychotherapist had recently joined the treatment team of an acute-care psychiatric unit of a general hospital that had a long-standing reputation as a training institution. The ambiance of the unit was one of respect among the professionals, in part due to their endorsement of a holistic view of treatment. However, in the past several years, the staff had been feeling a growing frustration with their sense that nothing of substance could be accomplished given patients' ever-diminishing lengths of stay. The average length of stay was 6 days, although some patients were hospitalized for only 2 to 3 days.

The patients were heterogeneous regarding ego functioning and diagnosis, although about half had a psychotic diagnosis. The other half had various types of character pathology. A psychodynamically oriented therapist, now departing, led a therapy group on the unit over several years and described the group as having an eclectic character. Staff reported that the therapist attempted to support members in modifying inappropriate social behaviors by gaining insight into the childhood roots of present problematic behaviors. Staff admitted to having had difficulty getting members to attend the group and expressed some puzzlement as to whether members' resistances were due to the inherently threatening nature of group therapy or to the therapist's approach. When a new therapist interviewed for the position, the unit administrator articulated a wish that she would run a group that patients would "like better." The previous group met four times weekly for hour-long sessions, a time frame available for the new therapist's group. The group was open ended, and membership changed on an almost daily basis. Members tended to enter the group immediately after admission to the unit. The new psychotherapist, who described herself as broadly psychodynamic, was faced with the task of identifying what model would be optimal in this setting with all its features.

Analysis

In this circumstance, the selection of an appropriate model would benefit not only the members of the group but also the unit at large. The therapist's demonstration of the value of a delimitation and concretization of goals would serve as an antidote to staff frustration and possibly provide an example for other modalities.

In selecting an approach, the therapist should consider the degree of empirical support each model has amassed. As the reader has seen, the empirical support varies considerably from model to model. However, for most of the models, the support for the model's application in IHPs, PHPs, and RTCs, specifically, is lacking. In addition to considering the empirical base of different approaches, the therapist should think about what demands different models make on the treatment context. A good beginning point is the set of fixed features of the setting because these features are maximally constraining to the therapist. Although these fixed features are often global aspects of the setting, this is not invariably the case. For example, member tenure in the group is a highly specific feature of the setting and is frequently not under the therapist's control given that it is linked to length of hospitalization. In our analysis, we begin with the more global variables, such as the philosophy of the institution, recognizing that some alternative order might be useful in other practitioners' settings.

In this example, because the practitioner's unit and possibly the institution embraced a holistic perspective, the therapist was minimally constrained in model selection philosophically. The caveat to this point is that staff's escalating frustration and sense of helplessness in relation to the demand to operate within a strict temporal frame might precipitate their adoption of a radically different perspective. Hence, the therapist must recognize that the frustration of the staff creates an unstable climate that must be taken into account in both selecting the model and planning its presentation to the treatment team.

Here, the group's embeddedness on the unit was a major force in the group dynamics. In any setting, a group on a unit is greatly affected by unit dynamics, events, issues, and so on. In such a circumstance, the therapist must anticipate the likelihood that staff's shared dissatisfaction will likely seep into the group sessions. The therapist must find a way to use this dissatisfaction to further members' well-being. As we have mentioned repeatedly, some models provide little opportunity for the group to deal with unit-level issues. Simply on the basis of the variables that have been considered, these models do not seem to be a good match for the practitioner's setting.

The temporal variables might be reviewed next. Because staff members were responding to one particular temporal feature, the average length of stay, one could anticipate that this feature would play a major role in the selection of an appropriate model. In this setting, members' tenures in the group were fairly brief. Of even greater import was the rather considerable segment of the admitted population that remained in the hospital for no more than two sessions. The brevity required that a single session be viewed as the length of the group. In other words, the therapist should not anticipate that members can transfer information from session to session. Moreover, the group should be designed so that each member can derive some benefit from each session. These considerations raise questions about the feasibility of the general psychodynamic, unstructured interpersonal, cognitive behavioral (with the exception of Freeman's (1990) theme-based cognitive behavioral model), IPT-G, DBT, schema-focused therapy, and problem-solving models, all of which require a member's tenure to be at least several sessions. ACT-G and mentalizing approaches could be offered only as psychoeducational group experiences with far more modest goals then typically would be pursued.

Compositional variables also might be considered in model selection. Patients on this unit were fairly heterogeneous in functioning. The therapist could respond to this heterogeneity in at least two ways. He could select a model that is conducive to the inclusions of members of radically different levels of functioning, or he could establish admission criteria for the group that would create greater homogeneity in functioning (e.g., the presence of a particular social skills deficit). These alternatives are not mutually exclusive. In a setting of this nature, a certain percentage of members probably would be so acutely disturbed that they would be unable to participate in any sort of group. The issue, then, is what degree of homogeneity is sought. One consideration in this regard is what other groups are present on the unit. For example, if activity groups having the earlier-cited characteristics of an effective group for low-functioning patients are available, the therapist might wish to design a group serving the special needs of the higher functioning patients. The great diagnostic variability might render the use of the cognitive behavioral model difficult, particularly given patients' typically brief hospitalizations.

From this analysis, three models emerge as being reasonably congruent with the features of the setting: the OR/S model and the interactional agenda and focus group versions of the interpersonal model. The interactional agenda group would be a good candidate if the needs of the lower functioning members could be served by either a focus group or, as suggested earlier, an activities therapy group. However, an advantage of the OR/S model over the interactional agenda group is its ability to focus systematically on unit dynamics. In this case, staff's high level of frustration makes unit dynamics particularly important. As indicated in Chapter 3, although the interactional agenda model can address individual member's idiosyncratic and maladaptive reactions to the unit, it has no mechanism to work with the reactions as the group as a whole. The interactional agenda format could, of course, be modified to address group-as-a-whole phenomena, and there are indications in the literature that some clinicians are making such modifications (e.g., Pollack et al., 2001; Taylor, Coombes, & Bartlett, 2002).

The OR/S model would also likely have a beneficial effect on the unit as a system. Because the model operates on the group in its status as a subsystem of the unit, any change in organizational features or affective tone of the group is likely to permeate through the broader community. The OR/S model would also be compatible with this particular therapist's theoretical orientation.

In summary, in this example, we see some advantage in the OR/S model over the interactional agenda group primarily because of the emotional tenor of the unit. However, the interactional agenda approach has a strength the OR/S model lacks: face validity from a staff perspective. In most institutions, the goals and methods of any interpersonal model are likely to be coherent to the staff. In contrast, staff members sometimes see the goals of the OR/S model as either elusive or counterintuitive. The goals of the model are at odds with the common assumption of the staff that their efforts should be directed at helping members overcome their proclivity for splitting. Given the perceived (if not real) failure of the previous group and the staff biases this failure created, if the therapist adopts an OR/S model, she must put substantial effort into staff education about the rationale and workings of the model.

Case 2: Partial Hospital Setting

Description

A large mental health facility had a PHP for individuals with severe and persistent mental illness. Many of these individuals entered this program on discharge from emergency crisis-oriented hospitalization. The PHP had a two-tier group psychotherapy system. One tier was a 5-day, week-long experience for individuals who had just entered the PHP (Level I group). Many of them were actively symptomatic. All of them were organized at either the lower borderline or psychotic level. The other group was for the graduates of this initial group experience (Level II group).

The staff member who had run this group left for a position at another institution. She had described her approach as "doing whatever works." Member satisfaction ratings taken on the group yielded mildly unfavorable results. Staff members hoped that a new group psychotherapist would reinvigorate the group. During the same period, Dr. Horne, one of the staff members, a psychiatric resident who had run psychotherapy groups in the past, began to contemplate what might be possible. In examining attendance statistics, Dr. Horne discovered that over 60% of the members did remain in the group for all five sessions and 80% remained for at least four.

Analysis

Dr. Horne began her analysis by recognizing that the two-tier system was a fixed feature of the setting, as was the length of stay of the Level I group. Therefore, a model that accommodates this time frame would be appropriate. Many models require longer tenures. For example, the social skills version of the behavioral model requires a longer period in the group for members to master the complex behaviors that will aid them in living successfully in the community. Interpersonal and psychodynamic models that involved a fairly low level of structure would lack the necessary efficiency in the face of such time constraints. However, more structured applications of each of these types might be suitable. The fact that members remained in the group for four or five sessions gave the therapist some flexibility. For example, the interactional agenda model can be difficult to implement when the therapist aims to have each member both set an agenda and do a significant amount of work in a given session. When members' returns are ensured, the therapist might vary which members obtain the most intensive attention in any one session. The therapist could also use a model in which one session could build on another. For example, participation in ACT over only four or five sessions has been observed to produce positive effects in patients with psychosis (Bach & Hayes, 2002; Martins, Castilho, Santos, & Gumley, 2016) and patients with chronic pain (McCracken, Sato, & Taylor, 2013).

The characteristics of the members should also influence model selection. The model would have to accommodate individuals who are experiencing high levels of stress yet occupy different levels of functioning. Most of the models in this text have the flexibility to address the needs of individuals at somewhat different levels of ego functioning. A few of the models—particularly the interpersonal focus group model—might serve well the needs of the members with psychosis but use insufficiently the resources of the higher functioning members, resources such as the ability to tolerate some anxiety in the group. Some models can be geared to different levels but not within the same group. For example, the social skills behavioral model can enable individuals at either the psychotic or borderline levels to improve their social skills. However, combining such individuals into a single group would not be feasible because individuals at each level have a different set of skills to master and refine.

A major issue with the prior group was that members did not see it as particularly useful. Apart from any other outcomes, member evaluation is important because negative views of the group can lead to dropping out and lack of participation. For members to commit to the group, they would have to see that the group's goals and processes address their extreme levels of discomfort. Some formats might do so more clearly and directly than others in members' perceptions. For example, the evidence that the problem-solving model produces symptom relief is strong. How such a model might support members in managing their levels of distress might not be obvious to members over their brief tenures. In contrast, for example, ACT speaks directly to members about their distress. Even though its primary aim is not to reduce distress, it does give members tools for understanding and accepting the distress. In this way, it might seem to members to be in alignment with their needs. Other models, such as CBT and DBT, also recognize that the patient is suffering. However, these latter models could not be easily delivered within the four- or five-session time frame.

In this vignette, the fact that Dr. Horne already has a background in group psychotherapy will serve her well in applying any of these models. Nonetheless, each one requires specific therapist competencies that Dr. Horne would have to acquire. Some models (e.g., DBT), ideally, would require that staff in the broader treatment environment learn their workings. Would staff be so motivated? Also, the therapist must contend with the orientation of the Level II group. The orientations of the two levels of group need not be identical, but they should be compatible. For example, ACT-G discourages members from using experiential avoidance. Imagine how disruptive it would be for a member to participate in an ACT group and then enter another group that provides techniques for experiential avoidance. Even if Dr. Horne has established the compatibility of her model with that used for the Level II group, it would behoove her to meet with the Level II group therapist so that the therapists can identify ways to make the continuity salient to members.

Case 3: Residential Treatment Center

Description

An RTC provided services to adolescents between the ages of 13 and 18 years. These male and female youth had a variety of emotional and behavioral problems, including anxiety, depression, comorbid substance abuse, and difficulty with anger management. The RTC did not publicly espouse a particular theoretical approach, but many staff members claimed to have a psychodynamic or interpersonal orientation or some combination of the two. The youth had available to them a wide variety of psychoeducational groups, such as assertiveness training, 12-step groups for drug and alcohol abuse, meditation, and stress-management groups. Family groups and recreational groups were also part of the programming.

The staff felt that some of the higher functioning youth might benefit from a more exploratory group. In fact, some of the residents themselves had lobbied for such a group, saying, for example, "We don't have enough of a chance to get into our issues." Staff stipulated that members should not begin the group until Week 2 both to allow adequate screening and to protect the group from those who might leave the RTC precipitously given that these departures tended to occur in the first few days as a resident. They hoped that once a member entered the group, he or she could remain for the duration of that individual's residency. Another expectation of staff was that 90-minute sessions would run 6 days a week.

Analysis

The group psychotherapist should take various contextual features into account in selecting a model for this setting. The fact that the staff wanted an exploratory opportunity for members was congruent with the staff members' theoretical bent, emphasizing interpersonal and psychodynamic psychotherapies. Given that the group was to meet six times a week, it was likely that a therapy team would staff the group rather than a single therapist. Therefore, it would be optimal to have a model that would be easily deliverable by many staff, provided they had a background in conducting psychotherapy groups. Both the frequency of meetings and the likely length of members' tenures in the group would lend themselves to a process-oriented group that either combined interpersonal or psychodynamic elements or that emphasized one of these orientations. To deliver such a model, the group therapist would have to carefully screen members for the group given that any less-structured approach would require members' tolerance of a moderate anxiety level. However, symptom heterogeneity could be easily accommodated by a process-oriented approach.

The approaches most consistent with this set of features are the unstructured psychodynamic or the unstructured interpersonal approach. These models easily accommodate the open-ended aspect of the group. Both models allow for transdiagnostic application. They benefit from member participation that lasts beyond a handful of sessions. Two more structured models that also would mesh with this setting are the mentalizing and IPT-G models. However, both these approaches would require considerable additional staff training, thereby necessitating staff willingness and site support. For IPT-G, some adaptation would be needed to accommodate the open-ended aspect of the model given that, each week, new members might enter and only some existing members might depart. The open-ended aspect would mute the unfolding of developmental stages that the approaches assume. Finally, all these approaches would demand some means for staff to communicate about the events of the session of each group.

FUTURE DIRECTIONS

The group psychotherapist aspiring to choose a workable approach for his or her setting will find the task challenging. As we consider the matrix in Table 2.1, listing all the contextual factors that influence whether a model will fit with the setting in light of the empirical findings presented in all the chapters, we cannot but be struck by the paucity of information on many matters. That is, currently, we know little about how most of the crucial contextual variables limit or enhance a given model's effectiveness in a particular site. Here, we briefly review the context variables again and consider what we do and do not know about the operation of each.

The philosophy and values of an institution or organization are often difficult to discern because not infrequently hidden beliefs contradict those that are stated. Despite this difficulty, accurately identifying a setting's philosophy and values is important because these elements shape what can happen in a group at a microscopic level (Karterud & Urnes, 2004). It appears to us that model builders are developing an increased appreciation of such broad systemic factors and at times comment on how certain intellectual stances, such as loyalty to the medical model, might hamper a model's delivery. Still, controlled studies on group climate and other broad features are difficult to carry out. Much insight might be gleaned from qualitative investigations in which researchers establish linkages between macroscopic aspects of the broader environment and microscopic aspects of group process. Qualitative methodologies have burgeoned over the last

2 decades and provide the research with many tools for discerning patterns (e.g., Denzin & Lincoln, 2005).

Time is one of the major limiting factors on what a group can accomplish and, as such, we need as much information as possible on what can be accomplished within different time frames. Some newer models, such as ACT, have been the object of so many research studies that we can see that this treatment produces positive outcomes across a range of time frames (including a mere two to three sessions). However, rarely is the length of group tenure investigated as a variable, much to the detriment of the various approaches. Without knowing what tenure is required for a particular type of change, the group psychotherapist is hindered from persuading third-party payers to make sound decisions about treatment reimbursement. Even conversations with hospital administration and treatment team members would be facilitated by the group psychotherapist's possession of such knowledge.

The study of member characteristics is similar to temporal variables in that we learn about who profits from what approaches simply by the findings yielded from studies that focus on a particular patient population. Rarely are outcomes of members with different psychological characteristics directly compared. Greene and Cole (1991) conducted the kind of study that would benefit the further development of the modality for IHP, PHP, and RTC settings. The member characteristic they examined was the level of functioning of the group member—whether he or she was organized at the psychotic or borderline level and whether the individual exhibited introjective or anaclitic pathology. With *introjective* pathology, the individual focuses on experienced insufficiencies of the self; *anaclitic* pathology involves a felt sense of interpersonal deprivation. Group structure was also varied, with some members participating in a relatively unstructured psychodynamic group and others in a structured activity-oriented group. Greene and Cole found complex interactions among the variables. Borderline-level patients perceived the self more positively, having participated in the less-structured group, and patients with psychosis made this same achievement more fully through membership in the structured group. The type of group was more important to the progress of anaclitic individuals, who saw themselves more favorably having participated in the psychodynamic group; introjective patients performed comparably in both conditions. Such research is consistent with a recently emerging transdiagnostic perspective emphasizing personality factors over symptoms (Kring & Sloan, 2009). Studies are also being conducted on how patients' characteristics affect the rate of change in IHPs, PHPs, and RTCs. For example, in a large-scale study, Allen et al. (2017) found that both anxious and depressed IHP patients show a pattern of rapid symptom reduction early in intensive treatment hospitalization (much of which is group based), with much slower but continuing change over an 8-week period. Such studies help group psychotherapists anticipate what level of change is likely via members' group participation.

As noted in Chapter 2, beyond the diagnostic and personality characteristics of the group members are identity variables that define individuals. Factors such as race, ethnicity, religious affiliation, ableness, sexual orientation, and gender identity (to name some) can shape a member's capacity to interact productively with other members of a psychotherapy group operating within the confines of a given theoretical approach. Models of group psychotherapy should attend to diversity factors (Lothstein, 2014). A member's status on some of these identities such as sexual orientation and gender identity can be linked to stigma, a force inextricably tied to an individual's state of psychological being. The importance of these factors intensifies when members differ on them and the differences are salient. Models should explicitly speak to how the therapist can work with differences to enable members to progress toward their treatment goals and avoid a circumstance in which group interactions reactivate past experiences of stigma. For example, writers on the social skills training model (e.g., Kopelowicz, Liberman, & Zarate, 2006) have pointed out that assertiveness training can aid individuals in coping with discrimination and stigma. In Table 9.1, we identify potential ways in which each of our models can identify diversity issues. In addition, research is needed to ascertain which identity and diagnostic variables might moderate the results from outcome studies performed on these models (Greene, 2017). For example, does ACT or CBT work equally well with individuals across races, ethnicities, and sexual orientations?

Admittedly, research on all member characteristics is extremely difficult to carry out, but group psychotherapy researchers could benefit from the use of methodologies other than the controlled experiment. For example, Greene (2017) described the considerable potential of case comparison studies in which the cases of two group members (both in the same group), one with a successful and another with a subpar outcome, are compared with attention to differences in personality styles and the microevents that characterize each individual's group trajectory.

Possibly the most neglected area of study concerns therapist characteristics. Little investment has been made in the discovery of what types and degrees of training are required to enable practitioners to use competently each of the different approaches. This neglect mirrors the broader inattention to training effects in the general group psychotherapy literature (Greene, 2017). It is encouraging, though, that some of the newer models such as ACT are providing empirical information about the training requirements

TABLE 9.1

Ways in Which Group Psychotherapy Models Provide
Opportunities for Multicultural Exploration

Model	Subtype	Multicultural processing opportunities
Interpersonal	General	The giver and receiver of communications can move toward mutual clarification of meaning of communications across cultural divides.
	Interactional agenda	Method enhances curiosity about others.
	Focus group	Treatment fosters feeling that interactions with others (including diverse others) can be warm and nourishing.
	Interpersonal psychotherapy–group	Highlights experiences that are universally challenging, accentuating features of the human condition that unite rather than divide.
Psychodynamic	General	Group members learn to tolerate those elements in themselves they project on others.
	Object relations/ systems	Group members learn to tolerate those elements in themselves they project on others.
	Mentalization	Members develop increased curiosity about one another and are less likely to develop assumptions about one another that are immune to disproving.
Cognitive behavior therapy		Therapists can support group members by refraining from questioning the validity of core cultural beliefs but, rather, exploring their helpfulness to the person's adaptation.
Acceptance and commitment therapy		Members have an opportunity to clarify whether behaviors that discriminate against others are consistent with their values and are conducive to the development of relationships that work. Members learn to defuse negative feeling toward others while recognizing that these feelings are transitory states rather than representations of reality.
Problem solving		When problems arise related to intergroup tensions, members systematically work out alternatives to solving the problem other than becoming dysregulated.
Social skills training		Members' sensitivity to one another is enhanced by mastering observational skills, which enable them to recognize others' reactions to their behaviors.

of model delivery (e.g., Eisenbeck, Scheitz, & Szekeres, 2016). Attention should also be given to the personality and intellectual characteristics of the therapist.

For all models, attention should be paid to minimal training requirements for a model's effective delivery. As Lothstein (2014) pointed out, group therapy requires attention to and use of group process. When therapists make interventions calling attention to group process, it is likely to raise members' anxiety levels. Therapists must have the requisite background to know how to manage members' elevated anxiety levels so that the treatment does not do more harm than good. Lothstein, speaking specifically about the inpatient group, questioned whether a credential such as the American Group Psychotherapy's Certified Group Psychotherapist designation (Bernard et al., 2008) might be appropriate at least for one therapist in the setting. We would extend his point to PHP and RTC groups as well. Of course, establishing such a credential would necessitate that institutions commit in substantial ways to training and provide reasonable remuneration for staff with such qualifications.

A FINAL NOTE

All group psychotherapy is contextual. The environment surrounding the group—be it the treatment environment, the economic climate, or the political atmosphere—has a bearing on what the psychotherapy group can accomplish. In some treatment circumstances, such as the private practice group, the influences of context might be subtle. However, in the treatment situations we have addressed in this book, the ways in which the context shapes the psychotherapy group are usually more evident. Therapists recognize when they are hampered in using a given approach because the size of the group is too large, the sessions too infrequent, or tenures of members too brief. Psychotherapy groups often founder in IHP, PHP, and RTC programs because the therapist does not take the context into sufficient account in model selection. When the fit is poor, all the efficacy evidence one could desire will not ensure the group's success. In this book, we have attempted to provide the kind of information about each model that will enable the group psychotherapist to engage in a more deliberative process of model selection. We are optimistic that in doing so, the therapist will be able to realize the potential of the model he or she selects for the benefit of group members served. With that in mind, we have presented a final table (Table 9.2) that broadly compares models across variables that might differ in the system in which each group therapist functions.

TABLE 9.2
Six Group Psychotherapy Models and Their Contextual Dimensions

Contextual dimensions model	Model philosophy that system must accept	Relation to treatment program	Staff participation	Minimum number of sessions for brief application and goal achieved	Ideal sessions for treatment effect of full model	Minimal and maximal sizes	Composition	Therapist characteristics	Cotherapist
Interpersonal	Relationship interactions are a core element of well-being	Can coexist with a variety of other activities and orientations	Not necessary	1 session Interpersonal goal for the day	1 or more	6–8	Wide range of ego functioning possible, but similarity more desired Wide range of symptom patterns	Capacity to be transparent within the here-and-now of the group	Not necessary
Psychodynamic	Well-being recognizes a range of conscious and unconscious determinants of experiences and behaviors	Incompatible with strong staff position that surface reactivity is only reality	Not necessary	1–2 sessions Can develop positive orientation toward exploratory work	12 (particularly for unstructured application)	6–10	Wide range of ego functioning and symptom patterns	Tolerance of a wide range of affects and impulses emerging in the group	Not necessary
Cognitive behavioral	Cognition affects emotion and behavior Dysfunctional cognitions increase symptomatology and reduce coping	Compatible with program that values skill acquisition and strengthening	Ideal to reinforce homework completion	1–2 sessions for teaching one skill (Rotating Theme Group)	6–12 48 for DBT 48 for schema	6–8	Symptom commonality enables treatment to proceed more efficiently	Must be technically skilled at CBT and able to operate within a collaborative empirical framework	Strongly preferred

(continues)

TABLE 9.2
Six Group Psychotherapy Models and Their Contextual Dimensions *(Continued)*

Contextual dimensions model	Model philosophy that system must accept	Relation to treatment program	Staff participation	Minimum number of sessions for brief application and goal achieved	Ideal sessions for treatment effect of full model	Minimal and maximal sizes	Composition	Therapist characteristics	Cotherapist
Acceptance and commitment therapy	Emphasizes personal growth rather than mere elimination of symptoms	Incompatible with strong approach to symptom relief only	Ideal	1–2 sessions for teaching concepts and exercises The longer a member's tenure in the group, the greater the exposure to and practice with hexaflex processes	8–12	6–15	Can accommodate a range of problems and symptoms Formats for symptomatically homogeneous groups are available	Therapist should have achieved a reasonable level of psychological flexibility	Not necessary
Interpersonal problem solving	Approach and skills of interpersonal problem solving exacerbate stress and psychiatric symptomatology	Compatible with treatment philosophy that values skill building to improve adaptive functioning	Ideal to encourage trying out of solutions	2 for standardized problems 3–4 to teach method of problem solving	12	8–12	Individuals should be at a comparable level of cognitive functioning	Therapist must be comfortable with high level of directiveness and know method of problem solving	Strongly preferred
Social skills training	Improvement of behavioral skills increases adaptive functioning	Works best in treatment environment that sees the important target of change as what can be behaviorally observed Incompatible with system that values only psychopharmacology	Necessary to encourage practice of learned skill	1–2 sessions for acquisition of single skill Booster sessions are useful far after the program is concluded	4–24	Chronically impaired: 3–5 members; otherwise, a larger number can be accommodated	All members must show well-defined social skill weakness that member has in common with other members	Therapist must be comfortable with high level of directiveness and provide strong support and encouragement	Strongly preferred

Note. Table specifications represent our estimations based upon the aggregate of the research, the observations and opinions of the model developers, and the inherent characteristics of the model. CBT = cognitive behavior therapy; DBT = dialectical behavior therapy.

REFERENCES

Alden, L. E., Wiggins, J. S., & Pincus, A. L. (1990). Construction of circumplex scales for the Inventory of Interpersonal Problems. *Journal of Personality Assessment, 55*, 521–536. http://dx.doi.org/10.1080/00223891.1990.9674088

Allen, J. G., Fowler, J. C., Madan, A., Ellis, T. E., Oldham, J. M., & Frueh, B. C. (2017). Discovering the impact of psychotherapeutic hospital treatment for adults with serious mental illness. *Bulletin of the Menninger Clinic, 81*, 1–38. http://dx.doi.org/10.1521/bumc.2017.81.1.1

American Psychiatric Association. (1994). *Diagnostic and statistical manual of mental disorders* (4th ed.). Washington, DC: Author.

Bach, P., & Hayes, S. C. (2002). The use of acceptance and commitment therapy to prevent the rehospitalization of psychotic patients: A randomized controlled trial. *Journal of Consulting and Clinical Psychology, 70*, 1129–1139. http://dx.doi.org/10.1037/0022-006X.70.5.1129

Bateman, A., & Fonagy, P. (2001). Treatment of borderline personality disorder with psychoanalytically oriented partial hospitalization: An 18-month follow-up. *The American Journal of Psychiatry, 158*, 36–42. http://dx.doi.org/10.1176/appi.ajp.158.1.36

Bateman, A., & Fonagy, P. (2003). Health service utilization costs for borderline personality disorder patients treated with psychoanalytically oriented partial hospitalization versus general psychiatric care. *American Journal of Psychiatry, 160*, 169–171. http://dx.doi.org/10.1176/appi.ajp.160.1.169

Bateman, A., & Fonagy, P. (2006). *Mentalization-based treatment for borderline personality disorder: A practical guide*. Oxford, England: Oxford University Press. http://dx.doi.org/10.1093/med/9780198570905.001.0001

Bateman, A., & Fonagy, P. (2008). 8-year follow-up of patients treated for borderline personality disorder: Mentalization-based treatment versus treatment as usual. *The American Journal of Psychiatry, 165*, 631–638. http://dx.doi.org/10.1176/appi.ajp.2007.07040636

Beck, A. T. (1976). *Cognitive theory and the emotional disorders*. Madison, CT: International Universities Press.

Beck, A. T. (1991). Cognitive therapy: A 30-year retrospective. *American Psychologist, 46*, 368–375. http://dx.doi.org/10.1037/0003-066X.46.4.368

Beck, A. T., & Steer, R. A. (1987). *Manual for the revised Beck Depression Inventory*. San Antonio, TX: Psychological Corporation.

Bernard, H., Burlingame, G., Flores, P., Greene, L., Joyce, A., Kobos, J. C., . . . Feirman, D. (2008). Clinical practice guidelines for group psychotherapy. *International Journal of Group Psychotherapy, 58*, 455–542. http://dx.doi.org/10.1521/ijgp.2008.58.4.455

Borge, F. M., Hoffart, A., Sexton, H., Clark, D. M., Markowitz, J. C., & McManus, F. (2008). Residential cognitive therapy versus residential interpersonal therapy for social phobia: A randomized clinical trial. *Journal of Anxiety Disorders, 22,* 991–1010. http://dx.doi.org/10.1016/j.janxdis.2007.10.002

Brabender, V., & Fallon, A. (1993). *Models of inpatient group psychotherapy.* Washington, DC: American Psychological Association.

Denzin, N. K., & Lincoln, Y. S. (Eds.). (2005). *The Sage handbook of qualitative research* (3rd ed.). London, England: Sage.

Derogatis, L. R., & Unger, R. (2010). *Symptom Checklist–90–Revised.* Hoboken, NJ: Wiley. http://dx.doi.org/10.1002/9780470479216.corpsy0970

Eisenbeck, N., Scheitz, K., & Szekeres, B. (2016). A brief acceptance and commitment therapy-based intervention among violence-prone male inmates delivered by novice therapists. *Psychology, Society & Education, 8,* 187–199.

Erickson, R. C. (1984). *Inpatient group psychotherapy: A pragmatic approach.* Springfield, IL: Charles C Thomas.

Ferencik, B. M. (1991). A typology of the here-and-now: Issues in group therapy. *International Journal of Group Psychotherapy, 41,* 169–183. http://dx.doi.org/10.1080/00207284.1991.11490642

Freeman, A. (1990). Cognitive therapy. In A. Bellack & M. Hersen (Eds.), *Handbook of comparative treatments for adult disorders* (pp. 64–87). New York, NY: Wiley.

Greene, L. R. (2017). Group psychotherapy research studies that therapists might actually read: My top 10 list. *International Journal of Group Psychotherapy, 67,* 1–26. http://dx.doi.org/10.1080/00207284.2016.1202678

Greene, L. R., & Cole, M. B. (1991). Level and form of psychopathology and the structure of group therapy. *International Journal of Group Psychotherapy, 41,* 499–521. http://dx.doi.org/10.1080/00207284.1991.11490677

Jang, K. L. (2005). *The behavioral genetics of psychopathology: A clinical guide.* New York, NY: Routledge.

Juarascio, A., Shaw, J., Forman, E. M., Timko, C. A., Herbert, J. D., Butryn, M. L., & Lowe, M. (2013). Acceptance and commitment therapy for eating disorders: Clinical applications of a group treatment. *Journal of Contextual Behavioral Science, 2,* 85–94. http://dx.doi.org/10.1016/j.jcbs.2013.08.001

Karasu, T. B. (1994). A developmental metatheory of psychopathology. *American Journal of Psychotherapy, 48,* 581–599.

Karterud, S., & Urnes, Ø. (2004). Short-term day treatment programmes for patients with personality disorders. What is the optimal composition? *Nordic Journal of Psychiatry, 58,* 243–249. http://dx.doi.org/10.1080/08039480410006304

Kibel, H. D. (1987a). Inpatient group psychotherapy—Where treatment philosophies converge. In R. Langs (Ed.), *The yearbook of psychoanalysis and psychotherapy* (Vol. 2, pp. 94–116). New York, NY: Gardner Press.

Kibel, H. D. (1987b). Contributions of the group psychotherapist to education on the psychiatric unit: Teaching through group dynamics. *International Journal of Group Psychotherapy, 37,* 3–29. http://dx.doi.org/10.1080/00207284.1987.11491038

Kibel, H. D. (2003). Interpretive work in milieu groups. *International Journal of Group Psychotherapy*, *53*, 303–329. http://dx.doi.org/10.1521/ijgp.53.3.303.42821

Kirchmann, H., Mestel, R., Schreiber-Willnow, K., Mattke, D., Seidler, K. P., Daudert, E., . . . Strauss, B. (2009). Associations among attachment characteristics, patients' assessment of therapeutic factors, and treatment outcome following inpatient psychodynamic group psychotherapy. *Psychotherapy Research*, *19*, 234–248. http://dx.doi.org/10.1080/10503300902798367

Kopelowicz, A., Liberman, R. P., & Zarate, R. (2006). Recent advances in social skills training for schizophrenia. *Schizophrenia Bulletin*, *32*, S12–S23.

Kring, A. M., & Sloan, D. M. (Eds.). (2009). *Emotion regulation and psychopathology: A transdiagnostic approach to etiology and treatment.* New York, NY: Guilford Press.

Lothstein, L. M. (2014). The science and art of brief inpatient group therapy in the 21st century: Commentary on Cook et al. and Ellis et al. *International Journal of Group Psychotherapy*, *64*, 228–244. http://dx.doi.org/10.1521/ijgp.2014.64.2.228

Martins, M. J., Castilho, P., Santos, V., & Gumley, A. (2016). Schizophrenia: An exploration of an acceptance, mindfulness, and compassion-based group intervention. *Australian Psychologist*, *51*, 1–10.

McCracken, L. M., Sato, A., & Taylor, G. J. (2013). A trial of a brief group-based form of acceptance and commitment therapy (ACT) for chronic pain in general practice: Pilot outcome and process results. *The Journal of Pain*, *14*, 1398–1406. http://dx.doi.org/10.1016/j.jpain.2013.06.011

McQuillan, A., Nicastro, R., Guenot, F., Girard, M., Lissner, C., & Ferrero, F. (2005). Intensive dialectical behavior therapy for outpatients with borderline personality disorder who are in crisis. *Psychiatric Services*, *56*, 193–197. http://dx.doi.org/10.1176/appi.ps.56.2.193

Meichenbaum, D. (2007). Stress inoculation training: A preventative and treatment approach. *Principles and Practice of Stress Management*, *3*, 497–518.

Neuhaus, E. C., Christopher, M., Jacob, K., Guillaumot, J., & Burns, J. P. (2007). Short-term cognitive behavioral partial hospital treatment: A pilot study. *Journal of Psychiatric Practice*, *13*, 298–307. http://dx.doi.org/10.1097/01.pra.0000290668.10107.f3

Piper, W. E., Rosie, J. S., Joyce, A. S., & Azim, H. F. (1996). *Two weeks in the life of the day treatment program.* Washington, DC: American Psychological Association. http://dx.doi.org/10.1037/10208-006

Pollack, L. E., Harvin, S., & Cramer, R. D. (2001). Inpatient group therapies for people with bipolar disorder: Comparison of a self-management and an interactional model. *Journal of the American Psychiatric Nurses Association*, *7*(6), 179–190. http://dx.doi.org/10.1067/mpn.2001.118418

Reisch, T., Thommen, M., Tschacher, W., & Hirsbrunner, H. P. (2001). Outcomes of a cognitive-behavioral day treatment program for a heterogeneous patient group. *Psychiatric Services*, *52*, 970–972. http://dx.doi.org/10.1176/appi.ps.52.7.970

Steil, R., Dyer, A., Priebe, K., Kleindienst, N., & Bohus, M. (2011). Dialectical behavior therapy for posttraumatic stress disorder related to childhood sexual abuse: A pilot study of an intensive residential treatment program. *Journal of Traumatic Stress, 24*, 102–106. http://dx.doi.org/10.1002/jts.20617

Taylor, R., Coombes, L., & Bartlett, H. (2002). The impact of a practice development project on the quality of in-patient small group therapy. *Journal of Psychiatric and Mental Health Nursing, 9*, 213–220. http://dx.doi.org/10.1046/j.1365-2850.2002.00478.x

Tyrberg, M. J., Carlbring, P., & Lundgren, T. (2017). Brief acceptance and commitment therapy for psychotic inpatients: A randomized controlled feasibility trial in Sweden. *Nordic Psychology, 69*, 1–16.

Westrup, D., & Wright, M. J. (2017). *Learning ACT for group treatment: An acceptance and commitment therapy skills training manual for therapists.* Oakland, CA: New Harbinger.

Wilberg, T., Karterud, S., Urnes, O., Pedersen, G., & Friis, S. (1998). Outcomes of poorly functioning patients with personality disorders in a day treatment program. *Psychiatric Services, 49*, 1462–1467. http://dx.doi.org/10.1176/ps.49.11.1462

Yen, S., Johnson, J., Costello, E., & Simpson, E. B. (2009). A 5-day dialectical behavior therapy partial hospital program for women with borderline personality disorder: Predictors of outcome from a 3-month follow-up study. *Journal of Psychiatric Practice, 15*, 173–182. http://dx.doi.org/10.1097/01.pra.0000351877.45260.70

INDEX

Clinical mission, *continued*
 and interpersonal approach, 99
 and organizational conflict, 33–36
 of problem-solving model, 344
 and psychodynamic models, 157–158
 of social skills training model,
  384–385
 and values, 33–34
Closed-ended groups, 39–40, 103
 and cognitive behavior therapy
  models, 193–194, 196–198
 for problem-solving training,
  345, 346
 for social skills training model, 385
Coaching, behavioral rehearsal
 with, 375
Coché, E., 42, 96, 304, 308, 315
Coché, J., 315
Cognition, 73
 and affect, 395–396
 affect and cognition continuum, 135
 and behavior, 180
 and behavioral models, 367
 and behavioral modification, 180–181
 and behavior patterns, 175
 and cognitive behavior therapy,
  175–179
 and psychodynamic approach,
  110–112
 as target for change in CBT models,
  180
Cognitive behavior therapy (CBT),
  171–240
 assessment, 190–192
 adapted approaches to, 200–210
 behavioral techniques, 196–197,
  235–237
 clinical illustration of, 210–223
 cognition and affect handled in, 395
 cognitive strategies, 196–197,
  232–235
 contextual dimensions of, 423
 demands of, 228–231
 and eating disorders, 97
 fundamentals of models, 172–173
 group exercises, 237–240
 homework, 195
 member composition, 188–190
 multicultural opportunities in, 421
 in partial hospital setting, 409–410

preparation for, 192–193
psychoeducational approach,
 173–174
and psychopathology, 178
research on, 223–228
in residential treatment settings, 410
rotating theme group, 200
structured agenda format, 193–195
theory of, 175–177
treatment goals, 178–182
variables in structure of, 182–200
Cognitive deficits, 180
Cognitive development, 302–303
Cognitive distortions, 176, 178–180
Cognitive distractions, 232
Cognitive fusion, 263
Cognitive Fusion Questionnaire, 283
Cognitive rehearsal, 235, 316
Cognitive restructuring, 203
Cognitive schemas, 176–179
Cognitive strategies
 and cognitive behavior therapy,
  232–235
 in cognitive behavior therapy
  models, 196–197
Cognitive therapy, 183–185
Cognitive triad, 175, 176
Cole, M. B., 42, 154, 419
Combinatorial entailment, 261
Committed action (in ACT-G),
  273–274
Community, 20–21
Comparative analysis of models,
  393–424
 case examples of, 411–418
 commonalities among, 394–397
 differences among, 397–402
 future directions of, 418–424
 group perspectives within system,
  402–406
 variation in settings, 407–411
Confianza, 161, 174
Conflict, 75–76
Conflict models, 398–400, 406
Constructive adaptive self-statements,
 232
Constructive behavior rules (in CBT
 models), 196–197
Contact with the present moment (in
 ACT-G), 269

Values
    and acceptance and commitment
        therapy–group, 270–273
    of care setting, and program
        selection, 33–34
    and clinical mission of care setting,
        33–34
Values Assessment Rating Form,
    272, 278
Values Narrative Form, 272
Vannicelli, M., 52
Verification, of solution
    implementation, 316–317
Vicarious learning, 98
Vinogradov, S., 84
Voelz, Z. R., 340–341
Von Wietersheim, J., 20

Wachtel, P., 282
Walden, S. L., 57
Watson, J. B., 360
Webber, M. A., 209
Web connecting exercise, 238
Weber, R., 157
"Weighing," of solutions, 315
Weishaar, M. E., 190
Weiss, B., 383
Weissman, M. M., 68, 90
Weisz, J. R., 383
Welch, R. R., 90
Wendel, S., 100
Wessler, R. L., 182

West, M. L., 47–48
Westrup, D., 260, 273
What-if technique, 234
What skills (DBT approach), 203
Wilberg, T., 409
Wilfley, D. E., 87, 90, 97, 100
Williams, J. M. G., 189
Wilson-Smith, D., 231
Wiseman, C. V., 227
Wise mind (DBT skill), 203
Wise mind exercise–expanding
    awareness, 239
Wise mind puzzle making exercise,
    239
Withdrawal, 72
Wolpe, J., 361, 366
Workability (in ACT-G), 265
Wrap-up steps (interactional agenda
    model), 81–82
Wright, M. J., 260, 273
Wright, N. P., 275, 276

Yalom, Irvin, 15, 20, 37, 42, 53, 68,
    69–73, 76, 77, 79, 80, 82, 84, 96,
    98, 100, 103
Yanos, P. T., 47–48
Young, J. E., 190, 206, 209
"Young anger," 76
Young Schema Questionnaire, 190

Zegarra, A., 73
Zum Vörde Sive Vörding, M. B., 284

ABOUT THE AUTHORS

Virginia Brabender, PhD, ABPP (Cl), is a faculty member in Widener University's Institute for Graduate Clinical Psychology. She is recognized by Widener as a Distinguished Professor (2017–2019) and is a fellow of Divisions 12 and 49 of the American Psychological Association, of the American Group Psychotherapy Association, and of the Society for Personality Assessment. She received her baccalaureate degree from the University of Dayton (1971) and a doctorate in psychology from Fordham University (1976). In addition to her work with Dr. April Fallon, she has authored *Introduction to Group Therapy* (2002), coedited *The Handbook of Gender and Sexuality in Psychological Assessment* (2016), and written numerous articles on ethics in professional psychology. She is on the Editorial Committee of the *International Journal of Group Psychotherapy*.

April Fallon, PhD, is a faculty member in clinical psychology at Fielding Graduate University and a clinical professor in psychiatry at Drexel College of Medicine. She received her baccalaureate degree from Allegheny College (1975) and a doctorate in psychology at the University of Pennsylvania (1981). She has received numerous awards for her teaching of psychiatry residents, including the Psychiatric Educator 2012 from the Philadelphia Psychiatric Society.

In addition to her work with Dr. Brabender, she has researched and written on the development of disgust in children and adults, body image and eating disorders, the effects of childhood maltreatment, and attachment and adoption. Along with her academic appointments, she maintains a private practice in Ardmore, Pennsylvania.

Virginia Brabender and April Fallon have coauthored four books: *Models of Inpatient Group Psychotherapy* (1993), *Essentials of Group Therapy* (2004), *Group Development in Practice: Guidance for Clinicians and Researchers on Stages and Dynamics of Change* (2009), and *The Impact of Parenthood on the Therapeutic Relationship: Awaiting the Therapist's Baby* (2nd ed., 2018). They coedited *Working With Adoptive Parents: Research, Theory, and Therapeutic Interventions* (2013).